PROGRESS IN BRAIN RESEARCH

VOLUME 35

CEREBRAL BLOOD FLOW

PROGRESS IN BRAIN RESEARCH

PROGRESS IN BRAIN RESEARCH
VOLUME 35

CEREBRAL BLOOD FLOW

Relationship of Cerebral Blood Flow and
Metabolism to Neurological Symptoms

EDITED BY

JOHN STIRLING MEYER

Department of Neurology,
Baylor College of Medicine,
Houston, Texas (U.S.A.)

AND

J. P. SCHADÉ

Central Institute for Brain Research,
Amsterdam (The Netherlands)

ELSEVIER PUBLISHING COMPANY
AMSTERDAM / LONDON / NEW YORK
1972

ELSEVIER PUBLISHING COMPANY
335 JAN VAN GALENSTRAAT,
P.O. BOX 211, AMSTERDAM, THE NETHERLANDS

AMERICAN ELSEVIER PUBLISHING COMPANY, INC.
52 VANDERBILT AVENUE, NEW YORK, N.Y. 10017

LIBRARY OF CONGRESS CARD NUMBER 73-168913

ISBN 0-444-40952-1

WITH 225 ILLUSTRATIONS AND 40 TABLES

PRINTED IN THE NETHERLANDS

List of Contributors

MANABU MIYAZAKI, Department of Internal Medicine, Osaka Municipal Kosai-in Hospital, Suita City, Osaka (Japan).

D. HADJIEV, Research Institute of Neurology and Psychiatry, Sofia (Bulgaria).

IAIN M. S. WILKINSON, The National Hospital, Queen Square, London W.C. 1 (U.K.).

CARL WILHELM SEM-JACOBSEN, Medical Director, The EEG Research Laboratory, Gaustad Sykehus, Vinderen, Oslo 3 (Norway).

OLE BERNHARD STYRI, Medical Director, Department of Neurosurgery, Rikshopitalet, Oslo (Norway).

ERIK MOHN, Norwegian Computing Center, Oslo (Norway).

CLIVE ROSENDORFF, Department of Physiology, and Department of Medicine, University of Witwatersrand, Johannesburg (South Africa).

JOHN C. KENNADY, Laboratory of Nuclear Medicine and Radiation Biology and the Department of Surgery/Neurosurgery, UCLA School of Medicine, Los Angeles, California 90024 (U.S.A.).

MARTIN REIVICH, Cerebrovascular Physiology Laboratory of the Department of Neurology, University of Pennsylvania, Philadelphia, Penna. 19104 (U.S.A.).

M. N. SHALIT, Department of Neurosurgery, Hadassah University Hospital, Jerusalem (Israel).

H. FLOHR, Department of Physiology, 53 Bonn and Department of Neurosurgery, University of Hannover, 3 Hannover-Buchholz (W. Germany).

M. BROCK, Department of Physiology, 53 Bonn and Department of Neurosurgery, University of Hannover, 3 Hannover-Buchholz (W. Germany).

W. PÖLL, Department of Physiology, 53 Bonn and Department of Neurosurgery, University of Hannover, 3 Hannover-Buchholz (W. Germany).

A. R. TAYLOR, Royal Victoria Hospital, Belfast (Northern Ireland).

H. A. CROCKARD, Royal Victoria Hospital, Belfast (Northern Ireland).

T. K. BELL, Royal Victoria Hospital, Belfast (Northern Ireland).

JOHN STIRLING MEYER, Department of Neurology, Baylor College of Medicine, Houston, Texas 77025 (U.S.A.).

K. M. A. WELCH, Department of Neurology, Baylor College of Medicine, Houston, Texas 77025 (U.S.A.).

J. C. DE VALOIS, Central Institute for Brain Research, Amsterdam (The Netherlands).

J. P. C. PEPERKAMP, Central Institute for Brain Research, Amsterdam (The Netherlands).

BRYAN JENNETT, Institute of Neurological Sciences, Glasgow, and The University of Glasgow, Glasgow (U.K.).

J. O. ROWAN, Institute of Neurological Sciences, Glasgow and The Regional Department of Clinical Physics and Bio-Engineering, Glasgow (U.K.).

SEYMOUR S. KETY, Harvard Medical School, Massachusetts General Hospital, Boston, Mass. (U.S.A.).

CESARE FIESCHI, Department of Neurology and Psychiatry, University of Rome and University of Siena (Italy).

LUIGI BOZZAO, Department of Neurology and Psychiatry, University of Rome and University of Siena (Italy).

J. DOUGLAS MILLER, Division of Neurosurgery, University of Pennsylvania, Philadelphia, Penna. 19104 (U.S.A.).

ALBERT STANEK, Division of Neurosurgery, University of Pennsylvania, Philadelphia, Penna. 19104 (U.S.A.).

THOMAS W. LANGFITT, Division of Neurosurgery, University of Pennsylvania, Philadelphia, Penna. 19104 (U.S.A.).

Other volumes in this series:

Volume 1: *Brains Mechanisms*
Specific and Unspecific Mechanisms of Sensory Motor Integration
Edited by G. Moruzzi, A. Fessard and H. H. Jasper

Volume 2: *Nerve, Brain and Memory Models*
Edited by Norbert Wiener† and J. P. Schadé

Volume 3: *The Rhinencephalon and Related Structures*
Edited by W. Bargmann and J. P. Schadé

Volume 4: *Growth and Maturation of the Brain*
Edited by D. P. Purpura and J. P. Schadé

Volume 5: *Lectures on the Diencephalon*
Edited by W. Bargmann and J. P. Schadé

Volume 6: *Topics in Basic Neurology*
Edited by W. Bargmann and J. P. Schadé

Volume 7: *Slow Electrical Processes in the Brain*
by N. A. Aladjalova

Volume 8: *Biogenic Amines*
Edited by Harold E. Himwich and Williamina A. Himwich

Volume 9: *The Developing Brain*
Edited by Williamina A. Himwich and Harold E. Himwich

Volume 10: *The Structure and Function of the Epiphysis Cerebri*
Edited by J. Ariëns Kappers and J. P. Schadé

Volume 11: *Organization of the Spinal Cord*
Edited by J. C. Eccles and J. P. Schadé

Volume 12: *Physiology of Spinal Neurons*
Edited by J. C. Eccles and J. P. Schadé

Volume 13: *Mechanisms of Neural Regeneration*
Edited by M. Singer and J. P. Schadé

Volume 14: *Degeneration Patterns in the Nervous System*
Edited by M. Singer and J. P. Schadé

Volume 15: *Biology of Neuroglia*
Edited by E. D. P. De Robertis and R. Carrea

Volume 16: *Horizons in Neuropsychopharmacology*
Edited by Williamina A. Himwich and J. P. Schadé

Contents

Studies on Cerebral Circulation by the Ultrasonic Doppler Technique — with Special Reference to Clinical Application of the Technique

MANABU MIYAZAKI

Department of Internal Medicine, Osaka Municipal Kosai-in Hospital, Suita City, Osaka (Japan)

INTRODUCTION

The ultrasonic Doppler technique is advantageous as compared with other techniques for the measurement of cerebral blood flow. The changes in the dynamics of cerebral circulation with various circulatory agents can be detected instantaneously and continuously as well as non-operatively by this technique. In addition, it is possible by this technique to measure blood flow individually in each vessel, *i.e.*, internal, external and common carotid arteries and internal and external jugular veins.

This paper deals with the principle and several clinical applications of the ultrasonic Doppler technique in the study of cerebral circulation and the useful characteristics of the method.

PRINCIPLE AND METHOD

The method was discussed by Satomura and Kaneko (1960), Miyazaki (1963) and Miyazaki and Kato (1965).

When an ultrasonic wave impinges upon a blood stream, the frequency of the reflected waves is altered due to Doppler's effect from the moving blood particles and turbulent (agitated) flow, especially from the former. A kind of noise is obtained by composing and demodulating the reflected waves and the direct wave. The frequency of the noise is proportional to the blood flow velocity.

When an ultrasonic wave impinges upon a moving subject, the frequency of the reflected waves (f') is converted as follows:

$$f' = \frac{c + u \cdot \cos \theta}{c - u \cdot \cos \theta} f$$

where f = frequency of direct wave
c = sound velocity
u = velocity of moving subject
θ = angle between the direction of ultrasonic wave and the direction of moving subject

References pp. 22–23

The frequency of the Doppler beat (fd) is obtained by composing and demodulating the reflected waves and the direct wave. The frequency of the Doppler beat (fd) is demonstrated as follows:

$$fd = f' - f = \frac{c + u \cdot \cos \theta}{c - u \cdot \cos \theta} f \doteqdot \frac{2\,u \cdot \cos \theta}{c} f = \frac{2\,u}{\lambda} \cos \theta \qquad (c \gg u)$$

λ = wave length

From the above formula, it has been postulated that the moving subject is converted to an audible sound, since the frequency of the Doppler beat is proportional to the velocity of the subject and that the Doppler's effect is theoretically minimum at $\theta = 90°$ and maximum at $\theta = 0°$.

Fig. 1 and Fig. 2 show the block diagram and the frequency characteristics of the

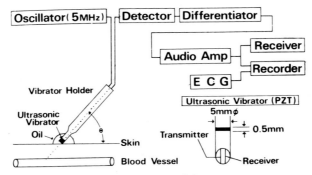

Fig. 1. Block diagram of the apparatus

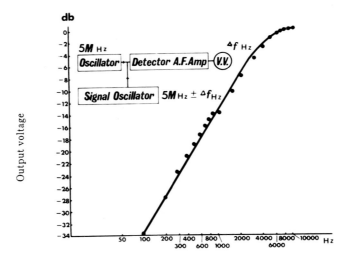

Frequency

Fig. 2. Frequency characteristics of the apparatus.

apparatus, respectively. The output voltage is proportional to the frequency between about 100 counts/sec and 6000 counts/sec. From these characteristics, the beat due to the Doppler's effect caused by the pulsation of the blood vessels (lower than about 100 counts/sec at arteries) is eliminated.

The rates of cerebral blood flow (ΔCBF), cerebral vascular resistance (ΔCVR) and cerebral oxygen consumption (ΔCMRO$_2$) are used as a measure of cerebral circulation and metabolism as follows (see Miyazaki, 1966 c; 1968 b).

Rate of cerebral blood flow (ΔCBF) (%) =

$$\frac{CBF' - CBF}{CBF} \times 100 = \frac{A'_{CBF} - A_{CBF}}{A_{CBF}} \times 100$$

Rate of cerebral vascular resistance (ΔCVR) (%) =

$$\frac{CVR' - CVR}{CVR} \times 100 = \left[\left(\frac{A_{CBF}}{A'_{CBF}} \times \frac{MAP'}{MAP} \right) - 1 \right] \times 100$$

Rate of cerebral oxygen consumption (ΔCMRO$_2$) (%) =

$$\frac{CMRO'_2 - CMRO_2}{CMRO_2} \times 100 = \left(\frac{A'_{CBF}}{A_{CBF}} \times \frac{C(A - V)O'_{2'}}{C(A - V)O_2} - 1 \right) \times 100$$

where CBF, A_{CBF}, CVR, CMRO$_2$, C(A-V)O$_2$ and MAP = cerebral blood flow, area of cerebral blood flow pattern, cerebral vascular resistance, cerebral oxygen consumption, cerebral arteriovenous oxygen content difference and mean artery pressure before maneuver, respectively. CBF', A'_{CBF}, CVR', CMRO$'_2$, C(A-V)O$'_2$ and MAP' = cerebral blood flow, area of cerebral blood flow pattern, cerebral vascular resistance, cerebral oxygen consumption, cerebral arteriovenous oxygen content difference and mean artery pressure after maneuver, respectively.

DYNAMIC OBSERVATIONS OF CEREBRAL CIRCULATORY CHANGE BY VARIOUS CIRCULATORY AGENTS

The change in the pulsatile diameter of the human common carotid artery which synchronizes with the cardiac cycle is so slight as to be negligible (Greenfield *et al.*, 1964; Miyazaki, 1968 a). Therefore, the blood velocity should change in proportion to the blood flow change in the human common carotid artery. From this principle, the changes in the dynamics of the cerebral circulation by various circulatory agents were observed by the ultrasonic Doppler technique as follows.

(1) Effect of low temperatures on cerebral circulation (Miyazaki, 1966 a)

The blood flow patterns in the internal carotid artery in the same subject observed at different seasons (in March and September) were hemodynamically compared. There were no significant differences between the blood flow patterns of March (room temp., 12 °C) and those of September (room temp., 30 °C), independent of the blood pressure change (Fig. 3). The constancy of the cerebral blood flow at the low

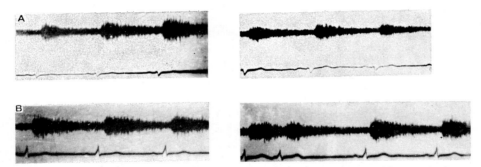

Fig. 3. Effect of low temperature on the blood flow patterns in internal carotid artery in the same subject. Left, indicates blood flow patterns of September and right, of March. (A) no change in blood pressure between two months. (B) markedly increased blood pressure in March (170/80–240/110).

temperature may well be based on the homeostasis of the extra- and intra-cranial circulation.

(2) *Effect of induced hypertension on cerebral circulation* (Miyazaki, 1966 a)

The blood flow patterns in the internal carotid artery before and after the administration of vasopressor drugs (adrenalin and noradrenalin) were hemodynamically compared.

The cerebral blood flow was markedly increased after the administration of adrenalin (Fig. 4). This phenomenon would mainly be due to increased cardiac output. On the other hand, two types of the cerebral blood flow were noted after the administration of noradrenalin (Fig. 5). One was a decrease in the blood flow accompanied by an increase in the blood pressure. The other was an increase in the

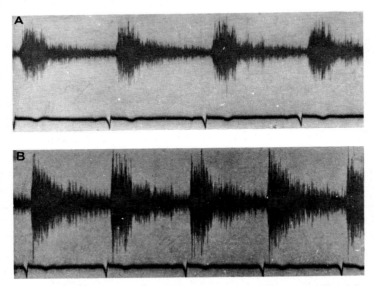

Fig. 4. Effect of induced hypertension by administration of adrenalin on the blood flow patterns in internal carotid artery. (A) control (B.P. 140/50). (B) after administration (B.P. 180/60).

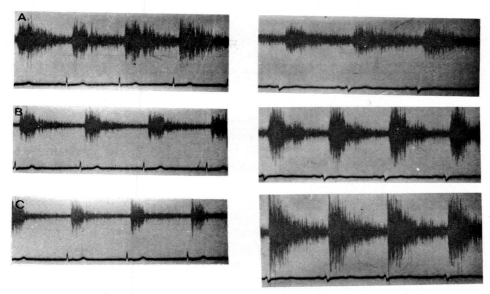

Fig. 5. Effect of induced hypertension by administration of noradrenalin on the blood flow patterns in internal carotid artery. Left, indicates blood flow patterns in a case of decreased blood flow and right, increased blood flow. (A) control, (B, C) after administration. Increasing rate of blood pressure moderate in B and severe in C.

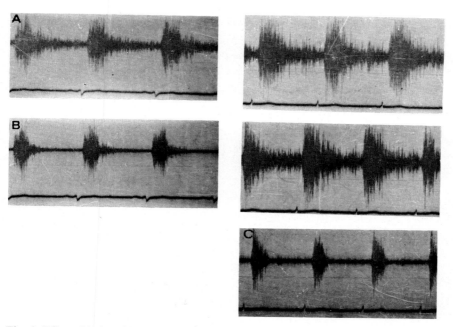

Fig. 6. Effect of induced hypotension on the blood flow patterns in internal carotid artery. Left, indicates blood flow patterns in severe cerebral arteriosclerosis and right, in mild cerebral arteriosclerosis. (A) control, (B) after antihypertensive drug, (C) after antihypertensive drug plus postural change. Decreasing rate of blood pressure moderate in B and severe in C.

blood flow. The latter type was prone to occur in the aged. This may mainly be due to the difference in the reactivity of the cerebral vessels to noradrenalin.

Thus, the effect of an induced hypertension on the cerebral circulation seems to be dependent on the hemodynamic correlation between the mechanism of hypertension and the reactivity of the cerebral vessel.

(3) *Effect of induced hypotension on cerebral circulation* (Miyazaki, 1965 a)

The blood flow patterns in the internal carotid artery were hemodynamically investigated during an induced hypotension by the intravenous infusion of an antihypertensive drug (hexamethonium) and during postural hypotension (supine→upright position) (Fig. 6).

In patients with severe cerebral arteriosclerosis, a decrease in the cerebral blood flow was observed by the intravenous infusion of the antihypertensive drug. On the other hand, in patients with mild cerebral arteriosclerosis, no such decrease was observed by the intravenous infusion of the antihypertensive drug. However, when both the intravenous infusion and the postural change were combined, a definite change in the cerebral blood flow was observed.

The findings suggest the presence of a trend for greater cerebral vascular insufficiency in patients with severe cerebral arteriosclerosis than in patients with mild cerebral arteriosclerosis due to disorder of the cerebral circulatory homeostasis (autoregulation).

(4) *Effect of arrhythmia on cerebral circulation* (Miyazaki, 1966 a)

The blood flow patterns in the internal carotid artery were investigated in patients with auricular fibrillation and premature beat (Fig. 7). Normal blood flow patterns were generally observed in cases of either auricular fibrillation or premature beat, *i.e.*, effective systole. However, in the presence of conspicuous arrhythmia such as severe auricular fibrillation or premature beat accompanied by a very short coupling,

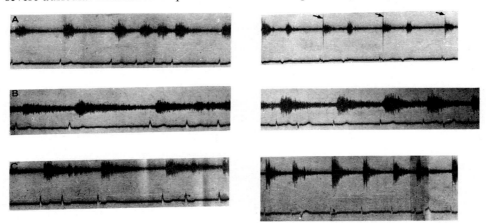

Fig. 7. Effect of arrhythmia on the blood flow patterns in internal carotid artery. Left, indicates blood flow patterns in auricular fibrillation and right, in premature beat. (↓) indicates the Doppler beat due to the pulsation of blood vessel.

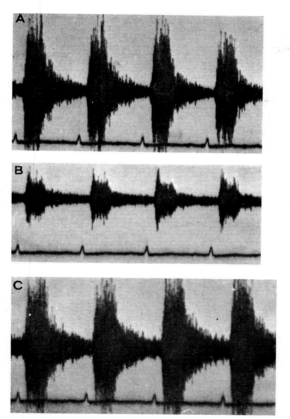

Fig. 8. Effect of aminophylline on the blood flow patterns in internal carotid artery, 81 years, B.P. 250/110. (A) control (B) during administration (C) after administration.

the cerebral blood flow was frequently decreased or completely ceased, *i.e.*, ineffective systole. The findings appear to be related to the elucidation of the mechanism of the Adams–Stokes syndrome.

(5) Effect of circulatory drugs on cerebral circulation (Miyazaki, 1966 b)

The ultrasonic Doppler technique is most appropriate for the investigation of the effect of cerebral circulatory drugs. For example, the effect of theophylline ethylenediamine and nicotinic acid on cerebral circulation were as follows.

First, the hemodynamic change in the internal carotid artery was investigated before, during and after the intravenous administration of theophylline ethylenediamine (250 mg) dissolved in a 5% glucose solution (20 ml). It was found that the effect of the drug on the cerebral circulation was dependent on the administration time, *i.e.*, cerebral vasoconstriction during administration and cerebral vasodilation after administration (Fig. 8). Theophylline ethylenediamine has been most widely used clinically for the treatment of cerebral vascular diseases. Two theories, however, have been presented as to the effect of the drug, *i.e.*, cerebral vasoconstriction and cerebral vasodilation. This experimental conflict as to the effect of theophylline

References pp. 22–23

ethylenediamine on the cerebral circulation may be partly derived from the above pharmacological characteristics of the drug.

Next, the hemodynamics of the extra- and intra-cranial arteries, *i.e.*, the external carotid artery and the internal carotid artery, were observed before, during and after the intravenous administration of nicotinic acid (20 mg) dissolved in a 5% glucose solution (20 ml). A contrasting circulatory effect between the extra- and intra-cranial arteries was observed dependent on the facial blushing in general, *i.e.*, when the facial blushing is conspicuous, there were observed an increase in the blood flow and a

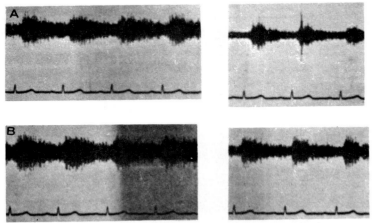

Fig. 9. Effect of nicotinic acid on cerebral circulation. A case with facial blushing (hemiplegic old man 60 years, B.P. 120/60). Left, indicates blood flow patterns in the internal carotid artery and right, in the external carotid artery. (A) control, (B) after administration.

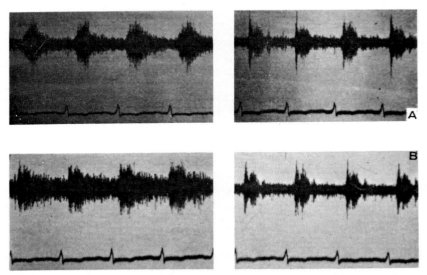

Fig. 10. Effect of nicotinic acid on cerebral circulation. A case without facial blushing (hypertensive old man 61 years, B.P. 210/80). Explanation of the patterns is the same as in Fig. 9. This case shows mild increase of blood flow in internal carotid artery without facial blushing.

decrease in the vascular resistance in the external and the internal carotid arteries, especially in the former; on the other hand, when facial blushing was absent, vasodilation in the external carotid artery was not observed and vasodilation in the internal carotid artery was not observed or if present, was very slight (Figs. 9 and 10).

It is generally said that nicotinic acid conspicuously increases the blood flow in the extracranial artery although the drug does not affect the blood flow in the intracranial artery. In other words, the results by the ultrasonic Doppler technique support the above concept.

(6) Effect of voluntary hyperventilation and the Valsalva maneuver on cerebral circulation (Miyazaki, 1968 b)

The hemodynamics in the internal carotid artery were investigated before, during and after voluntary hyperventilation and the Valsalva maneuver. The duration of a voluntary hyperventilation ranged from 2 to 3 min. The duration of the Valsalva maneuver, on the other hand, ranged from 30 to 40 sec. In addition, the blood pressure, pulse rate and blood gas content (PCO_2, PO_2, pH) were also determined.

During the voluntary hyperventilation, a decrease in the cerebral blood flow and an increase in the cerebral vascular resistance were observed (Fig. 11). This cerebral hemodynamic behavior reached the maximum level immediately after the maneuver (about 1 min) and the level was maintained or returned to the control level. The above results suggest that the cerebral hemodynamics reach a new steady state, rapidly and homeostatically, during the hyperventilation.

During the Valsalva maneuver, a decrease in the cerebral blood flow and an increase in the cerebral vascular resistance continued throughout the maneuver (Fig. 12). In

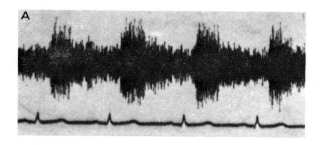

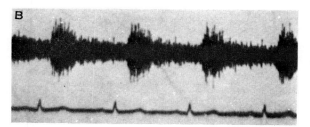

Fig. 11. Change of cerebral circulation during a voluntary hyperventilation (internal carotid artery). 62 years, B.P. 160/90. Bronchial asthma. (A) control, (B) during hyperventilation.

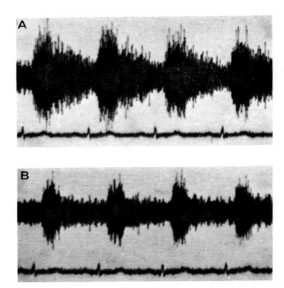

Fig. 12. Change of cerebral circulation during the Valsalva maneuver (internal carotid artery). 62 years, B.P. 145/95. Cerebral arteriosclerosis. (A) control, (B) during maneuver.

addition, the blood pressure was decreased, and the blood gas content was affected as follows: PO_2 and pH increased, although PCO_2 decreased. The above result suggests that decreases in the blood pressure and carbon dioxide pressure in the artery play an important role in the mechanism of the decreased cerebral blood flow during the Valsalva maneuver.

(7) *Effect of smoking on cerebral circulation* (Miyazaki, 1969)

The hemodynamics in the internal carotid artery were investigated before, during

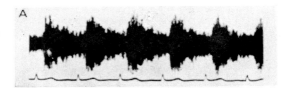

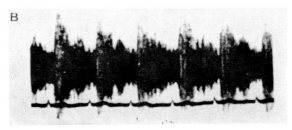

Fig. 13. Change of cerebral circulation in ordinary cigarette smoking (internal carotid artery). Normal young man, 27 years, B.P. 120/70. (A) control, (B) after smoking.

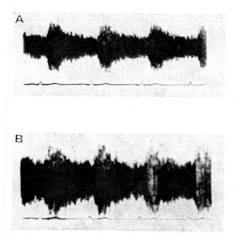

Fig. 14. Change of cerebral circulation in ordinary cigarette smoking (internal carotid artery). Bronchial asthma, 69 years, B.P. 140/85. (A) control, (B) after smoking.

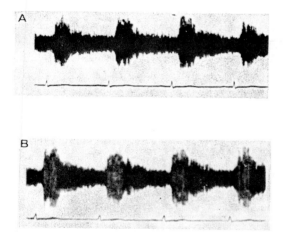

Fig. 15. Change of cerebral circulation in ordinary cigarette smoking (internal carotid artery). Coronary insufficiency, 67 years, B.P. 140/60. (A) control, (B) after smoking.

and after smoking in young and elderly smokers who were instructed to smoke cigarettes of the same type with ordinary and rapid inhaling speed. In addition, blood pressure and pulse rate were investigated throughout the smoking.

Ordinary smoking increased the cerebral blood flow and decreased the cerebral vascular resistance in all subjects following one to three inhalations (Figs. 13, 14 and 15). This state continued for about 10 to 20 min after smoking was stopped. On the other hand, blood pressure and pulse rate did not change or slightly increased. The cerebral circulatory effect of smoking with ordinary speed is mainly due to the direct effect of the chemical ingredients of tobacco (especially nicotine), since a significant correlation is not observed between cerebral hemodynamics and blood pressure.

References pp. 22–23

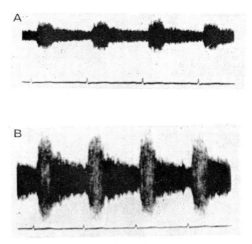

Fig. 16. Change of cerebral circulation in rapid cigarette smoking (internal carotid artery). Coronary insufficiency, 67 years, B.P. 140/60. Fig. 15 and Fig. 16 show the patterns in the same case.

By rapid smoking, changes in the cerebral hemodynamics, blood pressure and pulse rate were more conspicuous than by ordinary smoking (Fig. 16). Therefore, the secondary effect of the cardiocoronary hemodynamics on cerebral hemodynamics must be considered for understanding the increase of cerebral blood flow in rapid smoking.

To summarize the findings, ordinary slow smoking seems, at a glance, to have a favourable effect on cerebral hemodynamics, but habitual long-term smoking causes various pathological conditions within the body, including cerebral vascular disorders.

(8) Cerebral hemodynamics in patients with hypertensive encephalopathy (Miyazaki, 1965 a)

Hypertensive encephalopathy is divided into the following two forms by Oppenheimer and Fishberg (1954):

(i) The cerebral arterioles do not constrict strongly enough to counterbalance an abrupt and pronounced rise in the blood pressure. As a result, the pressure in the capillaries of the brain rises, transudation is favored and reabsorption hindered, and edema develops. This form develops more often in glomerular nephritis and toxemia of pregnancy than in essential hypertension. The clinical picture of this form is dominated by manifestations of increased intracranial pressure.

(ii) The cerebral arteries go into spasm with resultant ischemia of the territory supplied. This occurs especially in elderly patients with essential hypertension and cerebral arteriosclerosis. The clinical picture of this form is that of evanescent cerebral phenomena – faintness, aphasia, etc. – without increased intracranial pressure.

In the author's study, the pathophysiology of hypertensive encephalopathy was as presented in Table 1 and Fig. 17. In young subjects with hypertensive encephalopathy, a decrease in the cerebral blood flow due to an increased cerebral vascular resistance (namely, the second form of Oppenheimer's classification) was observed.

TABLE 1

MAIN CLINICAL FINDINGS IN YOUNG AND OLD PATIENTS
WITH HYPERTENSIVE ENCEPHALOPATHY

Age (yrs)	Young man 31	Old man 60
Blood pressure (mm Hg)		
During attack	230/130	230/130
Control	160/100	160/70
Subjective symptom	Headache, nausea, Tinnitus, Chest-discomfort	Headache, Palpitation
Renal function	15′ 12.5%	25%
(PSP test)	30′ 22.5%	38%
	60′ 35.0%	50%
	120′ 52.5%	60%
Urinary protein	±	—
Blood NPN (mg/dl)	36.4	26.4
Retinal finding		
Keith–Wagener	I	IIa
Scheie	I	II
CSF Pressure (mm H$_2$O)	250	280
Regitine test	—	

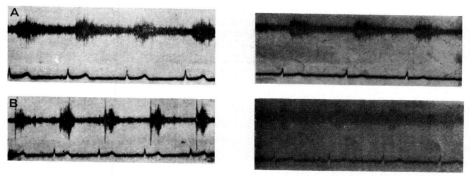

Fig. 17. Blood flow patterns in internal carotid artery in young and old patients with hypertensive encephalopathy. Left, indicates blood flow patterns in a young patient and right, in an old patient. (A) control, (B) during attack.

On the other hand, in elderly subjects with hypertensive encephalopathy, an increase of cerebral blood flow due to the increased blood pressure (namely, the first form of Oppenheimer's classification) was observed.

The cerebral blood flow patterns measured by the ultrasonic Doppler technique consist of the following three types: continuous pattern, discontinuous pattern and intermediate pattern. The cerebral vascular resistance in the continuous pattern is less potent than that in the discontinuous pattern. The intermediate pattern is in between the two (Fig. 18) (Miyazaki, 1967).

A significant correlation between the continuity grade of the cerebral blood flow pattern and the severity of the cerebral arteriosclerosis was observed. This suggests

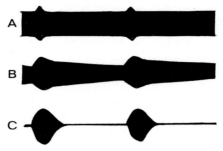

Fig. 18. Classification of cerebral blood flow pattern (internal carotid artery).
(A) continuous type, (B) intermediate type, (C) discontinuous type.

TABLE 2

CRITERIA FOR QUANTITATIVE DETECTION OF CEREBRAL ARTERIOSCLEROSIS BY
ULTRASONIC DOPPLER TECHNIQUE

Type of cerebral blood flow pattern	Severity of cerebral arteriosclerosis	Note
continuous type	both extracerebral atherosclerosis and intracerebral arteriolosclerosis are no or minimal.	pseudocontinuous type
discontinuous type	both extracerebral atherosclerosis and intracerebral arteriolosclerosis are severe. Among them, intracerebral arteriolosclerosis is much more severe than extracerebral atherosclerosis.	pseudodiscontinuous type
intermediate type	both extracerebral atherosclerosis and intracerebral arteriolosclerosis may belong to the continuous and discontinuous type.	pseudointermediate type

that the ultrasonic Doppler technique is also useful for the quantitative detection of cerebral arteriosclerosis, *i.e.*, anticipation of the cerebral vascular accidents. However, it is essential to consider several factors affecting the cerebral blood flow patterns for applications of this method. Table 2 gives rise to the criteria for quantitative detection of cerebral arteriosclerosis by this method.

PATHOPHYSIOLOGICAL OBSERVATIONS OF CEREBRAL CIRCULATION
IN SEVERAL PATHOLOGICAL SITUATIONS

Cerebral venous returns in various diseases (Miyazaki, 1965 c)

Cerebral venous return (blood flow in the internal jugular vein) mainly depends on vis a fronte based on cardiopulmonary function. In other words, the cerebral venous return for the thorax mainly depends on the respiratory pump action due to the decrease in the intrapleural pressure at the inspiratory phase and pressure–suction pump action due to the decrease in the intra-atrial pressure at the ventricular contraction. Therefore, the simultaneous measurement of cerebral venous return and cerebral blood supply are highly useful for the understanding of the pathophysiology, both of cardiopulmonary function and cerebral hemodynamics. However, the measurement of venous return has been controversial from the anatomical and physiological points of view.

In the author's study, cerebral venous return (blood flow in internal jugular vein) and cerebral blood supply (blood flow in internal carotid artery) were investigated by the ultrasonic Doppler technique in normal young subjects, hypertensive elderly subjects (healthy looking), very elderly subjects (healthy looking and normotensive) and patients with congestive heart failure (mitral stenosis), chronic pulmonary emphysema and severe anemia (no cardiopulmonary disease).

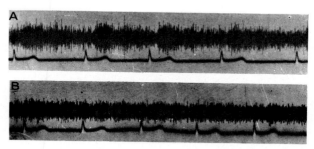

Fig. 19. Blood flow patterns in internal carotid artery (A) and internal jugular vein (B). Normal young man, 24 years.

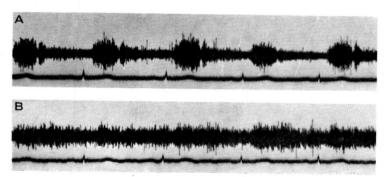

Fig. 20. Blood flow patterns in internal carotid artery and internal jugular vein. Hypertensive old man, 62 years, B.P. 200/120.

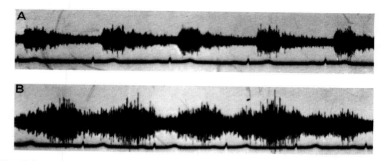

Fig. 21. Blood flow patterns in internal carotid artery and internal jugular vein. Very old man 84 years, B.P. 130/80.

References pp. 22–23

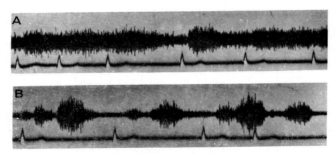

Fig. 22. Blood flow patterns in internal carotid artery and internal jugular vein. Patient with congestive heart failure (mitral stenosis). 60 years B.P. 115/60.

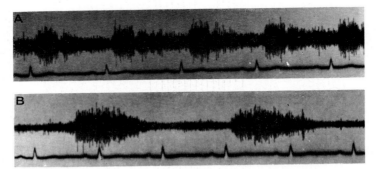

Fig. 23. Blood flow patterns in internal carotid artery and internal jugular vein. Patient with chronic pulmonary emphysema, 61 years, B.P. 150/80, VC 1800cc (51% of predicted normal) MBC 28.8 1/min (34% of predicted normal) FEV 1-0/FEV (%) 45%.

(i) Cerebral venous return in normal young subjects and hypertensive elderly subjects were continuous throughout the cardiac cycle (Figs. 19 and 20). From these results, it was suggested that the cerebral venous return in both groups was in a steady state.

(ii) Cerebral venous return in very elderly subjects was discontinuous in synchrony with the cardiac cycle (Fig. 21). The result indicates that the disorder of cerebral venous return was mainly due to heart failure (insufficiency of pressure–suction pump).

(iii) Cerebral venous return in patients with congestive heart failure was conspicuously discontinuous in synchrony with the cardiac cycle (Fig. 22). The result indicates that the disorder of cerebral venous return was mainly due to insufficiency of pressure–suction pump.

(iv) Cerebral venous return in patients with chronic pulmonary emphysema was observed only in the inspiratory phase and disappeared in the expiratory phase (Fig. 23). The result indicates that the disorder of cerebral venous return was mainly due to the respiratory insufficiency in these patients (insufficiency of respiratory pump).

Today, the following two theories as to the correlation between respiration and venous return have been presented, *i.e.*, inspiratory return and expiratory return (Brecher, 1956). The blood flow patterns in the internal jugular vein in patients with chronic pulmonary emphysema, in which the blood flow patterns were observed only

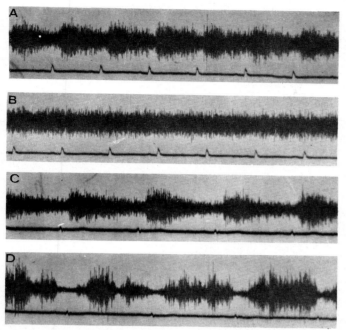

Fig. 24. Blood flow patterns in internal carotid artery (A, C) and internal jugular vein (B, D). Patient
with severe anemia (no cardiopulmonary diseases).
Top: 72 years, B.P. 110/50. Erythrocyte 200 $\times$ 10⁴, Leucocyte 2800 Hemoglobin 20% (Sahli).
Bottom: 75 years, B.P. 130/60, Erythrocyte 200 $\times$ 10⁴, Leucocyte 3000 Hemoglobin 20% (Sahli).

at the inspiratory phase and disappeared at the expiratory phase, support the inspiratory return theory.

(v) Cerebral venous return in patients with severe anemia consists of two types:
steady flow and unsteady flow (Fig. 24).

Focus detection of extracranial vascular lesions (Miyazaki, 1965 b)

The ultrasonic Doppler technique, similar to angiography, is useful for the focus
detection of extracranial vascular lesions. Fig. 25 shows the hemodynamic comparison
of both carotid arteries in one patient with tortuous common carotid artery of the
right side. A conspicuous difference was observed between the right and left blood
flow patterns of the common carotid artery in this case. The finding suggests that a
change in blood flow pattern occurs at the vascular focus in the case of extracranial
vascular lesions, *e.g.*, aortocranial arterial disease. In other words, the ultrasonic
Doppler technique may be used for detection of the extracranial vascular lesions.

Hemodynamic correlation between internal carotid artery and vertebral artery

Hemodynamic correlations between several vessels were investigated by the ultrasonic Doppler technique, *e.g.*, internal carotid artery and vertebral artery (Miyazaki,
1966 c), internal carotid artery and ophthalmic artery (Miyazaki, 1966 d), internal
carotid artery and peripheral artery *(ibid.)*, internal carotid artery and external

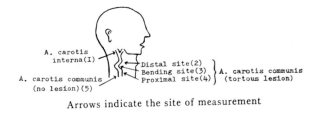

Arrows indicate the site of measurement

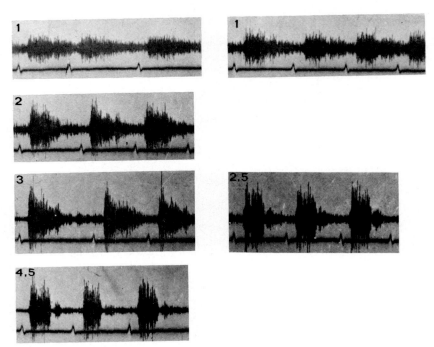

Fig. 25. The hemodynamic comparison of both carotid artery in one patient with tortuous common carotid artery of right side. Left, indicates blood flow patterns of right side and right, left side.

carotid artery (Miyazaki, 1963; Miyazaki and Kato, 1965), etc. In this paper, the hemodynamic correlation between internal carotid artery and vertebral artery is described as an example. The hemodynamic correlation of both the arteries before and after the intravenous administration of papaverine was investigated.

(i) A definitely significant correlation in vasodilation between both the arteries was observed (Fig. 26). The blood flow pattern in the vertebral artery was prone to be more discontinuous than that in the internal carotid artery in the aged regardless of the blood pressure or cerebral vascular disease. This suggests that cerebral vascular resistance in the territory of the vertebral artery was more increased compared to the internal carotid artery in the aged (see page 13).

As for the mechanism of the increased vascular resistance, anatomical characteristics and atherosclerosis of the vertebral-basilar artery must be considered. Of these, the latter factor is more important than the former since there is no significant

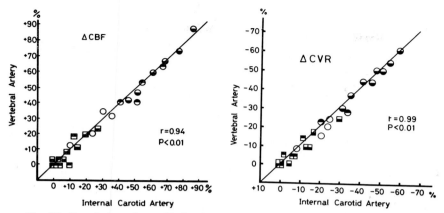

Fig. 26. Correlation of vasodilation in internal carotid artery and vertebral artery

○ normal young man

◕ young man ⎫
◔ old man   ⎬ hypertensive patient

◩ normotensive ⎫
◼ hypertensive ⎬ hemiplegic patient

difference between the blood flow pattern in the internal carotid artery and that in the vertebral artery in the younger age group.

(ii) Cerebral vasodilation in patients with cerebral vascular disease was prone to be less than that in those without the disease (Fig. 27 and Fig. 28). This suggests that the patients with cerebral vascular disease are more likely to fall into cerebral vascular insufficiency as the cerebral blood vessel is already in about maximal dilation, *i.e.*, failure of homeostatic regulation (autoregulation) of cerebral circulation.

For the measurement of cerebral blood flow by the ultrasonic Doppler technique, it is very important that the blood flow in a directed vessel, usually the internal

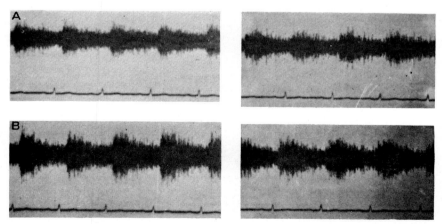

Fig. 27. Correlation of vasodilation in internal carotid artery and in vertebral artery, normal young man, 34 years, B.P. 125/75. Left, indicates blood flow patterns in internal carotid artery and right, in vertebral artery. (A) control, (B) after papaverine administration. Increasing rate of blood flow in both arteries completely coincident.

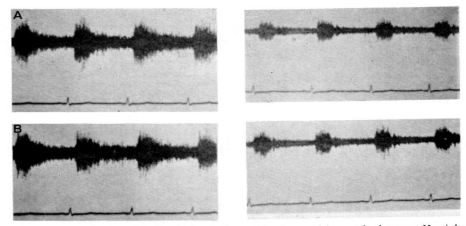

Fig. 28. Correlation of vasodilation in internal carotid artery and in vertebral artery. Hemiplegic old man (hypertensive), 60 years, B.P. 180/95. Explanation of patterns the same as in Fig. 27. No alteration of blood flow observed in both arteries.

carotid artery, is proportional to the whole cerebral blood flow. The significant correlation between the vasodilation of the internal carotid artery and that of the vertebral artery, on which the cerebral blood supply mainly depends, supports the usefulness of this technique except in such cases as complete occlusion of vessel.

A NEW APPROACH IN THE MEASUREMENT OF CEREBRAL BLOOD FLOW BY THE ULTRASONIC DOPPLER TECHNIQUE

The ultrasonic Doppler technique is a unique technique for the measurement of the blood flow compared with others. However, this method is still controversial from various points of view. Especially, the problems as to the probe is one of the most important points to be solved. The ordinary probe can be flexibly used but gives unstable data, i.e., optimum beat can be readily detected but the reproducibility of data is poor.

Rushmer (1967) has devised a new type of probe (Fig. 29). This probe may be stable since it is designed so as to adequately contact the skin. In this probe, both the

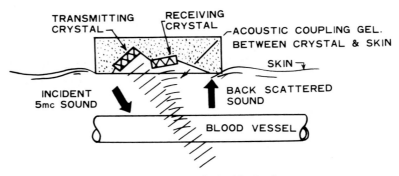

Fig. 29. New probe devised by Rushmer.

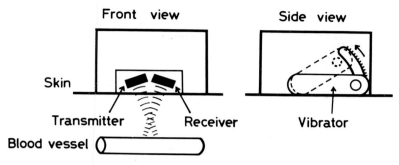

Fig. 30. Angle-variable probe devised by the author.

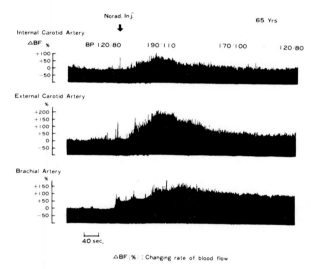

Fig. 31. Effect of induced hypertension (noradrenalin administration) on the blood flow in internal and external carotid arteries and brachial artery.
Although the blood flow was increased in these arteries, the changing rate and sustaining time of the increased blood flow was slightest in internal carotid artery. This fact suggests that the autoregulation and/or noradrenalin sensitivity are greater in internal carotid artery than in the others.

transmitter and receiver are fixed with the vibrator holder. Therefore, it may not always be appropriate for detecting the optimum beat because of the inflexibility. Recently, the present author has devised a new, more suitable probe (Fig. 30). This probe is not only stable but also flexible. Therefore, it is easy to detect the directivity of the ultrasound and the optimum beat. In addition, the data processing is carried out by means of on-line real-time system in the experiments using this probe.

This serial measurement will make it possible to carry out multiple and simultaneous blood flow measurements in men *in situ*, *i.e.*, the internal and external carotid arteries, peripheral artery and vein, etc. Fig. 31 shows one of the data. The blood flow change in the internal and external carotid arteries and brachial artery after the administration of circulatory agents is measured non-operatively, continuously and simultaneously (Miyazaki, 1971). In addition, the impedance of the cerebral circulation

References pp. 22–23

reflecting the cerebral vascular resistance may be obtained by a combination of both blood flow component and blood pressure component.

SUMMARY

The ultrasonic Doppler technique is advantageous as compared with other techniques for the measurement of cerebral blood flow. The changes in the dynamics of cerebral circulation with various circulatory agents can be detected instantaneously and continuously as well as non-operatively by this technique. In addition, it is possible by this technique to measure the blood flow individually in each vessel, *i.e.*, internal, external and common carotid arteries and internal and external jugular veins.

The principle and method as well as several clinical applications of the ultrasonic Doppler technique in the study of cerebral circulation are discussed. The technique has been used for dynamic observation of the changes in cerebral circulation with various circulatory agents and also for the pathophysiological observation of cerebral circulation in several pathological situations. Further, a new approach is described in the measurement of cerebral blood flow by the ultrasonic Doppler technique.

REFERENCES

BRECHER, G. A. (1956) *Venous Return*, Grune & Stratton, New York.

FISHBERG, A. M. (1954) *Hypertension and Nephritis*, Lea & Febiger, Philadelphia, p. 345.

GREENFIELD, J. C. JR. *et al.* (1964) Mechanics of the human common carotid artery *in vivo*. *Circulation Res.*, **15**, 240–246.

MIYAZAKI, M. (1963) Measurement of cerebral blood flow by ultrasonic Doppler technique. *Saishin-Igaku*, **18**, 1839–1851 (in Japanese).

MIYAZAKI, M. (1965 a) Mechanism of hypertensive encephalopathy and cerebral vascular insufficiency. *Jap. Circulation J.*, **29**, 109–112.

MIYAZAKI, M. (1965 b) Hemodynamic comparison of right and left carotid artery in patients with hemiplegia. *Jap. Circulation J.*, **29**, 383–386.

MIYAZAKI, M. (1965 c) Cerebral venous return in various diseases. *Jap. Circulation J.*, **29**, 103–108.

MIYAZAKI, M. (1966 a) Effects of low temperature, induced hypertension and arrhythmia on cerebral circulation. *Jap. Circulation J.*, **30**, 863–867.

MIYAZAKI, M. (1966 b) Effects of several vasodilators on cerebral circulation, with special reference to aminophylline, nicotinic acid and papaverine. *Jap. Circulation J.*, **30**, 1203–1209.

MIYAZAKI, M. (1966 c) Hemodynamic correlation of internal carotid artery and vertebral artery. *Jap. Circulation J.*, **30**, 981–985.

MIYAZAKI, M. (1966 d) Hemodynamic correlation between cerebral and peripheral-ophthalmic artery. *Jap. Circulation J.*, **30**, 1353–1358.

MIYAZAKI, M. (1967) Quantitative detection of cerebral arteriosclerosis. *Jap. Circulation J.*, **31**, 781–786.

MIYAZAKI, M. (1968 a) Pulsatile variation of vascular diameter of human common carotid artery. *Jap. Circulation J.*, **32**, 1003–1009.

MIYAZAKI, M. (1968 b) Cerebral hemodynamics during voluntary hyperventilation and the Valsalva maneuver. *Jap. Circulation J.*, **32**, 315–319.

MIYAZAKI, M. (1969) Circulatory effect of cigarette smoking, with special reference to the effect on cerebral hemodynamics. *Jap. Circulation J.*, **33**, 907–912.

MIYAZAKI, M. (1971) Multiple and simultaneous blood flow measurements by ultrasonic Doppler technique in man, with special reference to the circulatory effects of induced hypertension on internal, external carotid arteries and brachial artery. *Jap. Circulation J.*, **35**, 405–412.

Miyazaki, M. and Kato, K. (1965) Measurement of cerebral blood flow by ultrasonic Doppler technique. Theory. *Jap. Circulation J.*, **29**, 375–382.

Rushmer, R. F. *et al.* (1967) Clinical applications of transcutaneous ultrasonic flow detector. *J. Amer. Med. Assoc.*, **199**, 326–328.

Satomura, S. and Kaneko, Z. (1960) Ultrasonic blood rheograph: *3rd International Conference on ME, London*, p. 254–258.

Impedance Methods for Investigation of Cerebral Circulation

D. HADJIEV

Research Institute of Neurology and Psychiatry, Sofia (Bulgaria)

INTRODUCTION

During the last decade numerous methods have been developed for the study of cerebral circulation. Some of them, utilizing radioisotope indicators, made possible the quantitative determination of total and regional cerebral blood flow. Few techniques, however, yield painless, continuous and incessant information, with no risk for the patient, on circulation changes in different areas of the brain. Such information may be obtained by methods based on registration of impedance fluctuations occurring synchronously with cardiac activity and respiration, or by registering the total impedance changes of the head.

Schlüter (1921) attempted to localize brain tumors by determining cerebral impedance with the aid of an apparatus based on the bridge principle. Kedrov and Naumenko (1941) were the first to use alternating current of 279 kHz frequency and 30 mA strength for the study of brain circulation in experimental animals. Polzer and Schühfried (1950) for the first time applied cranial rheography (rheoencephalography) in man. They noted changes in the form of the rheoencephalogram with depression of its amplitude in carotid artery occlusion. The purpose of simultaneously assaying the circulation in both cerebral hemispheres led to the construction of a two-channel rheograph based on the bridge principle (Kaindl *et al.*, 1956).

With the bridge techniques for measurement of pulsatile variations in the impedance of the head (rheoencephalography I) the number of leads is limited and the possibility of interference between the electric current circles distributed in the different zones of the head cannot be ruled out. To remove this disadvantage Lechner and Rodler (1961) developed a method in which the current input electrodes are separated from the recording electrodes. This permits the performance of numerous simultaneous leads in a single electric current circle (rheoencephalography II). New techniques have recently been suggested for the measurement of cephalic impedance fluctuations: "guarded electrode system" (Lifshitz and Klemm, 1966), "monopolar rheoencephalography" (Namon and Markovich, 1967), registration of intracerebral impedance (Laitinen *et al.*, 1966), registration with DC amplifier–total impedance rheography (Lechner *et al.*, 1966), induction method (Rodler, 1969 a), utilization of very high current frequencies (Vaney, 1969), etc.

Efforts have been made recently for the quantitative evaluation by impedance techniques of the total and regional cerebral circulation by using some rheoencephalographic parameters (Hadjiev, 1968 a) or by registration of artificially induced changes in the electric conductivity of blood (Rodler, 1969 b).

Together with the technical progress in the field of impedance methods of examination of cerebral circulation, a series of problems pertinent to their electrochemical and biophysical principles were elucidated. However, some problems of the origin and nature of the rheoencephalographic wave are still debatable. The importance of some of its parameters still remains to be definitively clarified.

Opinions are conflicting concerning the facilities and limitations of the clinical application of impedance methods. Numerous investigations undertaken mainly with apparatus based on the bridge system for the measurement of cranial impedance changes proved the diagnostic value of the method in cerebral vascular diseases, in tumors, cranio-cerebral trauma and other pathologic processes (Jenkner, 1957, 1962; Pratesi *et al.*, 1957; Kunert, 1959, 1961; etc.). The diagnostic range of rheoencephalography substantially increases by making simultaneous hemispheric and regional recordings, using different tests for the evaluation of cerebral vascular reaction (Yarullin, 1967).

Some authors are sceptical about the usefulness of the impedance methods in the diagnosis of cerebral diseases. Perez-Borja and Meyer (1964), utilizing the bridge system, conclude that the method fails to give reliable clinical information on the diagnosis of cerebral vascular diseases since, in their opinion, an essential part of the rheoencephalographic wave originates from the extracranial vessels. Waltz and Ray (1967), using "monopolar rheoencephalography", never observed constant deflections in the impedance cephalograms in patients with cerebral vascular diseases; they conclude, therefore, that the method is not adequate for the assessment of cerebral circulation.

These conflicting data make a critical attitude toward the utilized impedance techniques necessary and require precise interpretation of the findings obtained.

A promising field for the application of impedance methods is the study of the effectiveness of vasoactive, metabolic-active and edema-controlling drugs on cerebral circulation. The continuous information on the state of the brain vessels and their reactivity which these methods provide attains major importance in prescribing treatment and controlling and its effectiveness in cerebral vascular diseases (Hadjiev, 1966 a).

THEORETICAL BASIS OF IMPEDANCE METHODS

It is known that tissue impedance consists of an active ohmic (R) and a reactive capacitance (X). Its magnitude may be calculated by the formula

$$(Z) = \sqrt{R^2 + X^2} \tag{1}$$

In the case of tissues, inductance is practically nonexistent and may be disregarded. X is therefore determined by the capacitance (C), and the relation between X_C and C is expressed by the equation:

$$X_c = \frac{1}{2\pi f C} \tag{2}$$

where f is the frequency of the alternating current. Therefore, the capacitance is inversely proportional to the frequency of the electric current and the magnitude of the capacitance. After reforming the first equation the impedance may be expressed with the formula:

$$(Z) = \sqrt{R^2 + \left(\frac{1}{2\pi f C}\right)^2} \tag{3}$$

Tissue electric resistance to constant current is quite high. For example, in the lower leg it amounts to 20000–60000 ohm/cm (Karellin, 1957). In this case a polarization resistance arises around the electrodes. When alternating current is passed the electric resistance of tissues falls with the increase in the current frequency.

TABLE 1

IMPEDANCE (Z) IN OHMS USING DIFFERENT ELECTRODES AND DIFFERENT
ALTERNATING CURRENT FREQUENCIES

Frequencies	2 cm² electrodes		15 cm² electrodes	
	Mean	Range	Mean	Range
30 kHz	620	900–480	150	180–130
120 kHz	400	530–300	130	160–110
500 kHz	340	450–250	110	130–91
1.5 mHz	330	450–220	97	130–83

In Table 1, modified after Lifshitz (1969), are given the overall impedance (Z) values of the skull for different frequencies of the electric current and varying fronto-mastoid localizations of the small and large electrodes. Investigations were carried out with 10 men from 23 to 50 years of age, without cerebral vascular disorders.

It may be clearly seen that with increasing frequency of the electric current the impedance of the skull decreases; it is lower when larger electrodes are used.

In view of their ability to penetrate into the butt, high frequency alternating currents are suitable for rheographic examination. In measuring the impedance changes of live tissues, however, the dependence of the electric conductivity of blood from the frequency of alternating current should be taken into consideration. With frequencies exceeding 200–250 kHz the difference between the electric conductivity of blood and of other tissues vanishes. The rheoencephalographic method is actually based on the determination of this difference (Lifshitz, 1963 a; Yarullin, 1967). Therefore, when measuring tissue electric resistance, alternating currents with frequencies from 20 kHz (Polzer and Schühfried, 1950) to 200 kHz (Nyboer, 1959) are most commonly used.

During the examination the tissues of the head practically do not change their electric resistance; the impedance changes occur synchronously with cardiac activity and the respiration phases. It may be suggested that impedance changes result from

amplifiers, permitting the registration of the total impedance changes (Lechner *et al.*, 1966). This "total impedance rheography" yields additional information on the blood volume in the tissue in various regions of the brain (Lechner and Martin, 1969; Lechner and Lanner, 1969).

To avoid that the record should depend from the position of the electrodes and the way they are placed, inductive methods have been developed for examining the magnetic field by means of a coil (Rodler, 1969 a).

(c) Three-terminal system ("Monopolar Rheoencephalography")

This is a modification of the tetrapolar method. With this approach one of the electrodes serving for the measurement of impedance fluctuations is connected with one of the current input electrodes. The reference electrode is 1.5 cm in diameter and the input electrodes have a diameter of 6 cm. Electric current with a frequency of 28–36 kHz and strength of 2 mA is used. Namon and Markovich (1967) believe that this measurement technique provides a more adequate localization of the pathologic process.

Thus, none of the methods known so far for measurement of cephalic impedance fluctuations has proved to be perfect, and therefore, efforts must be continued to further improve the impedance methods.

Our rheoencephalographic studies were carried out with two-channel and four-channel rheographs based on the bridge principle. We applied fronto-mastoid, occipito-mastoid, bitemporal and bimastoid leads. Electrodes measuring 9 cm^2 were used, attached to the skull by an electrode paste. For registration we used a polygraph apparatus with an appropriate time constant. Tracings were made in a horizontal position, in 45° Trendelenburg position and after performance of various tests.

Interpretation of the rheoencephalogram

The rheoencephalogram is a deflection from the baseline connecting the points of its systolic elevations due to changes in the impedance of the examined segment of the head. The normal rheoencephalogram consists of a steeply ascending branch which as a first peak reaches the maximum of the curve. It is followed by a descending limb which drops gradually to the baseline. A notch is seen on the descending branch localized usually at its middle third, and several, usually 2 or 3, additional peaks, lower than the first one.

The most important and still debatable question is whether and how far the rheoencephalogram reflects the state of the intracranial vessels. Proceeding from experimental and clinical observations, some authors contend that the rheoencephalogram is produced by pulsations of the external carotid artery and that predominating in it is the influence of extracranial vessels (Friedmann, 1955; Matzdorff, 1961).

It is known that owing to anatomical differences, it is impossible to conclude from animal studies on the vascular region from which the rheoencephalographic tracing derives. For this reason Bertha *et al.* (1955) studied 10 schizophrenic patients who had undergone prefrontal leucotomy. Comparing the tracings obtained with the

electrodes laid on the skin, bones, dura and pia mater, the authors judged that 10%
of the curves originated from the skin, 63% from the homolateral hemisphere and
27% from the contralateral one.

During a surgical approach to the carotid bifurcation, Jenkner (1962) using a
bipolar technique studied the influence of transient compression of the external and
internal carotid arteries on the rheoencephalogram. In the former case no changes
occurred, in the latter the rheoencephalogram was modified.

A personal observation (Hadjiev and Tzenov, 1966) confirmed Jenkner's finding
that the rheoencephalogram was not altered by digital compression on the common
carotid artery on the side of the occluded internal carotid artery, although the
simultaneously registered pulse of arteria temporalis superficialis disappeared. Seipel
et al. (1964) reported analogous data obtained by carotid compression on the side of
the occluded internal carotid artery.

Carotid artery compression provided evidence that the rheoencephalographic data
obtained by rheoencephalography II reflect intracranial impedance changes (Lechner
and Martin, 1969).

Yarullin (1965 a) established that compression of the vertebral artery (during
operation) at the site of its origine, results in an abrupt decrease in the amplitude of
the homolateral occipito-mastoid rheoencephalogram, suggesting that the latter
reflects the blood volume fluctuations in the vertebral artery basin.

The concept of the mainly intracranial origin of the impedance changes reflected
in the rheoencephalographic wave is confirmed also by the analysis of the relation
between the relative part of the anacrotic portion in the rheoencephalogram – giving
information on vascular tone – and the arterial and jugular CO_2 content assayed by
us in 45 patients with cerebral vascular lesions. Rheoencephalographic studies were
carried out with the bipolar technique, gas analysis was performed according to the
method of Natelson (1951).

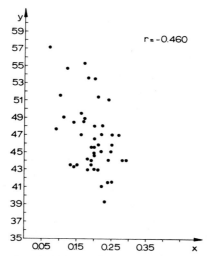

Fig. 1. Relationship between the relative part of the anacrotic section of the rheoencephalogram in
percentage *(x)* and the arterial CO_2 in volume % *(y)*.

References pp. 79–85

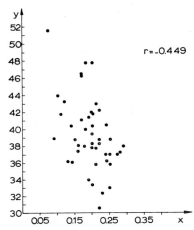

Fig. 2. Relationship between the relative part of the anacrotic section of the rheoencephalogram in percentage *(x)* and jugular CO_2 in volume % *(y)*.

Correlation analysis reveals a significant rectilinear negative correlation between the relative part of the anacrotic section in the rheoencephalogram and the CO_2 content of arterial and jugular blood (Figs. 1, 2).

The higher the carbon dioxide content in the arterial and jugular blood, the lower the cerebral vascular tone – a fact which is in keeping with the selective vasodilatory effect of carbon dioxide on cerebral blood vessels.

The data adduced present ample evidence of the decisive importance of intracranial vessels for the rheoencephalographic pattern. In some pathologic conditions, however (thrombosis of the internal carotid artery with collateral blood flow through the homolateral external carotid artery) the extracranial arteries may acquire a dominating role in the origin of the rheoencephalogram. In such cases compression of the extra-cranial arteries is followed by significant depression of the rheoencephalographic wave; nevertheless the wave continues to reflect the pulsatile fluctuations in the impedance of the brain.

Applying consecutive compressions of the superficial temporal and common carotid arteries, Seipel (1967) endeavoured to determine their involvement in the overall amplitude of the rest rheoencephalogram. In his hands, the method permits estimation in milliohms of the extracranial and intracranial circulation.

Whereas the importance of intracranial and extracranial arteries in the arousal of pulsatile fluctuations in the cephalic impedance has been the subject of numerous investigations, the role of the venous compartment of cerebral circulation has been insufficiently studied.

Venous waves in the rheoencephalograms were described early and late in the diastole. Wick (1955, 1962) observed venous wave in the rheoencephalogram of tricuspidal regurgitation in the early diastole, immediately after the end of the T wave in the electrocardiogram. The close proximity of the venous and arterial waves seems to be due to proximity of the skull to the central venous basins where abnormal fluctuations in the venous filling occur, rapidly transmissible to the cerebral venous system. Jenkner (1962) noted that the third wave in the rheoencephalogram which appears with the patient in Trendelenburg position immediately before the new systolic ascent of the curve reflects the changes in the venous blood filling of the brain. Seipel (1967) holds that the presystolic waves, common as they are, seem to be a normal finding.

To gain knowledge on the rheoencephalographic changes conditioned by the venous part of the cerebral circulation we carried out rheoencephalographic studies in situations which affect it (Hadjiev, 1965 a, 1966 b).

In normal persons placed in Trendelenburg position we observed characteristic changes in the rheoencephalogram – the amplitude shows intensive increase, with the second wave localized after the T wave of the electrocardiogram being highest. In most of these individuals a new wave appears before the systolic rise of the curve, before, synchronously with, or after the P wave of the electrocardiogram. The rheoencephalographic changes disappear after placing the subject in horizontal position.

To clarify the significance of cerebrospinal fluid dislocation for the changes in the pulsatile impedance fluctuations, rheoencephalographic tracings were made in the horizontal position and in Trendelenburg position before and after evacuation of cerebrospinal fluid. In a group of 5 patients with epilepsy the morphologic changes in the curve in Trendelenburg position before and after withdrawal of cerebrospinal fluid showed no essential differences. The second wave of the rheoencephalogram in Trendelenburg position kept increasing after evacuation of the cerebrospinal fluid; the presystolic wave was also seen clearly.

Thus, the removal of cerebrospinal fluid and the concomitant pressure changes are not responsible for the rheoencephalographic changes observed in Trendelenburg position.

A marked increase in the second wave of the rheoencephalogram is observed also after intravenous injection of nicotinic acid. This change is associated with elevation of the overall venous pressure and with the increasing pressure in the upper bulb of the internal jugular vein after administration of the drug.

Inverse changes in the rheoencephalogram with depression of its second peak occasionally arise after intravenous administration of Euphylline. These changes correlate well with the pressure fall in the upper bulb of the internal jugular vein after application of the drug.

These data suggest that the elevation of the second wave in the rheoencephalogram is associated with rising overall venous pressure and impeded venous outflow from the cranial space which arises in a variety of situations (Trendelenburg position, tricuspid regurgitation, overall venous pressure elevation under the influence of drugs).

The presystolic wave in the rheoencephalogram emerging in Trendelenburg position seems to have no direct association with the elevation in the overall venous pressure, because it is not invariably observed in cases of impeded venous outflow from the cranial space and in venous pressure elevation. This wave has obviously no relation to changes in cerebrospinal fluid pressure either. It may therefore be assumed that the presystolic wave lying before or synchronously with the P wave of the electrocardiogram reflects regional fluctuations in the filling of the cerebral veins. This assumption is supported by the presence of this wave in some disorders of cerebral circulation and its disappearance after intravenous administration of Euphylline (Hadjiev and Yarullin, 1967 a).

Thus, the impedance methods yield information not merely on the state of the brain arteries, but on cerebral venous circulation as well. Studies in Trendelenburg position may be used as a test for the assay of the venous brain circulation compartment; morphological changes in the rheoencephalogram associated with fluctuations in venous blood filling may serve to observe the effects of vaso-active drugs.

Nevertheless, the problem of how to eliminate the interference of extracranial vessels in the fluctuations of cephalic impedance has not been entirely solved. The influence of extracranial vessels on the impedance changes may be diminished by using larger electrodes or higher current frequencies.

Another possibility to attain this goal may be the "guarded electrode system" suggested by Lifshitz and Klemm (1966). This technique is claimed to create conditions for control and reduction of the electric current lines spreading along the cranial surface, and hence to diminish extracerebral tissue involvement in the pulsatile fluctuations of the cephalic impedance (Lifshitz, 1969).

In fact, difficulties in obtaining information on the intracranial circulation alone, due to its anatomical particularities, are attached to almost all the methods of examination of cerebral circulation.

Quantitative evaluation of cerebral blood flow by impedance methods

Quantitative information on the state of the cerebral circulation is of primary importance for an objective assessment of its disturbances, for their exact localization and pathogenesis and for discerning treatment.

A number of techniques have been developed recently for the assay of total and regional cerebral circulation, utilizing radioactive indicators either non-diffusible or diffusible through the vascular wall (Hedlund, 1966; Ingvar and Lassen, 1965). They give quantitative information on the circulation time of the indicator through the cerebral vascular bed and on the volume velocity of the cerebral blood flow. Some of these methods, however, are associated with trauma, have numerous disadvantages and require complex equipment, all of which limit their applicability.

For this reason, it seems attractive to use the impedance methods for quantitative assessment of the total and regional blood flow, as they are practicable and non-traumatic, although they do not yield quantitative information on cerebral circulation.

Recent studies have shown that the mean changes in the rheoencephalogram correlate with the changes of the cerebral blood flow occurring after inhalation of 5% carbon dioxide and 95% oxygen and after hyperventilation (Namon *et al.*, 1967). It was found that the relative part of the rheoencephalogram and the cerebral vascular resistance measured by a radioisotope venous dilution technique showed parallel changes (Hadjiev, 1968 a).

The attempt to use rheoencephalographic parameters for the quantitative assessment of cerebral blood flow therefore seems justifiable.

With that end in view we performed comparative studies of cerebral circulation in human subjects using rheoencephalography and the venous radioisotope dilution technique (Hadjiev, 1970 a).

Rheoencephalographic studies were done in supine position. We used aluminium electrodes, each one measuring 9 cm² which we fastened with an electrode paste over the glabella and in the area of the mastoid process. Fronto-mastoid rheoencephalogram and one-lead electrocardiogram were recorded with a three-channel electrocardiograph Galileo, at a paper speed of 25–50 mm/sec.

Five tracings free from artefacts were quantitatively analysed. The rheoencephalographic amplitude was measured in ohms and the mean rheoencephalogram (by planimeter) in mm²/sec. We measured the anacrotic section of the rheoencephalogram, from the start of the curve to its peak, and then calculated the part pertaining to one cardiac cycle. This parameter yields information on vascular tone and cerebral vascular resistance (Fasano et al., 1961; Yarullin, 1967).

Promptly after the rheoencephalographic examination we measured the cerebral blood flow (CBF) in the internal jugular vein of the surveyed hemisphere in the same patients using the venous radioisotope dilution method suggested by Solti et al. (1966) in the modification of Shillingford et al. (1962). The values found by this method and referred to 100 g of brain tissue are similar to those obtained by the method of Kety and Schmidt (1945). ^{131}I-labelled human serum albumin was used as indicator. The volume velocity of the cerebral blood flow was calculated by the formula:

$$\text{CBF (in ml/min)} = I_1 \left(\frac{C_1}{C_v} - 1 \right),$$

I_1 being the infusion rate in ml/min, C_1 – activity of infused isotope and C_v – mean isotope activity in blood samples from the internal jugular vein. By determining the mean arterial pressure (P_m) using a bloodless technique, we estimated also the cerebral vascular resistance by the formula:

$$\text{CVR} = \frac{P_m}{\text{CBF}}$$

We made correlation analysis of the relations between each of the three rheoencephalographic parameters and the cerebral vascular resistance measured by the venous radioisotope dilution technique. With regression analysis we evaluated the connection between the relative part of the anacrotic section of the curve and the cerebral vascular resistance (Hadjiev and Baikushev, 1969). We estimated also the coefficients for rectilinear and curvilinear correlation between the amplitude and the relative part of the anacrotic section of the rheoencephalogram.

A total of 32 patients with ischemic cerebro-vascular disorders were studied (10 women and 22 men between 47 and 87 years of age). In Fig. 3 are shown the values of the rheoencephalographic amplitude and the cerebral vascular resistance.

The correlation coefficient $r = 0.079$ does not essentially deviate from zero. Neither is the correlation between mean rheoencephalogram and cerebral vascular resistance significant: the correlation coefficient $r = 0.12$.

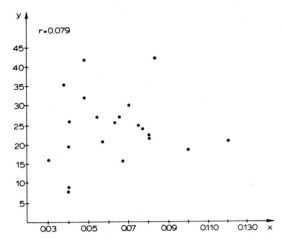

Fig. 3. Relationship between rheoencephalographic amplitude in ohms *(x)* and cerebral vascular resistance in dyn/sec/cm⁻⁵ *(y)*.

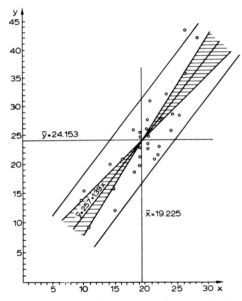

Fig. 4. Relationship between the relative part of the anacrotic section of the rheoencephalogram in percentage *(x)* and cerebral vascular resistance in dyn/sec/cm⁻⁵ *(y)*.

The values of the relative part of the anacrotic section in the rheoencephalogram and the cerebral vascular resistance are shown in Fig. 4. The correlation coefficient between these parameters is 0.84 and significantly deviates from zero ($P_{(t)} < 0.001$).

Using regression analysis, we found a rectilinear relationship between these parameters expressed by the equation $y = -2.57 + 1.39\ x$; 1.39 is the regression coefficient. The standard error of the regression coefficient is 0.16 and its maximal value (at a significance level = 0.05) is 0.34. Therefore, the regression line expressing the correlation between the analyzed parameters may lie between the straight lines $y^I = -2.57 + 1.05\ x$ and $y^{II} = -2.57 + 1.73\ x$, *i.e.* within the shaded range in the diagram.

The deviation of the separate results from the regression line ($S_{y\ 1,2}$) amounts to 4.25; the confidential regression zone at a level of significance $= 0.10$ is $y = (-2.57 + 1.39\ x) \pm 1.70 \times 4.25$.

The close correlation between the anacrotic section of the rheoencephalogram and the cerebral vascular resistance, and the absence of correlation between the rheoencephalographic amplitude and the cerebral vascular resistance make the absence of significant rectilinear and curvilinear correlation between these two rheoencephalographic parameters clear (Fig. 5).

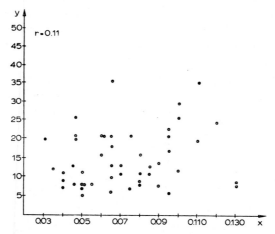

Fig. 5. Relationship between rheoencephalographic amplitude in ohms *(x)* and the relative part of the anacrotic section of the rheoencephalogram in percentage *(y)*.

These data indicate that the relative part of the anacrotic section of the rheoencephalogram is closely related to the cerebral vascular resistance. These two parameters undergo parallel changes. There is sufficient ground to assume that the cranial impedance changes reflect cerebral blood volume and blood redistribution changes in the brain, and to a much lesser extent the blood flow rate. These sources of impedance changes apparently depend on the resistance of the vessels upon the blood flow through the head. This means that the cephalic impedance changes, and hence the rheoencephalogram reflect the cerebral vascular resistance changes, thus making fluctuations in the blood flow and blood redistribution possible. This is confirmed also by the rise in the anacrotic section of the rheoencephalogram with elevation of the cerebral vascular resistance in cases of sclerosis of the brain vessels, marked intracranial hypertension and increased viscosity of the blood.

The parallelism between the anacrotic section of the rheoencephalogram and the cerebral vascular resistance permits (of quantitative measurement of cerebral blood flow with data derived from the rheoencephalographic method) using the formula

$CBF = P_m \times 60/CVR$. This yields rapid quantitative information on the volume velocity of the cerebral blood flow by a bloodless and non-traumatic procedure.

The marked deviation of the values obtained by us around the regression line and the width of the confidential zone require additional clarification; thus, the relative part of the anacrotic section in the rheoencephalogram seems a more accurate index of cerebral vascular resistance. One reason for this deviation may be the influence, however mild, of extracranial cerebral vessels on the course of the rheoencephalogram. It is desirable, therefore, to use a more perfect technique for recording pulsatile brain impedance fluctuations, or to introduce correction coefficients for the elimination of the extracranial impedance component. The latter possibility, however attractive, is difficult owing to the individual variations in the extracranial arteries, and hence, to the varying degree of their involvement in the cephalic impedance changes.

These difficulties do not rule out prospects for finding the most reliable rheoencephalographic parameter for quantitative measurement of the volume velocity of the cerebral blood flow. In this respect some parameters of the differential rheoencephalogram may appear useful. In addition, comparative investigations with other quantitative methods of measurement of cerebral blood flow may be more promising. A theoretically feasible approach to cerebral blood flow determination by impedance methods is to correlate impedance measured with brain-implanted electrodes with thermal clearance data which, as shown in the studies of Betz et al. (1966), may be calibrated by the ^{85}Kr clearance technique.

Another possibility for quantitative measurement of cerebral blood flow by impedance methods is the recording of "rheographic conductance" isolated from plethysmographic effects which is determined by the speed of blood flow (Lechner et al., 1965 a). This possibility has merely theoretical value.

The third approach in the use of impedance methods for quantitative assay of cerebral blood flow is based on principles analogous to those applied for determining circulation time and regional cerebral blood flow with radioactive indicators. Here the radioactive indicator is replaced by a substance altering blood conductivity, and the scintillation detectors by devices for the measurement and registration of impedance changes.

By injecting into the circulation substances reducing or increasing the electric conductivity of blood, the electric resistance of tissue is modified. This effect is maintained during the passage of blood with altered electric conductivity. When tracings are recorded with a DC amplifier, characteristic curves are produced with a steep ascending limb, peak, slowly declining to initial values. The curve may serve to appraise the blood circulation in the arterial, venous and capillary vessels of the brain (Rodler, 1960 a). With a similar injection technique Rodler (1969 b) claims that clearance curves can also be registered analogous to those obtained with diffusing radioisotopes, which can be analyzed similarly.

The following advantages of the impedance techniques for the determination of blood flow by recording artificially induced changes in electric conductivity of blood may be pointed out: simple equipment; ease of multiple simultaneous bilateral recording; and clearance of the radiation load (Rodler, 1969 b).

A disadvantage of this method is the need of absolute rest during the examination, which cannot be always controlled.

There is sufficient ground to believe that the impedance techniques will enable the obtention of continuous, non-stop quantitative information on cerebral blood flow and the following up of its changes under the influence of various factors. Future investigations must show which of the routes selected will be the most suitable for obtaining such information.

ABNORMAL RHEOENCEPHALOGRAMS

It is of great importance for the interpretation of the type of disturbed cerebral circulation to define the abnormal rheoencephalogram. The different impedance techniques, however, give different rheoencephalograms in cerebral vascular disorders (Markovich, 1969), which is one of the reasons for the conflicting opinions of the different authors regarding the clinical value of these methods.

According to Lugaresi *et al.* (1969) the characteristics of the abnormal rheo-encephalogram should depend not only on the morphology of the curve and the reaction to amyl nitrate inhalation, but also on the comparison of the curves on both sides of the head and assessment of the changes following carotid compression.

In addition, some of the differences in the rheoencephalographic parameters are age-dependent; for this reason the definition of theoretical abnormal rheoencephalo-gram is objectionable (Minz and Ronkin, 1967). On the other hand, the so-called "age"-conditioned changes have nothing specific and can hardly be distinguished from the changes caused by the pathologic processes.

Lugaresi *et al.* (1969) assume that the disappearance of dicrotism and the absence of changes following amyl nitrate inhalation are the most outstanding features of the abnormal rheoencephalogram. They regard the inclination of the ascending wave and a convex aspect of the descending wave to have minor diagnostic value.

Inasmuch as the rheoencephalogram reflects the cephalic impedance fluctuations conditioned by vascular resistance, the pathologic deviations would be manifested by signs of reduced or elevated vascular tone, and accordingly, by signs of dilated or narrowed vascular lumen. In addition, differences in the shape of the rheoencephalo-gram and its parameters may give information on the existence of vascular dystonia and cerebral venous congestion (Hadjiev, 1970 b).

(a) Reduced cerebral vascular tone

This is manifested by the following rheoencephalographic findings: steep rise of the anacrotic section of the curve, high amplitude, sharp peak, overt incisure with low localization (in the lower third of the curve or very close to the baseline), promi-nent post-incisure wave. These rheoencephalographic changes may be observed after inhalation of 5 to 7% CO_2 or cervical sympathectomy (Jenkner, 1962) resulting in dilation of the cerebral vessels. Analogous deviations may be induced by vasodilative drugs.

Under the influence of papaverine hydrochloride the elevated cerebral vascular

References pp. 79–85

tone is reduced; the curve becomes steeper, the amplitude height is increased, the peak becomes sharper, the incisure is localized low and the post-incisure wave is very marked. A presystolic wave appears occasionally; it reflects the increasing fluctuations in the blood filling of the venous compartments of the brain circulation, in connection with the inflow of a greater amount of blood secondary to cerebral vascular dilation.

These signs of reduced cerebral vascular tone may be observed also in a variety of pathologic conditions associated with cerebral hyperemia, such as contusion of the brain (Jenkner, 1962), following electroshock (Lifshitz, 1963 b), and others.

When the cerebral vessels are strongly dilated and venous blood outflow from the cranial space is impeded, a rise in the pre-incisure wave, attaining maximal height and merging with the peak of the curve, is observed in the rheoencephalogram together with the signs of vasodilation. Similar rheoencephalographic findings may be observed after intravenous injections of nicotinic acid which, in addition to cerebral vascular dilation, induces a rise in the total venous pressure thus impeding the venous outflow from the intracranial space (Hadjiev, 1965 b).

(b) Increased cerebral vascular tone

This is characterized by the following rheoencephalographic changes: slower rise in the anacrotic section of the curve, low amplitude, rounded peak, a poorly defined incisure localized in the upper one third of the descending branch, indistinct post-incisure wave. Similar alterations occur in the rheoencephalogram on stimulating the cervical sympathetic system and during hyperventilation (Jenkner, 1962).

High localization of the incisure and the post-incisure waves occasionally exceeding the peak may be observed in the non-sclerotic stage of arterial hypertension when arteriolar spasm is significant (Eninya, 1962).

The increased cerebral vascular tone is an obstacle to the blood inflow into the cranial space, which is gradually overcome. As a result, cranial impedance is altered more slowly which is manifested by a slow rise in the anacrotic portion of the curve. The pulsatile fluctuations of the contracted vessel are smaller, giving a lower amplitude in the rheoencephalogram.

Similar rheoencephalographic changes have been observed in organic stenosis of the cerebral vessels, secondary to atherosclerosis, vasculitis, etc. In these cases the ascending part of the curve slowly rises, the ascending branch is elongated, amplitude is low, the incisure and the additional waves are poorly defined or entirely absent. These changes in the form of the rheoencephalogram and its quantitative parameters are poorly, if at all, affected by vasodilating drugs. More significant changes in the curve after injection of vasodilating drugs have been observed accompanying vascular spasm; it is thus easy to differentiate functional components from organic ones of the vascular process (Hadjiev and Tzenov, 1964 a).

(c) Cerebral vascular dystonia

Cerebral vascular tone lability is manifested by alternating curves, modified according to elevated or reduced tone patterns. In the tracing one may observe normal rheoencephalograms as well. Cerebral vascular dystonia may be occasionally associated with transient disturbances of the venous circulation in the brain.

(d) Cerebral venous congestion

Venous outflow impediment from the intracranial space is manifested by a rise in the pre-incisure wave of the rheoencephalogram. The presystolic wave lying before, synchronously with or after the P wave of the electrocardiogram is not directly associated with the impeded blood outflow from the intracranial space. It probably reflects regional fluctuations in the filling of the cerebral veins.

In cases of mild cerebral venous congestion the descending branch of the curve is elevated with the convexity upwards.

Thus, the rheoencephalogram yields information on tone and lumen changes of the cerebral arteries, on the venous outflow from the intracranial space and the fluctuations in the blood volume of the cerebral veins. These changes may be manifested in subtle variation and manifold combinations on the abnormal rheoencephalogram. The method thus enables one to detect disorders in the arterial and venous vessels of the brain.

A number of cardiovascular and humoral factors affect the cephalic impedance and hence, the rheoencephalogram. The lumen and tone of the cerebral vessels are influenced by the arterial and venous pressure, the pulse rate and some metabolic factors. Additional information on these parameters is therefore required for the correct interpretation of the rheoencephalogram.

If as a result of miscellaneous influences the arterial pressure remains unchanged or declines, the amplitude of the rheoencephalogram increases and the relative portion of the anacrote diminishes – all these are signs of reduced cerebral vascular tone. Inverse relations are observed when vascular tone increases.

The correlation analysis between the basic rheoencephalographic parameters (amplitude, relative portion of the anacrote and mean rheoencephalogram) and the brachial arterial pressure (maximal, mean and minimal) made by us revealed a considerable negative rectilinear correlation ($r = -0.440$) between rheoencephalographic amplitude and mean arterial pressure.

With the increase of cardiac rate the amplitude of the rheoencephalogram decreases (Kaindl et al., 1959). This fact should be taken into consideration in evaluating the effect of stimuli inducing changes in the pulse rate.

The mean rheoencephalogram and the amplitude of the curve adequately correlate with the partial oxygen pressure in the arterial blood, with arterial pH, partial oxygen pressure in the jugular blood and the arterio-venous oxygen differences (Namon et al., 1967).

Our studies (Hadjiev and Marinova, 1970) on the effects of intravenous administration of 50 mg of cocarboxylase on cerebral hemodynamics and metabolism in patients with vascular lesions of the brain, carried out by using the venous radioisotope dilution technique, showed a significant decrease in the lactacidosis of the jugular blood and irregular changes in the cerebral blood flow. In some observations cerebral vascular resistance increased and the volume velocity of the blood flow diminished. In these cases rheoencephalographic symptoms of increased vascular tone were observed: the anacrotic portion of the curve was enlarged and, more seldom, the rheoencephalographic amplitude was depressed. Therefore, the variations in cerebral lactacidosis affect cerebral vascular tone, which can be visualized also by impedance methods.

These data suggest that changes in the metabolic parameters strongly affect the rheoencephalogram; in its interpretation, therefore, it is judicious to evaluate also the level of brain metabolism. Further correlation of the rheoencephalographic parameters with arterial and jugular pressure, the pulse rate and some indices of cerebral metabolism will probably contribute to a more thorough understanding of the mechanisms responsible for the abnormal rheoencephalogram.

FUNCTIONAL RHEOENCEPHALOGRAPHY

For the closer study of cerebral hemodynamics by impedance methods, different tests yielding information on the functional state of the cerebral vessels are of major practical and theoretical importance. A number of tests may serve to distinguish between organic and functional components of the vascular process, to provoke latent vascular insufficiency and to study collateral circulation. Simultaneous recording of cerebral impedance, arterial pressure, other cardiovascular phenomena and the electroencephalogram affords a more complete insight into the relationship between circulation and neuronal activity.

In performing functional rheoencephalography we used the following tests:

(a) Hyperventilation

Following hyperventilation for 3–5 min, the rheoencephalographic amplitude is depressed and the angle of inclination of the rising part of the curve is slightly decreased (Jenkner, 1962). These changes have been associated with a rise in the cerebral vascular resistance caused by the reduced partial CO_2 pressure in the arterial blood during hyperventilation. The test has value in studying the functional state of the cerebral vessels especially when vascular tone is reduced. Similar, but hardly perceptible changes in the rheoencephalogram occur when pure oxygen is breathed.

(b) Inhalation of CO_2

Inhalation of 5–7% CO_2 with air during 5–10 min induces a rise in the rheoencephalographic amplitude and in the angle of inclination of the ascending branch; the details of the curve, the waves of its descending part become more conspicuous (Jenkner, 1962). These changes are due to a fall of cerebral vascular resistance – as a result of the elevated partial CO_2 pressure in the arterial blood. The test is an important means for distinguishing between vascular spasm and organic stenosis of the vascular lumen.

(c) Changes of body position

The rheoencephalogram shows considerable changes when the position of the body is changed. Tracings should be obtained in horizontal and upright position, and in Trendelenburg position, using a tilting table.

With the orthostatic test some authors observed a decrease of the rheoencephalographic amplitude (Posteli *et al.*, 1957), while others (Dobner, 1958; Zenov, 1967) found it to increase.

Somewhat more uniform are the rheoencephalographic changes in Trendelenburg position: The amplitude and the anacrotic part of the curve considerably increases; a presystolic wave frequently appears (Jenkner, 1962; Lifshitz, 1963 b; Hadjiev, 1965 a). The rheoencephalographic amplitude increases because of a rise in the preincisure wave (Hadjiev, 1966 b; Zenov, 1967). In cases of increased cerebral vascular resistance due to cerebral atherosclerosis and high venous pressure these changes are less prominent (Hadjiev, 1965 a).

The tests associated with change of position, especially the Trendelenburg position, are of value for the assessment of the cerebral vascular reactivity and of the state of the cerebral venous vessels.

(d) Sideways turning of the head

Maximal sideways turning of the head renders the blood inflow difficult, especially from the occipital vertebral artery (Toole and Tucker, 1960; Bauer *et al.*, 1961). In normal subjects, this test produced a slight decrease in the amplitude of the occipito-mastoid rheoencephalogram contralaterally to the turning, and an increase ipsilaterally. Milder changes occurred in the occipito-mastoid tracings during occipital flexion of the head (Yarullin, 1967).

In our investigations, similar changes were observed in the bimastoid rheoencephalogram after sideways turning of the head. The fronto-mastoid rheoencephalogram showed milder deviations with this test. Thus, rheoencephalographic changes occurring with the head turned sideways and in occipital flexion may be utilized to assess the circulation in the vertebro-basilar system. More distinct changes were observed in the occipito-mastoid and bimastoid tracings.

(e) Compression of the common carotid artery

In normal individuals digital compression of the common carotid artery beneath the bifurcation lasting 20–30 sec leads to a sudden drop in the amplitude of the ipsilateral fronto-mastoid rheoencephalogram. In some cases the amplitude of the contralateral tracing is also slightly depressed. To control compression efficacy simultaneous palpation of the arteria temporalis superficialis or temporal pulsography may be used.

The common carotid artery compression test has great value for the diagnosis of carotid occlusion; it broadens the diagnostic utility of the rheoencephalographic technique (Lugaresi *et al.*, 1962; Yarullin, 1963; Hadjiev and Tzenov, 1966). It should be applied with caution because of the hazard of accidents – epileptic seizures, asystolia, etc.

The first to be compressed is the "damaged" artery and, if the rheoencephalographic amplitude decreases, compression of the "normal" artery should follow. Should "damaged" artery compression fail to change the tracing, it is desirable that the test be repeated with simultaneous performance of ipsilateral pulsography to control its adequacy.

(f) Compression of the superficial temporal artery

The artery is compressed before and above the auditory canal. In normal individuals the rheoencephalographic amplitude is barely, if at all, decreased (Hadjiev and Tzenov, 1964 b); in carotid stenosis or occlusion with collateral circulation through the ipsilateral carotid artery, the tracing is markedly depressed.

(g) Pharmacologic tests

A variety of drugs have been extensively used for functional assessment of the cerebral vessels (Auinger et al., 1953; Garbini et al., 1957; Posteli et al., 1957; Hadjiev and Tzenov, 1964 a).

A suitable drug for that purpose is *papaverine hydrochloride;* injected intravenously in a dose from 40 to 60 mg, it induces cerebral vasodilation. This effect of the drug may be used to distinguish vasospasm from organic constriction of the vascular lumen.

Intravenous administration of 20 mg of *nicotinic acid* also modifies the rheoencephalographic curve: there is a marked rise of the pre-incisure wave, and the descending branch is raised higher. These changes indicate increased blood filling of the venous vessels of the brain. Cerebral hemodynamics may deteriorate as a result of the marked venous congestion in the brain following nicotinic acid injection (Hadjiev, 1965 b).

Sublingual administration of *nitroglycerin* (0.00025–0.0005) is followed by an increase in the rheoencephalographic amplitude; the details of the descending branch become more distinct (Minz and Ronkin, 1967). This test has a serious disadvantage in the effect which nitroglycerin exerts directly on the heart (Fedorowsky, 1966).

For an adequate evaluation of cerebral vascular reactivity after pharmacologic tests it is necessary to take into consideration also the pulse rate and arterial pressure changes which may occasionally be induced by the drug used. The study of the effects of vasoactive drugs on the brain blood vessels is of major practical importance for a well motivated prescription of these drugs, especially in the acute period of cerebral stroke (Hadjiev, 1966). Information may thus be gained on brain vascular reactivity and objective data can be obtained on the adjustability of the cerebral circulation.

The rheoencephalograms in Fig. 6 illustrate a preserved and considerably reduced reactivity of the cranial vessels observed during the above described tests.

Simultaneous rheoencephalographic and electroencephalographic recording during carotid compression reveals the interrelation and sequence of deficient circulation and neuronal activity changes. Rheoencephalographic changes appear first, followed by electroencephalographic ones, indicating that the rheoencephalographic method is more sensitive in detecting circulatory failure than the electroencephalogram (Yarullin and Hadjiev, 1968; Geyer, 1969).

Therefore, tests of the functional state of the cerebral vessels yield more complete

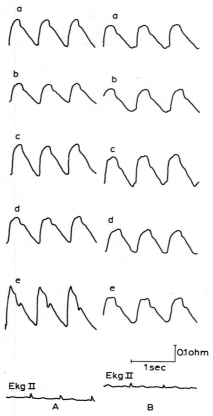

Fig. 6. Preserved (A) and considerably reduced cerebral vascular reactivity (B). Rest (starting) rheoencephalograms (a), after hyperventilation (b), after exercise (c), after intravenous administration of 20 mg of papaverine hydrochloride (d) and after sublingual application of 0.25 mg of nitro-glycerine (e).

information on the arterial vascular tone and lumen and venous cerebral vessels. The rheoencephalographic asymmetries appearing after change of body position, CO_2 inhalation and pharmacologic tests may be useful for the topical diagnosis of the vascular lesion.

Tests of sideways turning of the head and of compression of the common carotid and superficial temporal arteries yield valuable information on the site of the vascular damage and the pathways of collateral cerebral circulation, especially when multi-channel rheoencephalographic records are made.

RHEOENCEPHALOGRAPHIC CHANGES IN VASCULAR DISEASES OF THE BRAIN

The impedance methods are of great value in the diagnosis of vascular diseases of the brain. They yield information on the state of the vascular tone and the cerebral vascular resistance in these diseases which is of primary importance for the topical and pathogenetic diagnosis of circulatory disturbances of the brain and for their adequate therapy.

Rheoencephalographic studies of cerebral vascular lesions were performed mainly with rheoencephalography I. It is considered possible to detect focal circulatory disturbances with rheoencephalography II as well, although in a large number of lesions, especially those with deep localization, no specific rheoencephalographic changes have been found (Lechner *et al.*, 1965 b).

(a) Rheoencephalographic changes in atherosclerosis, arterial hypertension and vasculitis

Characteristic rheoencephalographic changes are demonstrable in atherosclerosis of the cerebral vessels. The form of the curve and its quantitative parameters are altered: amplitude is lower, the anacrotic section of the curve and its relative part increase, the angle of inclination becomes smaller, the additional waves disappear, the rheoencephalographic tracing becomes irregular and asymmetries of the curves for the left and right hemispheres are observed (Jenkner, 1957; 1962; Kunert, 1959; Schreiber, 1962; Tzenov and Hadjiev, 1964; etc.) In cases when atherosclerosis is accompanied by a rise of arterial pressure the inclination angle of the ascending branch of the curve may remain unchanged (Jenkner, 1962). Occasionally the curve forms a plateau or an arch.

The rheoencephalographic examination provides an objective assessment of cerebral atherosclerosis and yields conclusions on the severity of the process (Minz and Ronkin, 1967). We classified rheoencephalographic changes in cerebral atherosclerosis according to severity in three groups: changes characteristic of initial, moderate and severe atherosclerosis (Hadjiev, 1970 b).

In initial atherosclerosis the peak of the curve is slightly rounded, the post-incisure wave is indistinct, the anacrotic section of the curve increases, and its relative part amounts to 0.200. These changes are eliminated after intravenous administration of 40–60 mg of papaverine hydrochloride. Marked rheoencephalographic deviations accompany the change in the body position.

Moderate atherosclerosis is characterized by marked rounding of the peak, occasionally with slight plateau formation; the post-incisure wave is indistinct, the anacrote shows a stronger increase and its relative part is between 0.200 and 0.300. After intravenous administration of papaverine hydrochloride the rheoencephalogram fails to return toward normal, and reactions to change of body position are slight.

In severe atherosclerosis of the cerebral vessels, rheoencephalographic changes are the most marked: the peak is rounded, the curve has a distinct plateau or is arched; the post-incisure wave disappears, the ascending branch notably increases and usually amounts to more than 30% of a cardiac cycle. After intravenous administration of papaverine the rheoencephalogram remains unchanged or its amplitude is depressed. Change of body position usually provokes no essential abnormalities in the curve.

With increasing severity of the atherosclerotic process the rheoencephalographic amplitude is usually depressed, but these changes do not always run parallel. To a major degree they depend on arterial pressure values.

The rheoencephalographic method, therefore, helps in visualizing cerebral atherosclerosis and the extent to which it has developed. Thus, false conclusions caused by indirect methods of examination of cerebral vessels, such as the state of the retinal vessels, the aorta, etc., can be avoided. The method permits detection of early subclinical forms of cerebral atherosclerosis – an advantage which is of great practical importance.

Rheoencephalographic changes in arterial hypertension depend on the stage of the disease. In the absence of sclerotic changes in the cerebral vessels the anacrotic section of the curve is elongated during the phase of slow systolic filling – a manifestation of increased resistance in the arterioles. Signs of vascular dystonia are also observed in the anacrotic section corresponding to arteriolar filling. The additional waves of the descending branch are marked, and the pre-incisure wave may surmount the first peak of the curve. In the second and third stage of the disease amplitude is lower, the anacrotic section of the curve and its relative part increase. In the third stage of arterial hypertension these signs of increased cerebral vascular resistance are very strongly emphasized, and the curve may occasionally assume the form of an arch. These changes are more prominent during transient arterial pressure rise and during hypertonic cerebral vascular attacks; they may be associated with signs of regional angiospasm (Yarullin and Hadjiev, 1968).

With the fall of arterial pressure, the rheoencephalographic changes in the first and second stage of the disease disappear, and the rheoencephalograms tend to gain the normal pattern. In the sclerotic stage hypotensive treatment fails to induce notable improvement of the rheoencephalogram.

Similar rheoencephalographic changes indicating increased and labile cerebral vascular tone are also seen in vasculitis (Tzenov and Hadjiev, 1964). Significant rheoencephalographic deviations: depressed amplitude, increased anacrotic section of the curve and changes in its form may be seen in cerebral endarteritis.

It may therefore be stated that the rheoencephalographic changes in atherosclerosis, arterial hypertension and cerebral vasculitis reflect different stages of increased cerebral vascular resistance and a decrease in the pulsatile fluctuations of the cerebral vessels. They are not absolutely specific of any of these diseases and may be observed also in valvular disease, aortic stenosis in particular (Trautwein, 1963). Cerebral hemodynamic disorders arising secondary to acute disturbances of cerebral circulation should be added to the above described changes.

(b) Rheoencephalographic changes in pathology of the carotid arteries

Rheoencephalographic examination provides essential diagnostic aid in transient ischemic attacks and in cerebral infarction, arising in a variety of pathologic states of the carotid arteries: stenosis, kinking and occlusion.

Stenosis of the internal carotid artery The rheoencephalographic changes in stenosis of the internal carotid artery have been extensively studied by Yarullin (1967), Minz and Ronkin (1967), and others. Depressed amplitude, elongated anacrotic section of the curve and a larger relative part of the ascending branch are demonstrable on the side of the pathologic process in hemispheric fronto-mastoid leads. The post-incisure wave has a higher localization, but in some cases it lies low; in this latter situation, the peak is also somewhat more pointed. To summarize, in stenosis of the internal carotid artery cerebral vascular tone is increased, but may be occasionally decreased; symptoms of vascular dystonia may also be observed (Hadjiev and Wassileva, 1969). These changes are most conspicuous in the acute period of transient disturbances of cerebral circulation and in cerebral infarction (Hadjiev and Yancheva, 1970). Later, when adequate collateral circulation has been restored, the interhemispheric asymmetry diminishes and disappears. The regional leads: fronto-frontal, fronto-parietal and parieto-central usually reveal identical changes, the intensity of which may vary depending on the existence of additional stenosis and blood flow retardation in the basin of the anterior and medial cerebral artery.

Once the interhemispheric asymmetry has disappeared, during recovery and restoration after the stroke, functional tests, especially homolateral and contralateral compression of the common carotid artery, acquire diagnostic value. If the collateral circulation of the affected hemisphere passes through the circle of Willis, homolateral compression produces considerably milder depression of the rheoencephalographic amplitude of the ipsilateral hemisphere than does compression of the contralateral common carotid artery. In case the blood flow is re-established through the homolateral external carotid artery, compression of the homolateral common carotid artery is followed by a sharp depression of the rheoencephalographic amplitude. In these cases the amplitude is essentially depressed also after compression of the superficial temporal artery (Hadjiev, 1970 b).

Kinking of the internal carotid artery   The clinical manifestations of this type of pathology of the carotid arteries are similar to those observed in stenosis of the internal carotid artery. The hemispheric rheoencephalographic tracings show lower amplitude, elongation of the anacrotic section of the curve and its relative part and, in some cases, longer spreading time of the rheoencephalographic wave. Yarullin (1965 b) observed increase in the rheoencephalographic amplitude when the head was turned towards the side of the kinking; this is associated with correction of the kinking in this position resulting in improved blood flow in the affected hemisphere. Increase in the rheoencephalographic amplitude, though to a lesser degree, has also been observed after turning the head to the opposite side. Increase in the amplitude may likewise occur in any other position of the head leading to correction of the kinking; however, this has not been observed consistently, *i.e.* it is apparently associated with the type and degree of kinking (Hadjiev and Wassileva, 1969).

Occlusion of the internal carotid artery   A number of authors (Garbini and Picchio, 1957 b; Jenkner, 1959; Lugaresi *et al.*, 1962, 1964; Yarullin, 1963, 1967; Hadjiev, 1967 a; Minz and Ronkin, 1967; and others) emphasized the major diagnostic value of the rheoencephalographic examination in this type of pathology of the internal carotid artery. The acute period of thrombosis is characterized by a sharp depression of the amplitude and increase in the anacrotic section of the curve, elongation of the relative part of the anacrote toward a cardiac cycle, rounding of the peak and a higher position of the post-incisure wave in the rheoencephalogram. Prolonged spreading time of the rheoencephalographic wave was also observed. In more extensive cerebral infarction, the rheoencephalogram may show reduced vascular tone and venous congestion on the side of the lesion (Hadjiev and Wassileva, 1969).

According to Yarullin (1967) the diagnostic significance of the method substantially increases when regional rheoencephalography is applied; in addition to the depressed amplitude and deformation of the curve in the hemispheric tracing, similar changes were recorded in the fronto-frontal, fronto-parietal and parieto-temporal tracings.

With the restoration of efficacious collateral circulation the interhemispheric asymmetry may be lost. In these cases the functional tests acquire diagnostic significance. When collateral circulation is realized exclusively through the circle of Willis by the contralateral internal carotid artery or the vertebro-basilar system, compression of the common carotid artery on the side of the occluded internal carotid artery fails to induce changes in the rheoencephalographic tracing, although the pulse of the external carotid artery disappears in the pulsogram which serves as a criterion for the effectiveness of compression (Hadjiev and Tzenov, 1966). Compression of the contralateral common carotid artery in these cases frequently gives "le signe de la carotide".

When collateral circulation passes through the ipsilateral external carotid artery, compression of the homolateral common carotid artery is followed by a sharp depression of the amplitude. This occurs also after compression of the superficial temporal artery.

In our observations on internal carotid artery thrombosis just above the bifurcation, depressed amplitude and deformed curve are observed after digital compression of both the ipsilateral and the contralateral common carotid arteries. This indicates that collateral circulation may be channelled not only through Willis's circle, but also through the homolateral external carotid artery (Hadjiev, 1970 b).

According to Yarullin (1967) the test with the head turned sideways is essentially important for differentiating carotid thrombosis from stenosis and kinking. Turning the head to the side of the pathologic process in thrombosis is not accompanied by cerebral hemodynamic changes; in stenosis of the internal carotid artery the pulsation of the homolateral hemisphere decreases in kinking it increases.

Stenosis and occlusion of the common carotid artery In stenosis of the common carotid artery turning the head to the side of stenosis is manifested in depressing the amplitude of the hemispheric and temporal rheographic tracings (the latter reflecting pulsation of the external carotid artery). Compression of the occluded common carotid artery is not followed by changes in either the hemispheric or the temporal tracings (Yarullin, 1967).

Thus, rheoencephalographic examination utilizing functional tests and especially digital compression of the carotid and superficial temporal arteries is an aid in the diagnosis of carotid insufficiency and in the detection of the pathways of collateral circulation, which is of major practical importance for the therapeutic approach and, eventually, for sound indications and control of surgery.

In the acute period of the stroke with pathology of the carotid arteries, venous congestion and cerebral edema exert effect on the rheogram.

References pp. 79–85

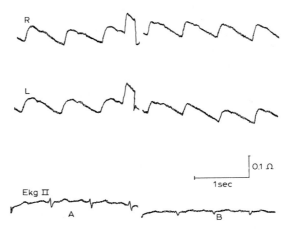

Fig. 7. Patient L.T., man aged 62. Chronic left-sided subdural hematoma. Fronto-mastoid rheoencephalograms before (A) and after (B) surgical evacuation of hematoma.

Once the hematoma was evacuated, all these rheoencephalographic changes disappeared (Fig. 7).

Therefore, apart from asymmetries in amplitude, symptoms of increased cerebral
vascular resistance may be observed on the side of the subdural hematoma.

(g) Rheoencephalographic changes in venous encephalopathy and cerebral edema

When venous outflow from the skull is impeded and intracranial pressure is raised,
the rheoencephalographic amplitude increases, the anacrotic section of the curve is
elongated and the descending branch is elevated and becomes more convex (McHenry,
1965). A presystolic wave is also observed, situated before or synchronously with the
P wave of the electrocardiogram. These changes are similar to those observed in
Trendelenburg position.

RHEOENCEPHALOGRAPHIC CHANGES IN BRAIN TUMORS

Several authors pointed out that brain tumors are usually unassociated with essential
rheoencephalographic changes (Orlandi *et al.*, 1957, Fasano *et al.*, 1961; and others).
Koecke (1961) recorded marked interhemispheric asymmetries in patients with
cerebral tumors when measured after extremes of inspiration and expiration. Jenkner
(1962) emphasized that there is no rheoencephalogram typical of brain tumor. The
pattern in tumors with poor blood supply is similar to that observed in cerebral
compression. Tumors with ample vascularization present themselves with a higher
rheoencephalographic amplitude on the side of the pathologic process.

Simultaneous electroencephalographic and multichannel hemispheric and regional
rheoencephalographic records were helpful in demonstrating cerebral circulatory
disorders in the zone of the tumor, and dislocation disturbances of cerebral hemodynamics in more remote regions of the brain. In hemispheric tumors the most
common findings are: depression of the rheoencephalographic amplitude, elongation

of the ascending branch and diminution of the slope of its inclination, especially in the zone of the artery compressed by the tumor (Majortchik and Yarullin, 1966).

Rheoencephalography has great diagnostic value in determining the degree of vascularization of the tumor. The rheoencephalographic amplitude on the side of the pathological process is higher in tumors with ample blood supply. This is associated, however, with symptoms of increased cerebral vascular resistance and venous congestion (Hadjiev, 1970 b).

Where marked venous congestion and cerebral edema mask the tumor-induced compression or intense blood supply, it is often difficult to interpret the rheoencephalograms. In these cases simultaneous hemispheric and regional rheoencephalographic investigations before and after vigorous treatment to control the edema have definite topical value. The changes caused by the tumor itself become more conspicuous (Hadjiev, 1970 b).

Interpretation of rheoencephalograms in patients with brain tumors, especially in advanced age, is difficult, all the more as frequently cerebral atherosclerosis contributes to the alteration of the rheoencephalographic pattern.

In arterio-venous angioma of the brain, the rheoencephalographic wave, escaping the capillary network, spreads at a higher rate and the peak of the curve appears more rapidly on the side of the angioma than on the side of the normal hemisphere. Moreover, rheoencephalographic amplitude on the side of the angioma is depressed (Jenkner, 1962).

Recording of intracerebral impedance, using implanted electrodes, makes it possible to study circulation in the brain tumor. Laitinen *et al.* (1969) established that circulation in the tumor differs from that of the adjacent tissues. Increased impedance was registered in deeply localized malignant tumors (Mori *et al.*, 1969), as well as in meningiomas (Organ *et al.*, 1968). According to the latter authors, impedance techniques are useful due to their capacity of precisely locating the tumor, thus permitting examination of biopsy specimens from deep-seated tumors.

RHEOENCEPHALOGRAPHIC CHANGES IN CRANIO-CEREBRAL TRAUMA

Rheoencephalographic examination in cranio-cerebral trauma yields information on the state of the cerebral vascular tone. This information is of particular importance for the therapeutic approach and prognosis.

In *cerebral contusion* Jenkner (1962) observed increase in the amplitude and the inclination angle of the ascending branch of the rheoencephalogram, which he interpreted as a sign of vascular dilation and hyperemia in the contused area. In addition to bilateral increase in the rheoencephalographic amplitude, rapid rise of the ascending branch and marked post-incisure wave, *concussion of the brain* is characterized by low tracings with rounded peak of the curve and high localization of the post-incisure wave (Lissitsa, 1967).

Evidence of reduced or increased cerebral vascular tone may, therefore, be demonstrated in cranio-cerebral trauma. Severe trauma is characterized by reduced vascular tone and signs of venous congestion, mild trauma by increased tone and evidence of cerebral ischemia (Yarullin, 1967).

The intracerebral or subdural hematomas which may accompany the trauma are manifested by distinct interhemispheric asymmetry and signs of increased cerebral vascular resistance on the side of the pathologic process.

In later periods following cranio-cerebral trauma, rheoencephalograms were obtained with low amplitudes, occasionally with interhemispheric asymmetry and changes in the shape of the curve similar to those observed in organic vascular lesions. Thus, follow-up rheoencephalographic studies in concussion of the brain reveal changes in the cerebral vascular tone and the development of organic processes in the cerebral vessels (Lissitsa, 1967).

RHEOENCEPHALOGRAPHIC CHANGES IN EPILEPSY AND MIGRAINE

Rheoencephalographic examinations in epilepsy and migraine may detect changes in the brain vascular tone during the epileptic or migraine attack; permanent asymmetries may be recorded during remission.

(a) Epilepsy

Rheoencephalographic changes have been described in the pre-paroxysmal, paroxysmal and interparoxysmal periods.

Ivanova (1969), from simultaneous rheoencephalographic and electroencephalographic records observed shortly before petit mal seizures rheoencephalographic changes indicating increased vascular tone and vascular dystonia (Fig. 8).

Merdjanov and Ivanova (1969) found marked rheoencephalographic changes during electroshock and cardiazol-shock seizures in curarized rabbits. They used needle-shaped electrodes implanted in the brain cortex and registered the pulsatile fluctuations of the cerebral impedance and the electrocorticogram, with parallel

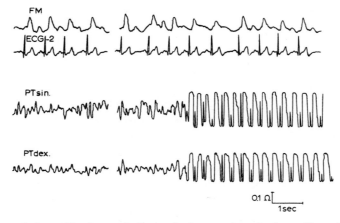

Fig. 8. Rheoencephalographic changes before and after a petit mal seizure. From the top: fronto-mastoid rheoencephalogram, electrocardiogram (II lead) and electroencephalograms (P-T left and right) (Ivanova, 1969).

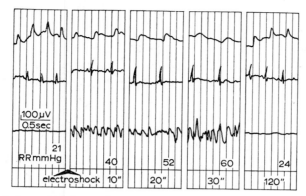

Fig. 9. Rheoencephalographic changes in a curarized rabbit during electroshock seizure. From the top: rheoencephalogram (fronto-occipital placing of electrodes), electrocardiogram (II lead), electro-corticogram from the right frontal area (bipolar lead), blood pressure in mm Hg (femoral artery) (Merdjanov and Ivanova, 1969).

records of the electrocardiogram and the femoral artery pressure. During electro-shock seizures the authors observed signs of increased cerebral vascular tone and venous congestion manifested by depression of the rheoencephalographic amplitude, increase in the relative part of the anacrotic section of the curve, rise of the dicrotic wave and of the descending branch and frequently, the appearance of pre-incisure and presystolic waves. Bradycardia and elevated arterial pressure were at the same time observed (Fig. 9).

During cardiazol-shock seizures the relative part of the rheoencephalogram in-creases simultaneously with the amplitude increase.

Interhemispheric asymmetry with signs of reduced vascular tone on the side of the focus was observed in Jacksonian seizures. The appearance of spike waves in the electroencephalogram was accompanied by sharpening of the rheoencephalographic peaks and increase in the amplitude and the post-incisure wave (Yarullin, 1967).

High rheoencephalographic amplitude, sharp peak of the curve and low localization of the post-incisure wave were observed also after electroshock (Mazzarella, 1961; Lifshitz, 1963 b).

Between seizures, high tracings, interhemispheric asymmetry and vascular dystonia are common findings.

It may therefore be stated that before and during seizure the rheoencephalographic methods disclose increased vascular tone and vascular dystonia which are rapidly replaced by cerebral vasodilation, probably induced by tissue acidosis, secondary to the neuronal activity in the epileptogenic focus. These studies support the importance which the impedance methods may have in the examination of cerebral circulation changes before, during and after the epileptic seizure.

(b) Migraine

Marked interhemispheric asymmetry with higher or lower amplitude on the side of the headache was observed during a migraine attack (Zbinden, 1962; Eninya, 1962).

In the majority of cases with migraine attacks Orioli *et al.* (1969) observed depression of the curve on the side of the headache. In some cases alternation of symptoms of increased and reduced vascular tone in the rheoencephalographic pattern was observed; this is attributed to a marked lability of tone (Minz and Ronkin, 1967).

Interhemispheric asymmetry in patients with migraine was recorded also during the free attack period (Zbinden, 1962).

Our (Hadjiev and Uzunov, 1969) rheoencephalographic studies in patients with migraine during the free attack period frequently present interhemispheric asymmetry and lability of vascular tone. We observed both increased and reduced vascular tone with signs of venous congestion. Intravenous administration of 0.25 mg of Deseryl during the period of remission was followed in some patients by cerebral vasodilation with the occasional appearance of a presystolic wave in the rheoencephalogram (Fig. 10).

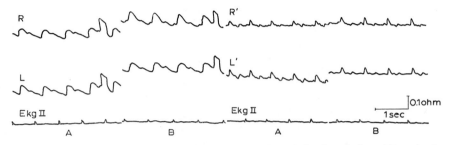

Fig. 10. Fronto-mastoid rheoencephalograms and their first derivatives before (A) and after (B) intravenous administration of 0.25 mg of Deseril.

We observed cerebral vasodilation after Deseryl injection in patients with initially increased vascular tone, whereas in cases of reduced tone a vasoconstrictive reaction usually occurred. These data prove the value of rheoencephalography for the precision of vascular tone in patients with migraine, which in turn underlies the prescription of adequate treatment.

RHEOENCEPHALOGRAPHIC CHANGES IN PARKINSONISM

Rheoencephalographic examination of patients with parkinsonian syndrome is difficult in the presence of hyperkinesis. When realizable, varying degrees of increased vascular tone may be observed. Vascular dystonia with symptoms of cerebral venous congestion is sometimes present in young individuals. Interhemispheric asymmetries have also been observed. These cerebral vascular disorders may be discussed from the etiological, pathogenetical and phenomenological aspect (Hadjiev, 1970 b).

Local vasomotor reactions in the deep structures of the brain were studied by means of impedance changes using implanted electrodes for the performance of stereotaxis operation (Birzis *et al.*, 1968). Impedance measurement in these structures may serve for precise localization of the areas considered for stereotaxic treatment (Tachibana *et al.*, 1967; Mori *et al.*, 1969).

RHEOENCEPHALOGRAPHIC INVESTIGATIONS INTO THE EFFECT
OF SOME VASOACTIVE AND METABOLIC-ACTIVE DRUGS

Extensive studies on the regional cerebral circulation by impedance and radioisotope clearance methods undertaken in the past few years revealed new aspects of the cerebral hemodynamic disturbances in vascular lesions of the brain. Ischemic and hyperemic foci, complete or partial loss of autoregulation were revealed in acute disturbances of the cerebral circulation (Hadjiev, 1966 a; Høedt-Rasmussen et al., 1967; Lassen and Paulson, 1969). This contributed to a more thorough pathogenetic analysis of cerebral lesions and, along with this, to a reevaluation of some extensively used vasodilating drugs. If cerebral blood flow and cerebral vascular reactivity in acute cerebral circulatory disturbances are disorganized, each new artificially induced deterioration of cerebral hemodynamics may have grave consequences. Thoroughly sound indications and control of the therapy in the acute phase of the stroke are therefore necessary.

Studies of Gottstein (1962) using the nitrogen oxide technique showed that intravenous administration of vasoactive substances usually fails to normalize cerebral vascular resistance and to substantially raise cerebral blood flow. Only slow and total changes of cerebral blood flow are detectable by the nitrogen oxide technique.

With the impedance methods it became possible to obtain information on the rapid and regional disorders of cerebral circulation occurring under the influence of a certain drug. For this reason, the impedance methods are particularly suitable for studying drug effects on cerebral circulation; in association with metabolic investigations they may provide additional knowledge on the effects of the vasoactive and metabolic-active drugs in a variety of cerebral circulatory disorders.

Our rheoencephalographic studies of drug effects were carried out in a group of 257 patients with disturbances of cerebral circulation. Investigations were performed in supine position. We used electrodes of 9 cm^2 each. After recording the initial rheoencephalograms, the electrocardiogram and bilateral brachial oscillograms, we injected the examined substance intravenously, and after 1, 3, 5, 10, 15 and 20 min new records were taken. Rheoencephalographic studies of the effect of orally administered vasoactive substances were made by double blind tests after a single dose and after a course of treatment. The effects of some of the intravenously applied drugs were studied by the venous radioisotope dilution method.

The data obtained by the rheoencephalographic and radioisotope studies were processed by stochastic analysis methods. The following rheoencephalographic parameters were assayed: amplitude, relative part of the anacrotic section of the curve, mean rheoencephalogram, expansion rate of cerebral vessels (expressed as the tangent of the inclination angle of the anacrote) and the spreading time of the rheoencephalographic wave (from the Q wave in the electrocardiogram to the beginning of the anacrotic section of the curve).

(a) Papaverine hydrochloride
Papaverine hydrochloride, the vasodilating effects of which are limited primarily

to the great blood vessels, has gained wide acceptance in the treatment of ischemic disturbances of cerebral circulation. Using the nitrogen oxide method in patients with cerebral circulatory disorders, some authors (Aizawa *et al.*, 1961) observed a rise in cerebral blood flow following intravenous administration of papaverine, while others (Shenkin, 1951) observed no significant changes in blood flow.

Few publications are available in the literature on rheoencephalographic studies of the effect of papaverine on cerebral circulation. The drug was shown to induce increase of the rheoencephalographic amplitude and a rise in cerebral blood flow (Kuwabara, 1959; Imadachi, 1960; Del Guercio, 1963).

Our (Hadjiev and Tzenov, 1964 a) rheoencephalographic studies in clinically normal individuals and patients with chronic insufficiency of cerebral circulation showed that intravenous administration of 40 mg of papaverine hydrochloride in normal individuals gives rise to a transient cerebral vascular dilation manifested by increased rheoencephalographic amplitude and expansion rate of the brain vessels. In patients with vascular lesions of the brain, vasodilation is milder, but lasts longer.

There are very few publications on rheoencephalographic studies of the effect of papaverine hydrochloride on cerebral circulation in the acute period of cerebral stroke. Del Guercio (1963) studied the rheoencephalographic and electroencephalographic changes following intramuscular administration of eupaverine in 10 patients with "cerebral vascular pathology", 5 of whom with lesions.

We (Hadjiev, 1969) studied the papaverine effects in 25 patients with cerebral stroke during the acute and subacute phases. Forty mg of papaverine were injected intravenously. Cerebral vasodilation was observed in 20 patients. The changes in the rheoencephalographic amplitude, the relative part of the anacrotic section of the curve, the expansion rate of the brain vessels and the pulse rate are illustrated in Fig. 11.

During the first minute the rheoencephalographic amplitude showed 10% increase,

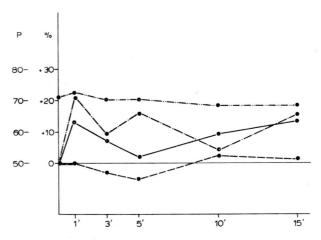

Fig. 11. Changes of: amplitude (———), relative part of the anacrotic section of the curve (———), vascular expansion rate (— · — · —) and pulse rate (— · · —) in patients with ischemic disturbances of cerebral circulation after 40 mg of i.v. papaverine hydrochloride. Abscissa: time following drug injection; ordinate: change in percentage and pulse rate.

as compared with the initial values ($p < 0.05$), followed by depression in the fifth minute and again increased at the end of the survey period. The relative part of the anacrotic section of the curve showed no important abnormalities. The expansion rate of the brain vessels increased by 21% during the first minute ($p < 0.05$) with slight subsequent variation, but without returning to normal level until the 15th minute. The pulse rate exhibited no apparent changes after the administration of papaverine.

The absolute initial amplitude values which normally vary from 0.060 to 0.150 ohms amounted to 0.080–0.206 ohms after the drug injection.

Simultaneous bilateral fronto-mastoid recording disclosed that amplitude changes and changes of the mean rheoencephalogram occurring after the administration of papaverine hydrochloride, were more marked on the side of the pathologic process; in the other hemisphere the changes were negligible, and the mean volume variations even tended to decrease. Other observations showed inverse changes with impaired circulation in the hemisphere injured by the pathologic process.

In addition to quantitative rheoencephalographic changes after the administration of papaverine hydrochloride, the peak of the curve becomes sharper and the incisure and additional peaks of its descending branch become more conspicuous.

The vasodilatory effect of papaverine hydrochloride is shown in Fig. 12.

No essential changes occurred in the systolic, mean and diastolic pressure in the surveyed group of patients after injecting papaverine hydrochloride. The oscillation

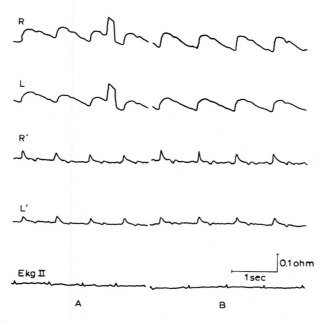

Fig. 12. Patient B.L., woman aged 66. Atherosclerosis of aorta, carotid and cerebral arteries. Hypoplasia of right vertebral artery. Transient ischemic attacks in the vertebro-basilar system. Fronto-mastoid rheoencephalograms and their first derivatives before (A) and 3 min after (B) of 40 mg i.v. papaverine hydrochloride.

index showed a more marked increase on the healthy side – by 23% of the initial values; on the paretic side the increase was less marked.

In the remaining 5 patients the rheoencephalographic changes indicated deteriorated cerebral circulation. Cerebral vasodilation following intravenous administration of 40 mg of papaverine hydrochloride in patients with cerebral stroke is much less effective than in the surveyed group of normal individuals. It is negligible also when compared with cerebral vascular relaxation in patients with chronic insufficiency of cerebral circulation. Acute disturbances of cerebral circulation apparently modify the reactivity of the brain vessels by reducing the intensity of their vasodilatory reaction.

Cerebral hypoxia accompanying cerebral infarction is associated with accumulation of carbon dioxide and other metabolic products in the brain tissue, thus inducing considerable dilation. In this way, the ability of the brain vessels to be further dilated is limited. The modified cerebral vascular reactivity in acute disturbances of cerebral circulation seems to be responsible also for the paradoxical reactions which occasionally occur after papaverine hydrochloride injection.

In addition to the modified cerebral vascular reactivity following papaverine injection, regional and interhemispheric differences underlie the intensity of the effect. Obviously these differences should be attributed to redistribution of the blood in the brain; they are a manifestation of "intracerebral steal syndrome".

The objective rheoencephalographic assessment of cerebral circulation changes following papaverine administration permits an individual approach to the indication of papaverine treatment; the latter is obviously contraindicated when cerebral vascular tone is clearly reduced and when paradoxical reactions with deteriorated cerebral circulation are observed.

(b) Halidor

Halidor (1-benzyl-1-(3′-dimethylaminopropoxycycloheptane fumarate), a compound of the Hungarian pharmaceutical industry, has a spasmolytic effect exerted directly on the smooth muscle fibres, and mild tranquilizing and local anesthesizing effects. Applied intravenously in carotid angiography, the drug causes cerebral vasodilation analogous to papaverine but without its side reactions (Vidovszky, 1965).

The rheoencephalographic changes following intravenous administration of 100 mg of Halidor were studied in 10 patients with arterial hypertension and 10 others with ischemic disorders of cerebral circulation (Hadjiev and Wassileva, 1967; Hadjiev, 1969). No important rheoencephalographic and blood pressure changes were observed in the hypertonic patients. In the ischemic patients, cerebral vascular relaxation and a mild decrease of systolic and mean arterial pressures were observed in response to the drug.

The changes in the rheoencephalographic amplitude, the relative part of the anacrotic section of the curve, the expansion rate of the brain vessels, the mean rheoencephalogram and the pulse rate are presented in Fig. 13.

In the first minute the amplitude slightly rises, the relative part of the anacrotic section of the curve increases with subsequent return toward initial values. The mean

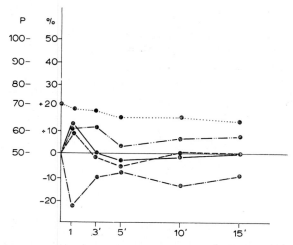

Fig. 13. Changes of amplitude (——), relative part of the anacrotic section of the curve (– – –), vascular expansion rate (–·–·–), mean rheoencephalogram (–··–··–) and pulse rate (···) in patients with ischemic disturbances of cerebral circulation after 100 mg of i.v. Halidor. Abscissa: the time following drug injection; ordinate: change in percentage and pulse rate.

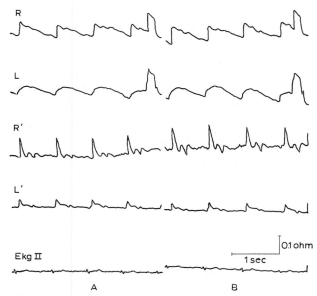

Fig. 14. Patient A.N., man aged 76. Atherosclerosis of aorta, carotid and cerebral arteries. Cerebral infarction in the basin of the left medial cerebral artery. Right-sided hemiparesis. Fronto-mastoid rheoencephalograms and their first derivatives before (A) and 3 min after (B) 100 mg of i.v. Halidor.

rheoencephalogram markedly increases ($p < 0.01$) and the expansion rate of the cerebral vessels declines.

The rheoencephalograms in Fig. 14 illustrate the vasodilatory effect of Halidor in a patient with cerebral infarction.

We carried out comparative investigations into cerebral hemodynamic and meta-

References pp. 79–85

TABLE 2

CHANGES OF CEREBRAL BLOOD FLOW, VASCULAR RESISTANCE, OXYGEN AND
GLUCOSE CONSUMPTION AFTER HALIDOR ADMINISTRATION

	Hemispheric blood flow ml/min	Cerebral vascular resistance dyn/sec/ cm^{-5} × 1332	Jugular pressure mm H_2O	Oxygen consumption ml/min	Glucose consumption mg/min
n	11	11	10	9	9
$\bar{x}$ before	243	28.5	169	24	24
$\bar{x}$ after	269	26.7	199	35	39
$p <$	0.05	0.05	0.01	0.01	0.01

bolic changes following intravenous administration of Halidor in 11 patients with ischemic disturbances of the cerebral circulation (Hadjiev and Ganev, 1968). The changes in the surveyed parameters and the results of statistical analysis are shown in Table 2.

After injecting Halidor, the cerebral blood flow in the affected hemisphere increases and cerebral vascular resistance diminishes. No important changes of blood flow and cerebral vascular resistance occurred in three patients with considerably reduced cerebral blood flow secondary to severe atherosclerosis and extensive cerebral infarction; however, oxygen consumption by the brain was increased in these cases. The mild effects of Halidor in patients with significantly reduced cerebral blood flow and severe atherosclerosis should be attributed to the limited ability of the cerebral vessels to dilate in these conditions. The increased oxygen and glucose consumption by the brain suggests that cerebral metabolism is improved after injecting the drug – manifested by increasing cerebral blood flow and by direct effects, as shown experimentally by Saratikov and Usov (1969).

Therefore, the rheoencephalographic changes observed after intravenous administration of Halidor agree with those demonstrated by the venous radioisotope dilution technique.

The mild venous pressure rise in the upper bulb of the internal jugular vein, parallel with the increase in the relative part of the anacrotic section of the curve and the second peak of the rheoencephalogram, does not interfere with cerebral hemodynamics when the initial venous pressure values are low; if they are high the incremental rise may have an unfavourable effect.

The beneficial effect of Halidor on cerebral hemodynamics and metabolism, the negligible arterial pressure changes and the absence of side reactions make this drug suitable for the treatment of ischemic disturbances of the cerebral circulation when cerebral edema is not marked. The results of our random clinical experiments assert the positive effect of Halidor.

(c) Nicotinic acid
Nicotinic acid is extensively used in the treatment of cerebral circulatory disturb-

ances. There are many reports on the beneficial effect of this drug in cerebral infarction, some mental disorders and atherosclerosis of the brain (Reisner, 1953; Murphy, 1956; Yochheim, 1962), while others claim to have noted unfavourable effect in cerebral stroke (Muratore, 1963).

The administration of nicotinic acid in cerebral infarction is based on its cerebral vasodilatory effect and its fibrinolytic (Imhof *et al.*, 1959) and hypolipemic properties (Mahl and Lange, 1963).

As regards the effect of the drug on the brain vessels, however, opinions are conflicting. Scheinberg (1950) and Aizawa *et al.* (1961), using the nitrogen oxide method, found that nicotinic acid does not much affect cerebral blood flow, cerebral vascular resistance and oxygen consumption by the brain. Feruglio and Micheli (1958) and Heyck (1962 a), using the same method, after intravenous administration of 100 mg of Ronicol observed increase of cerebral blood flow and diminution of the cerebral vascular resistance.

Rheoencephalographic studies on the influence of nicotinic acid on cerebral circulation are scanty. Auinger *et al.* (1953), Spunda (1955) and Zbinden (1962) observed increased rheoencephalographic amplitude after intravenous administration of Ronicol and Niconacid in normal individuals and in patients with lesions, migraine and vasomotor headache. Conversely, Imadachi (1960) observed no change or noted a decrease in the brain blood flow and significant rise of the peripheral blood flow after subcutaneous injection of 40 mg of nicotinic acid.

We (Hadjiev, 1965 b, 1969) studied the effects of 20 mg of i.v. nicotinic acid in 22 patients with ischemic disturbances of cerebral circulation. Control studies were undertaken in a group of 10 clinically normal individuals.

In normal individuals the administration of the drug resulted in significant increase ($p < 0.05$) of the rheoencephalographic amplitude, the relative part of the anacrotic section of the curve, the vascular expansion rate and the mean rheoencephalogram. Improvement of the cerebral circulation was noted in 18 of the surveyed patients after nicotinic acid injection. The amplitude showed maximal increase in the 3rd minute ($p < 0.05$) with a tendency to return slowly near the initial level until the 15th minute, without reaching it during that time. The relative part of the anacrotic section of the curve showed negligible changes. Cerebral vascular expansion rate increased significantly ($p < 0.05$). There was a marked increase in the mean rheoencephalogram ($p < 0.05$). All these changes were milder in patients than in normal subjects.

In four patients drug administration was followed by decrease in the rheoencephalographic amplitude, but the relative part of the anacrotic section of the curve was only slightly changed. In cases of impaired cerebral circulation following nicotinic acid injection, the starting rheoencephalogram usually presented a higher second peak and a large relative part of the anacrotic section of the curve.

The hypotensive effect of nicotinic acid is unstable. In some cases we observed biphasic arterial pressure changes – a fall after transient rise.

It should therefore be stated that intravenous administration of nicotinic acid in normal subjects leads not only to increased rheoencephalographic amplitude, and higher expansion rate of the vessels and of the mean rheoencephalogram; also, the anacrotic section of the curve increases at the expense of the slow systolic filling, with rounding of the peak. Similar changes may be observed in Trendelenburg position. These observations suggests that nicotinic acid is responsible for the increase in the pulsatile volume fluctuations due to enhanced blood filling in the venous system of the brain which, in turn, is caused by impeded venous outflow from the cranial space. These data are in agreement with the venous pressure rise in the upper bulb of the internal jugular vein after nicotinic acid injection. The effect of the drug on cerebral circulation should therefore be attributed to vasodilation in the terminal vessels – arterioles, capillaries and venules.

The effect of nicotinic acid on cerebral circulation in cerebral infarction is much milder. In the surveyed patients the relative part of the anacrotic section of the curve, being larger than in normal controls, considerably increases, probably because venous congestion in them does not become very intensive after the drug. As the arterioles and capillaries dilate, however, cerebral circulation improves; this is manifested in the rheoencephalogram by increased amplitude and mean rheoencephalogram. In the acute period of the attack this improvement is less conspicuous; the mean volume increase of the cerebral vessels is but limited.

Deteriorated cerebral circulation after nicotinic acid injection deserves special consideration. We observed such deterioration in cerebral infarction with rheoencephalographic evidence of severe cerebral venous congestion. The additional venous pressure rise in these patients obstructs venous outflow from the cranial space; as it is not accompanied by arteriolar and capillary dilation, cerebral circulation becomes impeded.

Rheoencephalographic studies on the effect of nicotinic acid on cerebral circulation support indications for the use of the drug as a dilator of the small cerebral vessels to improve the blood supply of the ischemic focus. This is one of the beneficial effects of this drug in cerebral infarction. The possibility that nicotinic acid may deteriorate cerebral circulation explains the unfavourable results of its use in cerebromalacia reported by Muratore (1963). The drug is therefore contra-indicated if cerebral hyperemic foci, venous congestion and increased venous pressure are observed – the latter usually accompanying latent or manifest heart failure – because of the hazard of transition of white cerebromalacia into red one. The effect of nicotinic acid on the small blood vessels makes its association with dilators of larger blood vessels (papaverine, etc.) useful.

(d) Complamin

Complamin (Xanthinol niacinate) has a vasodilating, fibrinolytic and cerebral metabolism-activating effect, which suggests its use in ischemic disturbances of cerebral circulation.

The effects of the drug on cerebral hemodynamics have been the subject of a few investigations. Schreiber (1960) observed increase in the rheoencephalographic amplitude and changes in the form of the curve in 9 out of 13 patients with vascular diseases of the brain. Increased cerebral blood volume is held responsible for these changes. In these studies arterial pressure changes have not been controlled. In a double blind experiment Lawrence (1969) observed that the rheoencephalograms were more readily improved in patients receiving Complamin treatment for 6 weeks than in those receiving placebo. Parallel with this the author observed improvement of the arm-to-retina fluorescein appearance time, which lead him to attributing rheoencephalographic improvement after Complamin treatment to increased circulation time.

In order to study the effects of Complamin on total and hemispheric cerebral circulation and to specify its therapeutic indications we followed up the rheoencephalographic changes occurring after intravenous administration of the drug in patients with cerebral vascular diseases (Yarullin and Hadjiev, 1970).

In 16 patients we studied the effect of intravenous administration of 150 mg of Complamin. The changes in rheoencephalographic amplitude, in the relative part of the anacrotic section of the curve and the mean rheoencephalogram recorded with bitemporal electrodes are demonstrated in Fig. 15.

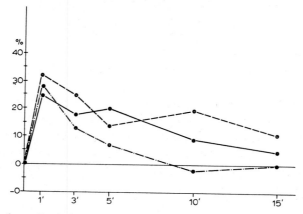

Fig. 15. Changes of: amplitude (———), relative part of the anacrotic section of the curve (– – –) and mean rheoencephalogram (–·–·–·–) in patients with ischemic disturbances of cerebral circulation after 100 mg of i.v. Complamin. Abscissa: time following drug injection; ordinate: change in percentage.

The amplitude shows a maximal increase during the first minute after injecting the drug, but the changes are insignificant. The relative part of the anacrote increases during the first minute ($p < 0.05$) and thereafter tends to decrease. The mean rheoencephalogram also shows maximal increase during the first minute ($p < 0.05$) and up to the 15th minute declines toward the initial values.

Fronto-mastoid rheoencephalograms on the side of the ischemic lesion show a significant increase in the amplitude, the relative part of the anacrotic section of the curve and the mean rheoencephalogram. On the opposite hemisphere the changes are insignificant, and sometimes amplitude and mean rheoencephalogram tend to decrease.

There was no change in the spreading time of the rheoencephalographic wave following Complamin injection. This fact does not support the assumption that improvement of the rheoencephalogram after the drug is due to circulation time changes.

References pp. 79–85

Arterial pressure in some of the surveyed patients was slightly reduced. Its changes were transient and tended to return toward the initial level by the 15th minute. It may therefore be stated that the influence of Complamin on total cerebral hemodynamics evaluated by bitemporal rheoencephalography in patients with ischemic disturbances of cerebral circulation is important only during the first minute after administering the drug. A transient increase in the amplitude and in the relative part of the anacrotic section in the rheoencephalogram occurs because of retardation of the slow systolic filling. These effects are similar to the rheoencephalographic changes following nicotinic acid injection. They are attributable to arteriolar, capillary and venular dilation.

The greater intensity of changes on the side of the ischemic lesion recorded by fronto-mastoid rheoencephalography and the appearance of opposite changes in the other hemisphere may be attributed to a peculiar "intracerebral steal syndrome", resulting from blood redistribution in the brain.

Dilation of the small cerebral vessels, including the venules, after Complamin injection cautions against the use of the drug where cerebral hyperemic foci and marked venous congestion are present. In these situations cerebral circulation may be impaired as a result of increasing vascular hypotonia and venous congestion, or of redistribution of blood toward other areas of the brain where the capacity of the cerebral vessels to dilate has been preserved.

Complamin should be considered contra-indicated in patients with ischemic disorders of cerebral circulation and low arterial pressure. Additional pressure fall which the drug may cause, might impair cerebral circulation. Our rheoencephalographic studies suggest that Complamin may be used for the treatment of cerebral ischemia associated with high arterial pressure, increased cerebral vascular tone and absence of cerebral venous congestion.

(e) Hydergin

According to Rothlin (1950), hydrated alkaloids of secale cornutum exert inhibitory effect on the vasoconstrictive centers and adreno-sympathicolytic drugs have gained acceptance in the treatment of arterial hypertension (Kappert et al., 1948; Brandt and Winter, 1954; Lasch and Moritz, 1955) and cerebromalacia (Lazorthes, 1961).

There are only few studies on the effect of these drugs on cerebral circulation in man, dealing with their competent application in cerebral vascular disorders. Using the nitrogen oxide method, Gottstein (1962) found no cerebral circulation changes following Hydergin infusion. Heyck (1962 b), however, found that intravenous or intramuscular administration of Hydergin in patients with reduced cerebral blood flow substantially increases it by reducing cerebral vascular resistance.

Using rheoencephalography I, Spunda (1955) observed a limited increase in the amplitude following intravenous administration of 0.3 mg of Hydergin in normal subjects and in patients with cerebral stroke, whereas Auinger et al. (1953) observed a considerable increase in the rheoencephalographic amplitude. By means of rheoencephalography II, Lechner et al. (1965 c) established that intravenous administration of Hydergin improves the circulation in various regions of the brain; moreover, differences were observed in the degree of changes.

We (Hadjiev, 1967 b, 1969) studied the rheoencephalographic changes following intravenous administration of 0.3 mg of Hydergin in 20 patients with disturbances of cerebral circulation. Control investigations were carried out in 5 clinically normal subjects.

In normal individuals the rheoencephalographic amplitude and the mean rheoencephalogram were markedly increased ($p < 0.05$), while the relative part of the anacrotic section showed only minor changes. Therefore, intravenous administration of Hydergin leads to cerebral vasodilation without significant arterial pressure change.

Hydergin injection in patients gave rise to rheoencephalographic changes indicative of cerebral vasodilation: elevation of the amplitude of the curve, increased expansion rate of cerebral vessels and mean rheoencephalogram, and shortened relative part of the anacrotic section of the curve. Fig. 16 is a graphic illustration of the changes in

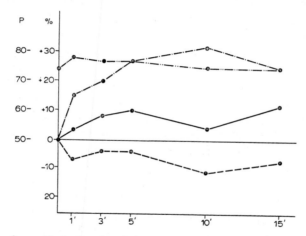

Fig. 16. Changes of: amplitude (——), relative part of the anacrotic section of the curve (---), vascular expansion rate (—·—) and pulse rate (—··—) in patients with ischemic disturbances of cerebral circulation after 0.3 mg of i.v. Hydergin. Abscissa. time following drug injection; ordinate: change in percentage and pulse rate.

the amplitude, the anacrotic section of the curve, the cerebral vascular expansion rate and the pulse rate in these patients. Maximal elevation of the rheoencephalographic amplitude is found in the 15th minute, highest expansion rate of the brain vessels in the 10th minute, and the most explicit shortening of the anacrotic section of the curve in the 5th minute. Changes of the amplitude and of the mean rheoencephalogram are statistically significant ($p < 0.05$).

Hydergin injection in patients markedly decreases the systolic, mean and diastolic pressures, and the effect lasts beyond the 15th minute. Accordingly, cerebral vasodilation and a marked decrease of systolic pressure were observed in the surveyed patients after Hydergin injection; the former effect was more marked than in normal

References pp. 79–85

subjects. Cerebral vasodilation following Hydergin injection may be associated with the adrenolytic action of the drug which is slower and stands out clearly against the background of the stress accompanying cerebral stroke.

The rheoencephalographic changes following intravenous administration of Hydergin are a sound basis for its use in the treatment of cerebral infarction associated with high arterial pressure, since in the pathogenesis of these conditions cerebral angiodystonia and catecholamine discharge play a prominent role. Treatment with hydrated alkaloids of secale cornutum should be discouraged in focal ischemic disturbances of cerebral circulation arising as a result of arterial hypotonia, because additional arterial pressure fall might aggravate cerebral ischemia.

(f) Euphylline

After the communication of Mainzer (1949) on the treatment of cerebral stroke with Euphylline a series of reports appeared on its beneficial effect, especially during the first few hours of the stroke (Meninger-Lerchenthal, 1953; Weihs, 1954; Quandt and Julich, 1959). Other authors (Gianoli, 1956; Hangarter and Henssge, 1956) claim to have never observed such favourable effects or consider the drug with scepticism. Hadorn (1960), observed 705 cases of cerebral infarction, hemorrhage and vascular insufficiency, and failed to find any improvement in the prognosis of the acute stroke attributable to Euphylline therapy. Mortality rate was not lower than in control patients who did not receive Euphylline treatment. Recently, some authors, dealing with the question of discriminative application of Euphylline noted that its effect was better in transient disturbances of cerebral circulation (Levin, 1963).

Investigations with the nitrogen oxide method in normal subjects and in patients with vascular diseases of the brain have shown that Euphylline reduces cerebral blood flow and increases cerebral vascular resistance (Wechsler *et al.*, 1950; Gottstein *et al.*, 1961; Fazekas and Alman, 1963). Heyck (1962 b), however, using the same method in patients with reduced cerebral blood flow claims that it is substantially increased following Euphylline injection while cerebral vascular resistance diminishes.

Rheoencephalographic studies of the effect of Euphylline are scanty and contradictory. Spunda (1955) observed a slight increase in the rheoencephalographic amplitude, Jenkner (1962) found it to decrease, while Imadachi (1960) reported a slight reduction of cerebral blood flow after administration of Euphylline.

Because of the contradictory data on the therapeutic effect of this drug in cerebral stroke and the conflicting results of studies on its influence on cerebral circulation, we studied the rheoencephalographic hemodynamics following intravenous administration of Euphylline (Hadjiev, 1967 c). Fifty-six patients – 19 with brain hemorrhage, 28 with cerebral infarction and 9 with transient focal disturbances of cerebral circulation – were studied after 0.24 g of i.v. Euphylline. Controls were 5 clinically normal subjects.

The effect of Euphylline on the rheoencephalogram in normal subjects consisted of slight transient cerebral vasoconstriction without essential changes of the systolic, mean and diastolic arterial pressure. In some patients, cerebral vascular tone increased after Euphylline injection, similar to the effect observed in normal individuals. The

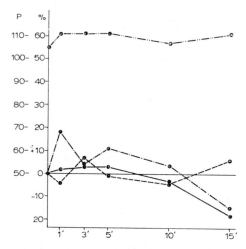

Fig. 17. Changes of: amplitude (——), relative part of the anacrotic section of the curve (———), vascular expansion rate (—·—) and pulse rate (—··—) in patients with disturbances of cerebral circulation after 0.24 mg of i.v. Euphylline. Abscissa: time following drug injection: ordinate: change in percentage and pulse rate.

changes of amplitude, anacrotic part of the curve, expansion rate of the cerebral vessels and of the pulse rate in this group of patients are shown in Fig. 17.

At the end of the survey period the amplitude was markedly decreased. The relative part of the anacrotic section of the curve showed equivocal changes, and the vascular expansion rate, after an initial rise, tended to decrease at the end of the observation period. Maximal decrease of the mean rheoencephalogram was reached in the 15th minute.

In another group of patients Euphylline had an inverse effect. Cerebral vascular tone was depressed, the amplitude and expansion rate of the cerebral vessels were markedly increased, the relative part of the anacrotic section of the curve and the mean rheoencephalogram were diminished.

It may therefore be concluded that in the surveyed group of patients Euphylline was shown to both increase and decrease cerebral vascular tone. The nature of the cerebral vascular reaction appeared to be related to the initial state of the tone: when it was increased it usually declined, and conversely.

In addition to these hemispheric changes of cerebral hemodynamics we studied the influences on the regional cerebral circulation (Hadjiev and Yarullin, 1967) in 15 patients with pathology of the carotid and vertebral arteries (10 of them verified by angiography). We found that the regional effects of Euphylline on cerebral hemodynamics were not only of different intensity, but sometimes of different nature. The rheoencephalograms in Fig. 18 may serve to illustrate the regional effects of Euphylline on cerebral circulation.

The more marked effect on the vertebro-basilar area should be pointed out; obvious asymmetries were observed that were not revealed by the routine rheoencephalogram. These data illustrate the beneficial effect of the drug on some brain stem symptoms

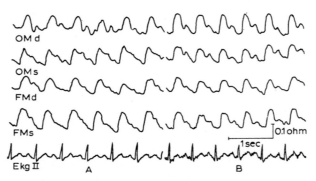

Fig. 18. Patient B.F., man aged 56. Atherosclerosis of aorta, carotid, vertebral and cerebral arteries. Transient ischemic attacks in the basin of the vertebro-basilar system. Occipito-mastoid and fronto-mastoid rheoencephalograms before (A) and after (B) 0.24 mg of i.v. Euphylline.

(Cheyne-Stokes breathing, etc.) in vascular diseases of the brain. The regional changes of vascular tone may be associated with the varying functional state and degree of atherosclerotic lesion of the brain or may be considered a manifestation of "intra-cerebral steal syndrome". Euphylline effects may also be clearly distinguished in the venous compartment of cerebral circulation. Disappearance of the presystolic wave after injecting the drug is an evidence of such effect. The improved venous outflow observed in the vertebro-basilar system is another explanation for the favourable drug effect. The regional effects of Euphylline show that it influences cerebral hemo-dynamics not only by means of changes in total circulation and respiration, but also by its effect on cerebral vascular tone. These data do not agree with the concepts of other authors who attribute the effects of Euphylline to its cardiotonic action (Gott-stein *et al.*, 1961). Cerebral vascular constriction occasionally caused by the drug is apparently desirable in cases of pathologic vasodilation and congestion which characterize the hyperemic cerebral foci.

(g) Adenosine triphosphate

Adenosine triphosphate (ATP) is an important source of energy for supplying the metabolic demands of the brain. It has been experimentally demonstrated that ATP synthesis in the brain is disturbed in ischemic and anoxic situations (Cohen, 1962) and its concentration rapidly falls (Kirsch and Leitner, 1967).

Studies with the nitrogen oxide method showed that intravenous administration of 20 mg of ATP dissolved in 40 ml of a 40% glucose solution increases oxygen con-sumption by the brain and the cerebral blood flow (Aizawa *et al.*, 1961). Using the same method, Gottstein (1962) failed to observe any significant changes in the cerebral blood flow after intravenous administration of adenosine monophosphate and adenosine triphosphate.

To gain insight into the effect of ATP on cerebral hemodynamics we studied the rheoencephalographic effects of this compound in 15 patients with ischemic disturb-ances of cerebral circulation, alone and in combination with papaverine hydrochloride (Hadjiev *et al.*, 1969 a). Twenty mg of ATP were injected intravenously, while the

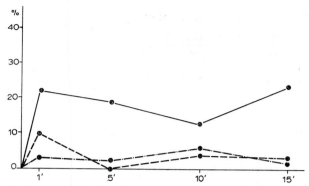

Fig. 19. Changes of: rheoencephalographic amplitude in percentage after i.v. papaverine hydrochloride (– – –), Atriphos (–·–·–) and the two drugs simultaneously (———). Abscissa: time following drug injections; ordinate: change in percentage.

combination of the two medicines (20 mg of ATP and 40 mg of papaverine hydrochloride dissolved in 50 ml of glucose–saline solution) was applied by intravenous infusion.

Fig. 19 illustrates the rheoencephalographic amplitude changes after intravenous administration of ATP, papaverine hydrochloride and the combination of the two drugs.

The amplitude changes following Atriphos administration were moderate; maximum increase 6% in the tenth minute was non-significant. Papaverine hydrochloride injection resulted in a notable amplitude increase ($p < 0.05$). Major and persistent deviations in this parameter occurred after injecting both drugs. In the first minute the amplitude showed 22% increase in comparison with the initial values; after a slight decrease in the 10th minute, the level rose to 24% in the 15th minute.

Similar but milder changes were observed in the right hemisphere as well. Here also, the effect on the rheoencephalographic amplitude of ATP–papaverine combined was stronger than that of each of the two drugs alone.

After ATP administration the mean rheoencephalogram was increased by 11% compared with the initial values; these changes persisted until the end of the study period. A major increase in this parameter by 23% in the first minute was observed after papaverine hydrochloride administration. The mean rheoencephalogram changes after ATP–papaverine infusion were found to be significant ($p < 0.05$), reaching a maximum of 11% against the initial values in the 15th minute. The changes following ATP and ATP–papaverine were most explicit at the end of the survey period.

The rheoencephalograms in Fig. 20 illustrate the beneficial effect of ATP–papaverine infusion on cerebral hemodynamics. The systolic, mean and diastolic pressure following ATP–papaverine administration is negligible. Therefore, the simultaneous intravenous infusion of 20 mg of Atriphos and 40 mg of papaverine hydrochloride substantially increases the maximal and mean volume fluctuations of the cerebral blood vessels. The effects of this complex medicine are stronger and persist longer than the effect of Atriphos or papaverine hydrochloride alone.

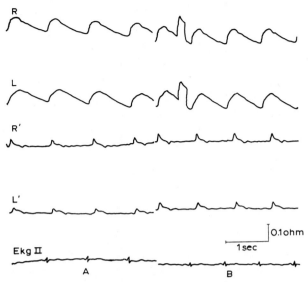

Fig. 20. Patient T.K., man aged 69. Atherosclerosis of aorta, carotid and cerebral arteries. Cerebral infarction in the basin of the right medial cerebral artery. Left-sided hemiparesis. Fronto-mastoid rheoencephalograms and their first derivatives before (A) and 15 min after (B) i.v. infusion of 40 mg of papaverine hydrochloride and 20 mg of Atriphos.

The regional, interhemispheric differences in the intensity of these effects must be associated with the localization of the pathologic process. The pathologic focal area becomes the site of the more significant changes in cerebral hemodynamics.

Although the cerebral hemodynamic changes following ATP and ATP–papaverine injection are more marked on the side of the pathologic process, circulation is improved in the other hemisphere as well. The more marked cerebral vasodilation observed after ATP–papaverine injection seems to be the result of the effect of papaverine on the smooth muscles of the cerebral vessels as well as of effect on cerebral metabolism in which ATP interferes.

To investigate this problem we studied the cerebral hemodynamic and metabolic changes induced by 20 mg of ATP injected intravenously with 10 ml of physiologic saline in 19 patients with cerebral circulatory disturbances (Hadjiev et al., 1969 b, c).

Hemispheric blood flow was determined by the venous radioisotope dilution technique before and 10 minutes after injecting the drug. We obtained blood samples before and at the 10th and 15th minute from the upper bulb of the internal jugular vein and from the femoral artery, and measured oxygen and carbon dioxide content in volume percentage, using a micro-gasometric technique and glucose concentration by the reductometric method (Natelson, 1951; Ceriotti, 1963). Then we calculated the respiratory quotient of the brain and its glucose–oxygen ratio.

After the drug injection, in some patients the hemispheric cerebral blood flow was increased and the cerebral vascular resistance fell; in others blood flow was reduced and vascular resistance increased (Table 3).

Hemispheric cerebral blood flow was found to significantly increase when its initial values were low, and to slightly decrease with normal initial values.

TABLE 3

CHANGES OF CEREBRAL BLOOD FLOW AND VASCULAR RESISTANCE AFTER
ATP ADMINISTRATION

	Increased cerebral blood flow group		Reduced cerebral blood flow group	
	Hemispheric blood flow ml/min	Cerebral vascular resistance dyn/sec/ $cm^{-5} \times 1332$	Hemispheric blood flow ml/min	Cerebral vascular resistance dyn/sec/ $cm^{-5} \times 1332$
n	5	5	6	6
$\bar{x}$ before	255.6	28.8	347.6	22.1
$\bar{x}$ after	370.4	19.4	257.0	27.7
$p <$	0.025	0.10	0.10	0.10

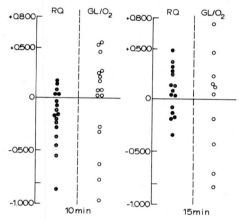

Fig. 21. Changes of respiratory quotient and glucose–oxygen ratio in the 10th and 15th min after i.v. administration of 20 mg of adenosine triphosphate.

The respiratory quotient of the brain is substantially reduced in the 10th minute after ATP administration and, along with this, there is an insignificant increase in the glucose–oxygen ratio. In the 15th minute the respiratory quotient rises above the initial values, while the glucose–oxygen coefficient returns toward the initial values (Fig. 21).

It may, therefore, be assumed that in the 10th minute after ATP administration anaerobic glycolysis becomes more intensive and in the 15th minute, the respiratory quotient rises, although insignificantly, *i.e.* CO_2 output from the brain increases, without being accompanied by significant changes in the arterial jugular oxygen level. These data are in agreement with the hemodynamic effects of ATP observed by rheoencephalography. They are most prominent in the 15th minute. Presumably ATP, by activating the glycolytic process, causes CO_2 accumulation in the brain tissue which, in turn, produces secondary vasodilation and improves the blood supply to the ischemic area. The stronger effect of the employed drug complex on brain

References pp. 79–85

hemodynamics observed by the rheoencephalographic technique may be explained by the cumulative vasodilatory effect of ATP and the direct relaxing effect of papaverine hydrochloride on the cerebral vessels. The metabolic processes activated by ATP run a longer course, which explains the long lasting effect of the employed drug complex.

As in ischemic disturbances of cerebral circulation it is expedient to improve oxygen and glucose supply to the ischemic area and to regulate metabolic disorders, the administration of vasodilating agents and substances influencing cerebral metabolism will improve the prospects for the treatment of cerebral ischemia.

(h) Cinnarizin

According to pharmacological data, Cinnarizin (Stugeron), a preparation of Janssen Pharmaceutica (Belgium) is a potent and long-acting vasodilating drug.

The favourable effect of Cinnarizin in patients with cerebral circulatory disturbances has been established in clinical studies (Behrens, 1966). In a group of 52 patients with cerebral atherosclerosis, cranio-cerebral trauma and migraine Wilcke (1966) observed shortly after the institution of Cinnarizin treatment remarkable improvement of the constitutional symptoms; after many weeks of treatment with this compound using a radioisotope method he demonstrated improvement of the cerebral blood flow.

In a randomized clinical experiment we (Hadjiev and Maximov, 1968) studied by rheoencephalography the effects of Cinnarizin in 21 patients with ischemic disturbances of cerebral circulation. The patients received one Cinnarizin tablet three times daily or placebo in the same dose. We followed up the constitutional symptoms and the neurologic and psychopathologic disturbances. Control examination was undertaken after 15 days of Cinnarizin treatment.

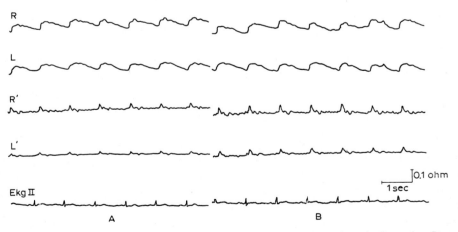

Fig. 22. Patient A.S., man aged 56. Atherosclerosis of aorta, carotid and cerebral arteries. Stenosis of right internal carotid artery. Cerebral infarction in the basin of the right medial cerebral artery. Left-sided hemiparesis. Fronto-mastoid rheoencephalograms and their first derivatives before (A) and 15 days after (B) Cinnarizin treatment.

The therapeutic effect of Cinnarizin on the neurologic disorders was good: not only were the constitutional symptoms improved, but also the motor and sensory disturbances.

Control rheoencephalographic investigations performed after 15 days of Cinnarizin treatment failed to disclose changes in the amplitude and the relative part of the anacrotic section of the curve, markedly differing from those observed in patients who received placebo. Differential rheograms in some Cinnarizin-treated patients showed increased amplitude for which the rise of vascular wall expansion rate was responsible. These changes are illustrated by rheograms in Fig. 22.

Whereas the rheoencephalographic curve reflecting major cerebral hemodynamic changes is a less sensitive criterion for the evaluation of the ensuing changes, its first derivative already shows reduced cerebral vascular tone.

These data suggest that improvement of clinical symptoms may be associated with Cinnarizin-induced decrease of cerebral vascular tone, which is detectable by rheoencephalography in some patients. The use of Cinnarizin in ischemic disturbances of cerebral circulation manifested by increased vascular tone and reduced cerebral blood flow is therefore justified.

(i) Agyrax

In recent years a group of synthetic agents designated as "vasorelaxants" have gained acceptance in the treatment of cerebral ischemia. They abolish smooth muscle spasm, but have no sympathicolytic effect and do not cause general vasodilation and hypotonia. Some of these drugs stimulate the heart muscle, give rise to tachycardia and raise the stroke and minute volume of the heart (Whittier, 1964). To these agents belongs Nylidrine.

Experimental studies in rabbits have shown that Nylidrine raises the blood flow in the internal carotid artery (Winsor et al., 1960). In an acute experiment this drug was shown to prevent the appearance of slow wave activity after hyperventilation. Moreover, the effect of a single dose persists for 2 hours (Whittier, 1964). Reports were published on the favourable effect of Nylidrine in ischemic disorders of cerebral circulation. If this drug is combined with tranquilizing agents its effects may be potentiated. Agyrax is such a combined medicine (Histamethizine dichlorhydrate 12.5 mg, Nylidrine 3 mg, Hydroxyzine dichlorhydrate 10 mg), produced by the firm Ucepha (France). It has gained wide acceptance in the treatment of labyrinthic vertigo attacks of vascular or other origin.

We studied the rheoencephalographic changes after Agyrax in 12 patients with ischemic disorders of cerebral circulation. The patient was given one Agyrax pill after records of the starting rheoencephalograms and oscillograms were completed. New rheoencephalographic and oscillographic tracings were made in the 15th, 30th and 45th minute at full rest and without changing position of electrodes and cuffs.

Agyrax intake was followed by a notable rise of the rheoencephalographic amplitude and the mean rheoencephalogram and this effect of the drug did not expire before the 45th minute. Inverse changes occurred with the relative part of the anacrotic section of the curve which was considerably reduced.

During the entire follow-up period, no changes in the minimal, mean and maximal brachial pressure were observed.

These data suggest that Agyrax causes cerebral vasodilation which, in the absence of total arterial pressure changes should be associated with a direct effect of the drug on vascular smooth muscles, manifested by increase of the maximal as well as of the mean volume fluctuations of the cerebral vessels. These effects should be attributed primarily to Nylidrine whose vasodilating effect in man has been confirmed indirectly, by electroencephalography.

The vasodilating effect of Agyrax makes this drug suitable for the treatment of ischemic disorders of cerebral circulation, in particular of the non-obstructive ones where angiodystonia is definitely of pathogenetic importance; the drug, however, is not indicated in vasodilation and paresis of the cerebral vessels (Hadjiev and Yarullin, 1970 e).

(j) Deserile

There are numerous reports in the literature on the favourable therapeutic effect of antiserotonin compounds, Deserile in particular, on migraine. The mechanism of their effect has not been fully elucidated. With this end in view we studied by the rheoencephalographic method the effect of Deserile on the cerebral circulation in patients with migraine in free attack period.

A total of 15 patients with migraine were studied; 0.25 mg of Deserile dissolved in 10 ml of a 10% glucose solution was administered by slow intravenous injection. Total cerebral hemodynamics evaluated by bitemporal rheoencephalography showed no change after injecting the drug. Analyzing the hemispheric rheoencephalograms, however, two groups of patients were discerned according to the Deserile-induced changes. In the first group there was a notable decrease of cerebral vascular tone, being strongest in the 10th minute after Deserile injection; in the second group vascular tone was increased.

The cerebral vasodilation observed in group I in response to Deserile should be associated with the antiserotonin effect of the drug, causing the smooth musculature of the vessels to relax.

In group II, the mean amplitude values following Deserile injection showed only a negligible decrease. Meanwhile, there was a rise in the mean values of the relative part in the anacrotic section of the curve. In this group of patients, therefore, Deserile produced an increase of cerebral vascular tone.

The comparison of these two groups of patients displaying opposite reactions (vasodilation and vasoconstriction) to Deserile reveals essential differences in the initial state of their vascular tone: where the initial vascular tone had been increased, the patients reacted with vasodilation and where it had been reduced, the reaction was vasoconstriction. This dependence of vascular reactions to Deserile from the initial state of cerebral vascular tone merits further extensive investigation. Similar dependence was recorded also for other drugs acting on cerebral vascular tone. Heyck (1962 b), using the nitrogen oxide technique, found that the higher the initial values of cerebral vascular resistance, the stronger its decrease after intravenous administration of Hydergin. A study of the dependence of cerebral vascular tone from its starting state following Deserile injection would have both theoretical and practical importance for motivated Deserile treatment.

The different manner in which cerebral vessels react to Deserile treatment throws light on the causes of the equivocal therapeutic results reported by various authors. To obtain good results, the drug should therefore be prescribed after studying the initial state of the vascular tone, to appraise the changes which the drug might induce. The impedance methods for the study of cerebral circulation are suitable for that purpose (Hadjiev and Usunov, 1969).

CONCLUSION

The impedance methods of examination of total and regional cerebral circulation have a sound theoretical basis, but a number of problems pertaining to their technical improvement, to the origin of impedance fluctuations and the elimination of extracranial vascular interference, the interpretation of rheoencephalographic curves, etc., require further elucidation. These methods are, therefore, in the developing stage.

It may be suggested that changes of blood volume and blood redistribution in the vascular system and, to a lesser extent, blood flow velocity are the factors responsible for the pulsatile fluctuations of cephalic impedance. These sources of impedance fluctuations depend on the resistance which cerebral vessels exert to the blood passage through them.

Under normal conditions of recording the rheoencephalographic curve, the impedance fluctuations conditioned by intracranial vessels are of decisive importance. The rheoencephalogram reflects both the arterial and venous compartments of cerebral circulation. By changing the body position and raising the pressure in the upper bulb of the internal jugular vein, it was demonstrated that the increase in the pre-incisure wave of the rheoencephalogram is a manifestation of impeded outflow from the intracranial space, whereas the presystolic wave reflects regional fluctuations in the blood volume in cerebral veins.

The impedance methods permit of the quantitative measurement of cerebral blood flow. Significant positive direct correlation between cerebral vascular resistance – measured by a venous radioisotope dilution technique – and the relative part of the anacrotic section of the rheoencephalogram provides conditions for the quantitative measurement of the volume velocity of cerebral blood flow. There are also other ways for obtaining quantitative information on cerebral blood flow by impedance methods. With their realization, the impedance methods of examination of cerebral circulation will gain even greater utility.

Abnormal rheoencephalograms reflect reduced or elevated vascular tone, vascular dystonia, cerebral venous congestion or a combination of these deviations. In addition to arterial and jugular pressure levels and the pulse rate, abnormal rheoencephalographic patterns are also influenced by CO_2 and lactate concentrations in the arterial and jugular blood.

References pp. 79–85

Functional rheoencephalography using different tests allows the evaluation of vascular tone and of the pathways of collateral circulation.

Significant rheoencephalographic changes may be observed in vascular diseases of the brain. This is helpful for an objective assessment of cerebral atherosclerosis and its severity, in the diagnosis of carotid obstruction and stenosis, etc. The changes observed are not specific for a definite type of impaired cerebral circulation, but impedance methods may aid in localizing ischemic or hyperemic foci in a particular area of the brain, which has great importance for the pathogenetic diagnosis of stroke.

Impedance methods are also helpful in disclosing circulatory disturbances in brain tumors, cranio-cerebral trauma, epilepsy, migraine and parkinsonism.

Rheoencephalographic studies on the effects of a series of vasoactive and metabolic-active drugs in patients with impaired cerebral circulation are of major theoretical and practical importance. The surveyed medicines were shown to exert effects of varying nature and duration on the arterial and venous vessels of the brain. The substances used exert regional, occasionally inverse effects on cerebral circulation and give rise to "intracerebral steal syndrome". Therefore, the impedance methods provide continuous and incessant information on the rapid and regional cerebral circulatory changes occurring under the influence of a drug. This lends considerable value to impedance techniques for adequate treatment and for the control of its effectiveness, especially in acute disorders of cerebral circulation where the principle of "primum non nocere" should be strictly observed.

SUMMARY

A number of problems pertaining to the theory and practical application of methods for measuring pulsatile fluctuations of cephalic impedance and total impedance changes are still unsolved. Nevertheless, there is sufficient ground to admit that these methods provide information on cerebral circulation and on the state of the arterial and venous vessels of the brain. Recent studies suggest that the impedance methods are capable of providing qualitative information on total and regional cerebral blood flow. Thus their importance in the study of cerebral circulation is expected to grow.

Impedance techniques are of great value for the diagnosis of cerebral vascular diseases and for the detection of circulatory disturbances in brain tumors, cranio-cerebral trauma, etc. These methods, especially combined with different tests, may gain importance for the early diagnosis of cerebral atherosclerosis running an a-symptomatic course or manifested by scanty and non-specific psychopathologic disturbances. This, in turn, will contribute to the prevention of grave vascular lesions of the brain.

Impedance methods may be used extensively to study the effects of a variety of drugs on total and regional circulation, thus making possible the prescription of well-motivated treatment in patients with cerebral circulatory disorders and the control of its effectiveness. This has practical importance in particular in the acute period of cerebral stroke when any additional deterioration of cerebral hemodynamics may have unfavourable and even fatal consequences.

REFERENCES

AIZAWA, T., TAZAKI, J. AND GOTHO, F. (1961) Cerebral circulation in cerebrovascular disease. *World Neurol.*, **2**, 635–648.

AUINGER, W., KAINDL, F. AND NEUMAYR, A. (1953) Über die Brauchbarkeit der Schädelrheographie am Menschen, insbesondere zur Beurteilung des Effektes therapeutischer Massnahmen auf das Verhalten der Gefässe. *Z. Kreislaufforsch.*, **42**, 104–111.

BAUER, R., SHEEHAN, S. AND MEYER, J. (1961) Arteriographic study of cerebrovascular disease. *Arch. Neurol.*, **4**, 113–131.

BEHRENS, E. (1966) Medikamentöse Beeinflussung der Hirndurchblutung durch Stutgeron. *Med. Welt*, **17**, 2029–2031.

BERTHA, H., HEPPNER, F., JENKNER, F. L., LECHNER, H. AND RODLER, R. (1955) Untersuchungen zur Deutung des Schädelrheograms. *Zbl. Neurochir.*, **15**, 257–262.

BETZ, E., INGVAR, D. H., LASSEN, N. A. AND SCHMAHL, F. W. (1966) Regional blood flow in the cerebral cortex, measured simultaneously by heat and inert gas clearance. *Acta physiol. scand.*, **67**, 1–9.

BIRZIS, L., AGUILAR, J. A. AND TACHIBANA, S. (1968) Cerebral hemodynamics revealed by electrical impedance changes. *Confinia Neurol.*, **30**, 1–16.

BRANDT, I. AND WINTER, H. (1954) Zur Hochdruckbehandlung mit Hydergin. *Ärztl. Wochschr.*, **31**, 724–730.

CERIOTTI, G. (1963) Microdetermination of blood glucose. *Clin. Chim. Acta*, **8**, 157–158.

COHEN, M. M. (1962) The effect of anoxia on the chemistry and morphology of cerebral cortex slices in vitro. *J. Neurochem.*, **9**, 337–344.

DEL GUERCIO, R. (1963) Considerazioni sull' emodinamica cerebrale attraverso l'esame comparativo reografico ed electroencefalografico. Nota II, Attività della papaverina in soggetti affetti da vasculopatie cerebrale. *Riforma Med.*, **77**, 911–914.

DOBNER, E. (1958) Die Schädelrheographie als Methode zur Diagnose orthostatischer Kreislaufstörungen, *Electromedizin*, **5**, 169–174.

ENINYA, G. I. (1962) Cranial rheography in some vascular diseases. *Klinick. Med.*, **40**, 89–94.

FASANO, V. A., ANGELINO, P. E., BRAGUZZI, E. AND BROGGI, G. (1961) Considerations sur la rheographie cranienne. *Neuro-chirurgie*, **7**, 202–207.

FAZEKAS, J. F. AND ALMAN, R. W. (1963) Vasodilatators in cerebral vascular insufficiency. *Amer. J. Med. Sci.*, **246**, 410–416.

FEDOROWSKY, YU. N. (1966) *Rheoencephalography in Some Psychiatric Diseases*, Moscow, p. 41.

FERUGLIO, F. S. AND MICHELI, B. (1958) Modifications produites par le "Ronicol compositum" sur l'hémodynamisme et le métabolisme du cerveau dans les vasculopathies cérébrales aigues. *Cardiologia*, **32**, 317–326.

FRIEDMANN, G. (1955) Der Wert der Schädelrheographie, *Ärztl. Wochschr.*, **10**, 553–556.

GARBINI, G. C., DE MARCHIE, R. AND VANNINI, P. (1957) Valutazione reografica della componente funzionale spastica nelle cerebropatie vascolari mediante farmaco vasodilatore. *Riv. Med. Bologna*, **3**, 459–470.

GARBINI, G. C. AND PICCHIO, A. A. (1957) *La Reografia. Fisiopatologica e Clinica*, Bologna Med., Bologna.

GEYER, N., RODLER, H. AND LECHNER, H. (1965) Experimental investigations aiming at the interpretation of the rheogram. In: MARTIN, F. AND LECHNER, H. (Eds.), *Rheoencephalographia*, Verlag der Wiener Medizinischen Akademie, Vienna, p. 33–41.

GEYER, N. (1969) Simultaneous deduction from EEG, classical and recording REG signal over a D.C. channel. In: LECHNER, H., GEYER, N., LUGARESI, E., MARTIN, F., LIFSHITZ, K. AND MARKOVICH, S. (Eds.), *Rheoencephalography and Plethysmographical Methods*, Excerpta Med. Foundation, Amsterdam, pp. 104–108.

GIANOLI, A. C. (1956) Die Frühbehandlung des Schlaganfalls. *Schweiz. Med. Wochschr.*, **86**, 235–239.

GOTTSTEIN, U., BERNSMEIER, A., SEBENING, H. AND STEINER, K. (1961) Zur Behandlung zerebraler Durchblutungsstörungen mit Euphyllin (Theophyllin-Aethylendiamin). Der Einfluss von Euphyllin auf die Hirndurchblutung und zerebralen Stoffwechsel des Menschen. *Med. Klin.*, **56**, 1589–1592.

GOTTSTEIN, U. (1962) *Der Hirnkreislauf unter dem Einfluss vasoaktiver Substanzen*, Dr. Alfred Hüthig Verlag, Heidelberg.

HADJIEV, D. AND TZENOV, A. (1964 a) Rheographische Untersuchung der Papaverinwirkung auf die

Hindurchblutung bei Gefässerkrankungen des Grosshirns, *Psychiat. Neurol. Med. Psychol. (Lpz.)*, **16**, 242–244.

HADJIEV, D. AND TZENOV, A. (1964 b) Cranial rheography. *Neurol. Psychiat. Neurosurg. (Sofia)*, **3**, 97–104.

HADJIEV, D. (1965 a) Cerebrovascular insufficiency and the role of the cerebral vasomotor reactions for its development. *Neurol. Psychiat. Neurosurg. (Sofia)*, **4**, 339–345.

HADJIEV, D. (1965 b) Einfluss der Nikotinsäure auf die zerebrale und die periphere Durchblutung bei Insulten (Rheoenzephalographische und oscillographische Untersuchungen). *Psychiat. Neurol. Med. Psychol. (Lpz.)*, **17**, 291–296.

HADJIEV, D. (1966 a) Rheoencephalographic studies of the influence of some vasoactive drugs on the cerebral circulation in cerebral stroke. *Dissertation*, Sofia.

HADJIEV, D. AND TZENOV, A. (1966) An attempt to extend the diagnostical possibilities of skull rheography in vascular diseases of the brain. *Bull. Res. Inst. Neurol. Psychiat. (Sofia)*, **10**, 223–228.

HADJIEV, D. (1966 b) Rheoencephalographic assessment of the brain venous circulation. *Works of the Institute for Neuropsychiatric Research (Sofia)*, **12**, 39–43.

HADJIEV, D. AND YARULLIN, H. (1967) Rheoencephalographic studies on the influences of Euphylline on regional cerebral circulation. *Neurol. Psychiat. Neurosurg. (Sofia)*, **6**, 69–76.

HADJIEV, D. (1967 a) Der Wert der rheoencephalographischen Methode bei Gefässerkrankungen des Gehirns. *Psychiat. Neurol. Med. Psychol. (Lpz.)*, **19**, 304–309.

HADJIEV, D. AND WASSILEVA, J. (1967) Rheoencephalographic investigations regarding the effect of Halidor on cerebral blood flow in ischaemia. *Therapia Hung.*, **15**, 1–3.

HADJIEV, D. (1967 b) L'influence du rédergame sur la circulation cérébrale chez les malades atteints d'apoplexies. *Zh. Nevropatol. Psikhiat.*, **67**, 33–37.

HADJIEV, D. (1967 c) The effect of Euphylline on cerebral and peripheral circulation in cerebro-vascular insults. *Zh. Nevropatol. Psikhiat.*, **67**, 538–542.

HADJIEV, D. (1968) A new method for quantitative evaluation of cerebral blood flow by rheoence-phalography. *Brain Res.*, **8**, 213–215.

HADJIEV, D. AND GANEV, G. (1968) Halidor hatása az agy haemodynamikájára és anyagcseréjére ischaemiás agyi keringési zavarokban szenvedő betegeknél. *Orv. Hetilap*, **102**, 37–40.

HADJIEV, D. AND MAXIMOV, K. (1968) Therapeutical effectiveness of Cinnarizin in ischemic disorders of the cerebral circulation. *Works of the Institute for Neuropsychiatric Research (Sofia)*, **14**, 119–123.

HADJIEV, D. AND BAIKUSHEV, B. (1969) Analysis of the relationship between the relative section of the anacrotic part of the rheoencephalogram and the cerebrovascular resistance, determined by radio-isotope venous dilution method. *Bull. Res. Inst. Neurol. Psychiat. (Sofia)*, **13**, 28–32.

HADJIEV, D. AND UZUNOV, N. (1969) The effect of Deserile on cerebral blood circulation in patients with migraine in the interval between attacks. *Bull. Res. Inst. Neurol. Psychiat., (Sofia)*, **13**, 24–31.

HADJIEV, D. AND WASSILEVA, J. (1969) Rheoencephalographic investigations in ischemic disorders of the brain circulation. *Works of the Institute for Neuropsychiatric Research (Sofia)*, **15**, 43–51.

HADJIEV, D. (1969) *Vasoactive Drugs in Cerebral Stroke*, Medicina i Fiskultura, Sofia.

HADJIEV, D., YARULLIN, H. AND WASSILEVA, J. (1969 a) Rheoencephalographic studies of the effects of Atriphos and papaverine on the cerebral circulation in patients with ischaemic disorders of cerebral circulation. *Neurol. Psychiat. Neurosurg. (Sofia)*, **8**, 145–151.

HADJIEV, D., VICHEV, E. AND MARINOVA, Z. (1969 b) Influence of adenosine triphosphate on the cerebral blood flow and carbohydrate metabolism in ischemic disorders of the cerebral circulation. *Works of the Institute for Neuropsychiatric Research (Sofia)*, **15**, 17–23.

HADJIEV, D., VICHEV, E. AND MARINOVA, Z. (1969 c) ATP influences on cerebral hemodynamic and metabolism in patients with ischaemic cerebral disturbances. In: BROCK, M., FIESCHI, C., INGVAR, D. H., LASSEN, N. A. AND SCHÜRMANN, K. (Eds.), *Cerebral Blood Flow. Clinical and Experimental Results*. Springer-Verlag, Berlin-Heidelberg-New York, pp. 149–151.

HADJIEV, D. (1970 a) Quantitative evaluation on cerebral blood flow by rheoencephalography. *Ann. N.Y. Acad. Sci.*, **170**, 622–626.

HADJIEV, D. (1970 b) Rheography. In: GANEV, G. (Ed.), *Clinical Electrophysiology*, Medicina i Fiskultura, Sofia, pp. 223–251.

HADJIEV, D. AND MARINOVA, Z. (1970) Influence of cocarboxylase upon the cerebral hemodynamic and metabolism in ischemic disturbances of cerebral circulation. *Bull. Res. Inst. Neurol. Psychiat., (Sofia)*, **14**, 43–49.

HADJIEV, D. AND YANCHEVA, ST. (1970) Transient cerebral circulation disorders. *Bull. Res. Inst. Neurol. Psychiat.*, (Sofia), **14**, 50–56.

HADJIEV, D. AND YARULLIN, H. (1970) Rheoencephalographic investigations on the effect of Agyrax in patients with ischemic disorders of the cerebral circulation. *Bull. Res. Inst. Neurol. Psychiat.*, (Sofia), **14**, 21–25.

HADORN, W. (1960) Berichterstattung über die Euphyllin-Behandlung des Hirnschlags auf Grund der statistischen Verarbeitung von 705 Fällen. *Schweiz. Med. Wochschr.*, **90**, 1301–1302.

HANGARTER, W. AND HENSSGE, J. (1956) Zur Behandlung von apoplektischen Insulten mit gefässerweiternden Mitteln. *Deut. Med. Wochschr.*, **81**, 937–939.

HEDLUND, S. (1966) Hemodynamics of the cerebral blood circulation studied by means of radioactive isotopes. *Acta Neurol. Scand.*, **41**, 299–303.

HEYCK, H. (1962 a) Der Einfluss der Nikotinsäure auf die Hirndurchblutung und den Hirnstoffwechsel bei Cerebralsclerosen und anderen diffusen Durchblutungsstörungen des Gehirns. *Schweiz. Med. Wochschr.*, **92**, 226–231.

HEYCK, H. (1962 b) Über die Beeinflussbarkeit der Hirndurchblutung und des Hirnstoffwechsels durch Medikamente. Ergebnisse quantitativer Messungen am Menschen. *Therap. Umschau*, **19**, 62–67.

HØEDT-RASMUSSEN, K., SKINHOJ, E., PAULSON, O., EWALD, J., BJERRUM, J. K., FAHRENKRUG, A. AND LASSEN, N. A. (1967) Regional cerebral blood flow in acute apoplexy. The "luxury perfusion syndrome" of brain tissue. *Arch. Neurol.*, **17**, 271–281.

IMADACHI, T. (1960) Studies on cerebral circulation by means of rheography; especially the effect of various drugs. *J. Kurume Med. Assoc.* (Kurume, Nippone), **23**, 6849–6869.

IMHOF, P., IMHOF, M., EICHENBERGER, E. AND LAUNER, H. (1959) Über die Aktivierung der Fibrinolyse durch Verabreichung von Nikotinsäure. *Schweiz. Med. Wochschr.*, **28**, 736–740.

INGVAR, D. H. AND LASSEN, N. A. (1965) Methods for cerebral blood flow measurements in man. *Brit. J. Anaesthesiol.*, **37**, 216–224.

IVANOVA, L. (1969) Recherches rheoencephalographiques au cours de crises de petit-mal. In *International Symposium on the Pathogenesis of Epilepsy, Summaries, Varna, Bulgaria, 7–9 October, 1969*, pp. 35–36.

JENKNER, F. L. (1957) Über den Wert des Schädelrheogramms für die Diagnose zerebraler Gefässstörungen. *Wien. Klin. Wochschr.*, **69**, 619–624.

JENKNER, F. L. (1962) *Rheoencephalography. A Method for the Continuous Registration of Cerebrovascular Changes*, Ch.C Thomas, Springfield, Ill.

KAINDL, F., POLZER, K. AND SCHUHFRIED, F. (1956) Mehrfach- und Differential-Rheographie. *Verh. Deut. Ges. Kreislaufforsch.*, **21**, 451–458.

KAINDL, F., POLZER, K. AND SCHUHFRIED, F. (1959) *Rheographie. Eine Methode zur Beurteilung peripherer Gefässe*, Verlag Dr. Steinkopff, Darmstadt.

KAPPERT, A., BAUMGARTNER, P. AND RUPP, F. (1948) Über die blutdrucksenkende Wirkung neuer dihydrierter Mutterkornalkaloide. *Schweiz. Med. Wochschr.*, **78**, 1265–1269.

KARELLIN, W. A. (1957) Rheovasography in the diagnosis of endarteriitis obliterans. *Dissertation*, Moscow, 1957.

KEDROV, A. A. AND NAUMENKO, A. I. (1941) Some specific regulations of the cerebral circulation. *Fiziol. Zh. (Mosk.)*, **27**, 431–438.

KETY, S. S. AND SCHMIDT C. F. (1945) The determination of cerebral blood flow in man by the use of nitrous oxide in low concentration. *Am. J. Physiol.*, **53**, 143–147.

KIRSCH, W. M. AND LEITNER, J. W. (1967) Glycolytic metabolites and cofactors in human cerebral cortex and white matter during complete ischemia. *Brain Res.*, **4**, 358–368.

KOECKE, K. (1961) Erweiterung der schädelrheographischen Diagnostik durch Registrierung in den extremen Respirationsphasen. *Elektromedizin*, **6**, 73–74.

KOECKE, K. (1962) Theoretische Grundlagen der Schädelrheographie in besonderer Beziehung zur Zerebralsklerose. *Wien. Med. Wochschr.*, **112**, 227–230.

KUNERT, W. (1959) Über die Grundfrage der Schädelrheographie. *Z. Klin. Med.*, **156**, 94–116.

KUNERT, W. (1961) Fortschritte der Schädelrheographie. *Z. Kreislaufforsch.*, **50**, 572–580.

KUWABARA, T. (1959) Study of cerebral circulation by impedance plethysmography. *Brain and Nerve (Tokyo)*, **11**, 647–660.

LAITINEN, L. V., JOHANSSON, G. G. AND SIPPONEN, P. (1966) Recording of regional cerebral circulation by an impedance method. A preliminary report. *Brain Res.*, **2**, 184.

LAITINEN, L. V., JOHANSSON, G. G. AND SIPPONEN, P. (1969) Intracerebral impedance method for investigation of regional cerebral blood flow. In: LECHNER, H., GEYER, N., LUGARESI, E., MARTIN, F., LIFSHITZ, K. AND MARKOVICH, S. (Eds.), *Rheoencephalography and Plethysmographical Methods*, Excerpta Med. Foundation, Amsterdam, pp. 145–149.

LASCH, F. AND MORITZ, E. (1955) Weitere Untersuchungen zur blutdrucksenkenden Wirkung des Hydergin. *Deut. Med. Wochschr.*, **31**, 1137–1139.

LASSEN, N. A. AND INGVAR, D. H. (1961) The blood flow of the cerebral cortex determined by radioactive krypton 85. *Experientia*, **17**, 62–69.

LASSEN, N. A. AND INGVAR, D. H. (1963) Regional cerebral blood flow measurement in man. *Arch. Neurol.*, **9**, 615–624.

LASSEN, N. A. AND PAULSON, O. B. (1969) Partial cerebral vasoparalysis in patients with apoplexy: dissociation between carbon dioxide responsiveness and autoregulation. In: BROCK, M., FIESCHI, C., INGVAR, D. H., LASSEN, N. A. AND SCHÜRMANN, K. (Eds.), *Cerebral Blood Flow. Clinical and Experimental Results*, Springer-Verlag, Berlin-Heidelberg-New York, pp. 117–119.

LAWRENCE, R. M. (1969) A double-blind study comparing xanthinol niacinate (Complamin) with a placebo using rheoencephalographic data, electroencephalographic studies and arm-to-retina fluorescein appearance time. In: LECHNER, H., GEYER, N., LUGARESI, E., MARTIN, F., LIFSHITZ, K. AND MARKOVICH, S. (Eds.), *Rheoencephalography and Plethysmographical Methods*, Excerpta Med. Foundation, Amsterdam, pp. 204–207.

LAZORTHES, G. (1961) *Vascularisation et Circulation Cérébrales*, Masson et Cie, Paris.

LECHNER, H. AND RODLER, H. (1961) Eine neue Methode zur Registrierung intrakranieller Kreislaufveränderungen. *Elektromedizin*, **2**, 75–77.

LECHNER, H., RODLER, H. AND GEYER, N. (1965 a) Theorie der Entstehung der rheographischen Kurve. In: MARTIN, F. AND LECHNER, H. (Eds.), *Rheoencephalographia*, Verlag der Wiener Medizinischen Akademie, Vienna, pp. 19–29.

LECHNER, H., GEYER, N. AND RODLER, H. (1965 b) Present possibilities of detecting a localized vascular disturbance by rheoencephalography. In: MARTIN, F. AND LECHNER, H. (Eds.), *Rheoencephalographia*, Verlag der Wiener Medizinischen Akademie, Vienna, pp. 259–267.

LECHNER, H., GEYER, N., RODLER, H. AND MAYR, F. (1965 c) The influence of vaso-active drugs on the rheogram. In: MARTIN, F. AND LECHNER, H. (Eds.), *Rheoencephalographia*, Verlag der Wiener Medizinischen Akademie, Vienna, pp. 195–204.

LECHNER, H., RODLER, H. AND GEYER, N. (1966) The technical development of field rheography, *J. Instrument. Life Sci.*, **4**, 150–154.

LECHNER, H. AND MARTIN, F. (1969) Introduction to rheoencephalographic methods. In: LECHNER, H., GEYER, N., LUGARESI, E., MARTIN, F., LIFSHITZ, K. AND MARKOVICH, S. (Eds.), *Rheoencephalography and Plethysmographical Methods*, Excerpta Med. Foundation, Amsterdam, pp. 3–9.

LECHNER, H. AND LANNER, G. (1969) On the question of possible differentiation: various supply areas with recording rheographic signals over a D.C. channel. In: LECHNER, H., GEYER, N., LUGARESI, E., MARTIN, F., LIFSHITZ, K. AND MARKOVICH, S. (Eds.), *Rheoencephalography and Plethysmographical Methods*, Excerpta Med. Foundation, Amsterdam, pp. 99–103.

LEVIN, G. Z. (1963) Diagnosis and therapy in the acute phase of cerebrovascular insult. *Works of the Research Institute of Neurology and Psychiatry (Leningrad)*, **32**, 5–54.

LIFSHITZ, K. (1963 a) Rheoencephalography: I. Review of the technique. *J. Nervous Mental Disease*, **136**, 388–398.

LIFSHITZ, K. (1963 b) Rheoencephalography: II. Survey of clinical applications. *J. Nervous Mental Disease*, **137**, 285–296.

LIFSHITZ, K. AND KLEMM, K. (1966) The use of electrode guarding in rheoencephalography. *Proc. 19th Ann. Conf. Engng. in Med. Biol.*, **8**, 39.

LIFSHITZ, K. (1969) An investigation of electrode guarding and frequency effects in rheoencephalography. In LECHNER, H., GEYER, N., LUGARESI, E., MARTIN, F., LIFSHITZ, K. AND MARKOVICH, S. (Eds.), *Rheoencephalography and Plethysmographical Methods*, Excerpta Med. Foundation, Amsterdam, pp. 10–16.

LIFSHITZ, K. (1970) Electrical impedance cephalography (rheoencephalography). In: CLYNES AND MELSUM (Eds.), *Biomedical Engineering Systems*, Chapter 2, McGraw Hill, New York.

LISSITSA, F. M. (1967) La dynamique des indices rhéoencéphalographiques au cours du traumatisme cranio-cérébral fermé. *Zh. Nevropatol. Psikhiat.*, **67**, 343–347.

LUGARESI, E., REBUCCI, G. G. AND COCCAGNA, G. (1962) Il valore diagnostico della compressione della carotide: contributo reografico, EEG et clinico. *G. Psichiatol. Neuropatol.*, **4**, 1–15.

LUGARESI, E., REBUCCI, G. G., COCCAGNA, G., GIOVANARDI, P. AND ORIOLI, G. (1964) La reoencefalografia: contributo semeiologico e fisiopatologico. *Sist. Nerv.*, **16**, 69–81.

LUGARESI, E., ORIOLI, G. AND SABATTINI, L. (1969) The abnormal REG. In: LECHNER, H., GEYER,

N., LUGARESI, E., MARTIN, F., LIFSHITZ, K. AND MARKOVICH, S. (Eds.), *Rheoencephalography and Plethysmographical Methods*, Excerpta Med. Foundation, Amsterdam, pp. 136–139.

MAHL, M. AND LANGE, K. (1963) A long term study of the effect of nicotinic acid medication on hypercholesteremia. *Amer. J. Med. Sci.*, **246**, 673–676.

MAINZER, F. (1949) Frühbehandlung des Schlaganfalls mit Aminophyllin *Schweiz. Med. Wochschr.*, **79**, 108–110.

MAJORTCHIK, V. E. AND YARULLIN, KH. KH. (1966) L'importance de l'enrégistrement simultané du rhéoencéphalogramme (REG) et de l'électroencéphalogramme (EEG) pour la localisation de l'atteint focal du cerveau d'origine vasculaire et tumoreuse. *Z. Nevropatol. Psykhiat.*, **66**, 1148 -1156.

MARKOVICH, S. E. (1969) Clinical rheoencephalography. In: LECHNER, H., GEYER, N., LUGARESI, E., MARTIN, F., LIFSHITZ, K. and MARKOVICH, S. (Eds.), *Rheoencephalography and Plethysmographical Methods*, Excerpta Med. Foundation, Amsterdam, pp. 133–135.

MATZDORFF, F. (1961) Experimentelle rheographische Untersuchungen am Modell. *Elektromedizin*, **6**, 68–70.

MAZZARELLA, B., DEL GUERCIO, R. AND DE NATALE, L. (1961) Comportamento della reografia cranica e periferica durante terapia elettro-convulsivante. *Rivista "L'Ospedale Psichiatrico" (Napoli)*, **4**, 449–456.

MCHENRY, L. C. (1965) Rheoencephalography. A clinical appraisal. *Neurology*, **15**, 507–517.

MENINGER-LERCHENTHAL, E. (1953) Gesellschaft der Arzte in Wien. *Wien. Med. Wochschr.*, **103**, 119–122.

MERDJANOV, CH. AND IVANOVA, L. (1969) Rheoencephalographic studies at the time and after epileptiform seizures. In: *Intern. Symp. on the Pathogenesis of Epilepsy, Summaries, Varna, Bulgaria*, 7–9 October, 1969, pp. 54–55.

MINZ, A. YA. AND RONKIN, M. A. (1967) *Rheographic Diagnosis of Cerebrovascular Diseases*, Zdorovja, Kiev.

MORI, K., ITO, M. AND SHIMABUKURO, H. (1969) Electrical impedance method for localizing brain structures (second report). *Brain and Nerve (Tokyo)*, **21**, 123–128.

MOSKALENKO, YU. E. AND NAUMENKO, A. J. (1964) Hemodynamics of cerebral circulation. In: SIMONSON, E. AND MCGAVACK, TH. H. (Eds.), *Cerebral Ischemia*, Ch. C. Thomas, Springfield, Ill.

MURATORE, F. (1963) Terapia medica degli accidenti vascolari cerebrali nella fase acuta. *Minerva Med.*, **54**, 2317–2327.

MURPHY, I. P. (1956) Recent advances in the investigation and management of cerebrovascular disease. *Circulation*, **5**, 281–293.

NAMON, R. AND MARKOVICH, S. E. (1967) Monopolar rheoencephalography. *Electroencephalog. Clin. Neurophysiol.*, **22**, 272–274.

NAMON, R., GOLLAN, F., SHIMOJYO, S., SANO, R. M., MARKOVICH, S. E. AND SCHEINBERG, P. (1967) Basic studies in rheoencephalography. *Neurology*, **17**, 239–252.

NATELSON, S. (1951) Routine use of ultramicro methods in the clinical laboratory. *Amer. J. Clin. Pathol.*, **21**, 1153–1172.

NYBOER, J. (1959) *Electrical Impedance Plethysmography*, Ch. C. Thomas, Springfield, Ill.

ORGAN, L. W., TASKER, R. R. AND MOODY, N. F. (1968) Brain tumor localization using an electrical impedance technique. *J. Neurosurg.*, **28**, 35–44.

ORIOLI, G., PAZZAGLIA, P. AND MANTOVANI, M. (1969) A rheographic and polygraphic study on migraine. In: LECHNER, H., GEYER, N., LUGARESI, E., MARTIN, F., LIFSHITZ, K. AND MARKOVICH, S. (Eds.), *Rheoencephalography and Plethysmographical Methods*, Excerpta Med. Foundation, Amsterdam, pp. 164–169.

ORLANDI, G., GARBINI, G. C. AND GENTILI, C. (1957) Criteri reografici differenziali fra affezioni vascolari e neoplastiche del cervello. *Minerva Med.*, **48**, 3225–3228.

PEREZ-BORJA, C. AND MEYER, J. S. (1964) A critical evaluation of rheoencephalography in control subjects and in proven cases of cerebrovascular disease. *J. Neurol. Neurosurg. Psychiat.*, **27**, 66–72.

POLZER, K. AND SCHÜHFRIED, F. (1950) Rheographische Untersuchungen am Schädel, *Wien. Z. Nervenheilk.*, **3**, 295–298.

POSTELI, T., GARBINI, G. C. AND MONTALI, M. (1957) Rilievi sfigmici reografici cerebrali. *Riv. Med. Bologna*, **3**, 435–458.

PRATESI, F., NUTI, A. AND SCIAGRA, A. (1957) Reografia cranica prove funzionale nella diagnostica delle vasculopatie cerebrale. *Minerva Med.*, **79**, 3223–3224.

PRATESI, F., DEIDDA, C., CARAMELLI, L. AND DABIZZI, R. P. (1969) Original method of selective rheography of the carotids and the vertebral arteries. In: LECHNER, H., GEYER, N., LUGARESI, E., MARTIN, F., LIFSHITZ, K. AND MARKOVICH, S. (Eds.), *Rheoencephalography and Plethysmographical Methods*, Excerpta Med. Foundation, Amsterdam, pp. 109–114.

QUANDT, J. AND JULICH, H. (1959) Prophylaxe und Therapie der zerebralen Kreislaufstörungen. In: J. QUANDT (Ed.), *Die zerebralen Durchblutungsstörungen des Erwachsenenalters*, VEB Verlag Volk und Gesundheit, Berlin, p. 624.

RATNER, N. A., DENISSOVA, E. A. AND SMASCHNOVA, N. A. (1958) *Hypertensive Crisis*, Medgiz, Moscow, p. 113.

REISNER, H. (1953) Klinik und Therapie des zerebralen Insultes, *Klin. Med. Wien*, 9, 385–402.

RODLER, H. (1969 a) Methods for rheoencephalography II and their further development. In: LECHNER, H., GEYER, N., LUGARESI, E., MARTIN, F., LIFSHITZ, K. AND MARKOVICH, S. (Eds.), *Rheoencephalography and Plethysmographical Methods*, Excerpta Med. Foundation, Amsterdam, pp. 17–23.

RODLER, H. (1969 b) Rheographic recording techniques of rheography II possible at the present time. In: LECHNER, H., GEYER, N., LUGARESI, E., MARTIN, F., LIFSHITZ, K. AND MARKOVICH, S. (Eds.), *Rheoencephalography and Plethysmographical Methods*, Excerpta Med. Foundation, Amsterdam, pp. 96–98.

ROTHLIN, E. (1950) Pharmakologie und Klinik der hydrierten Mutterkornalkaloide, *Wien. Klin. Wochschr.*, 62, 893–895.

SARATIKOV, A. AND USOV, L. (1969) Effect of chloracizin, no-spa and Halidor upon cerebral circulation and metabolism. In: *International Cerebral Blood Flow Symposium, Abstracts, Mainz, April 10–12, 1969*, p. 38.

SCHEINBERG, P. (1950) The effect of nicotinic acid on the cerebral circulation with observation on extracerebral contamination of cerebral venous blood in the nitrous oxide procedure for cerebral blood flow. *Circulation*, 1, 1148–1154.

SCHLÜTER, A. (1921) Apparat zur Bestimmung des elektrischen Widerstandes im Gehirn, *Zbl. Chir.*, 48, 1827–1828.

SCHREIBER, H. (1960) Untersuchungen über die Änderungen der Durchblutungsgrösse des Gehirns unter 3-(Methyl-oxyäthylamino)-2-Oxypropyl-Theophyllin-nicotinat mit Hilfe der Schädel-rheographie. *Med. Klin.*, 55, 509–511.

SCHREIBER, H. (1962) Zur Diagnose der Zerebralsklerose. Untersuchungen mittels Schädelrheographie. *Med. Welt. (Stuttg.)*, 32, 1643–1649.

SEIPEL, J., ZIEMNOWICZ-RADVAN, S. AND O'DOHERTY, D. S. (1964) Cranial impedance plethysmo-graphy-rheoencephalography as a method of detection of cerebrovascular disease. In: SIMONSON, E. AND MCGAVACK, TH. H. (Eds.), *Cerebral Ischemia*, Ch. C. Thomas, Springfield, Ill.

SEIPEL, J. H. (1967) *The Biophysical Basis and Clinical Applications of Rheoencephalography*, Federal Aviation Administration, Office of Aviation Medicine, Georgetown Clinical Research Institute, Washington.

SHENKIN, H. A. (1951) Effect of various drugs upon cerebral circulation and metabolism in man. *J. Appl. Physiol.*, 3, 465–471.

SHILLINGFORD, J., BRUCE, TH. AND GABE, I. (1962) The measurement of segmental venous flow by an indicator dilution method. *Brit. Heart J.*, 24, 157–165.

SIGMAN, E., KOLIN, A., KATZ, L. N. AND YOCHIM, K. (1937) Effect of motion on the electrical con-ductivity of the blood. *Amer. J. Physiol.*, 118, 708–719.

SOLTI, F., KRASZNAI, M., ISKUM, M., REV, J. AND NAGY, J. (1966) Measurement of blood flow in the brain and lower extremities in man. *Cor et Vasa (Praha)*, 8, 178–184.

SPUNDA, CH. (1955) Über Wert und Anwendung der Schädelrheographie. *Wien. Klin. Wochschr.*, 67, 788–792.

TACHIBANA, S., KURAMOTO, S., INANAGA, K. AND IKEMI, Y. (1967) Local cerebrovascular responses in man. *Confinia Neurol.*, 29, 289–298.

TOOLE, J. F. AND TUCKER, S. H. (1960) Influence of head position upon cerebral circulation. *Arch. Neurol.*, 2, 616–623.

TRAUTWEIN, H. (1963) Schädelrheographie und Arteriosclerose. *Med. Welt*, 14, 1307–1413.

TZENOV, A. AND HADJIEV, D. (1964) The significance of rheoencephalography in studying the cerebral circulation in neurological patients. *Works of the Institute for Neuropsychiatric Research (Sofia)*, 10, 35–43.

VANEY, P. (1969) Impedance changes in the brain at very high frequencies. In: LECHNER, H., GEYER,

N., LUGARESI, E., MARTIN, F., LIFSHITZ, K. AND MARKOVICH, S. (Eds.), *Rheoencephalography and Plethysmographical Methods*, Excerpta Med. Foundation, Amsterdam, pp. 91–95.

VIDOVSZKY, T. (1965) Untersuchung der gefässerweiternden Wirkung der i.v. Halidor-Injection mittels zerebraler Angiographie. In: *Vereinigte Heil- und Nährmittel-Werke*, Budapest, pp. 1–8.

WALTZ, A. G. AND RAY, C. D. (1967) Inadequacy of "Rheoencephalography". A clinical study of impedance cephalography for evaluation of cerebrovascular disorders. *Arch. Neurol.*, **16**, 94–107.

WECHSLER, R. L., KLEISS, L. M. AND KETY, S. S. (1950) The effects of intravenously administered aminophylline on cerebral circulation and metabolism in man. *J. Clin. Invest.*, **29**, 28–30.

WEIHS, E. (1954) Euphyllin in Prophylaxe, Therapie und Nachbehandlung des apoplektischen Insultes. *Münch. Med. Wochschr.*, **16**, 1453–1454.

WHITTIER, J. R. (1964) Vasorelaxatant drugs and cerebrovascular disease. *Angiology*, **15**, 82–87.

WICK, E. (1955) Über die Form der rheoencephalographischen Kurve bei Trikuspidal Klappen-insuffizienz. *Z. Kreislaufforsch.*, **44**, 857–865.

WICK, E. (1962) Die venöse Nebenwelle im Rheogramm. *Wien. Med. Wochschr.*, **9**, 192–195.

WILCKE, O. (1966) Ergebniss der Behandlung zerebraler Durchblutungsstörungen mit Cinnarizin. *Med. Welt*, **17**, 1472–1477.

WINSOR, T., HYMAN, C. AND KNAPP, F. M. (1960) The cerebral peripheral circulatory action of nylidrin hydrochloride. *Amer. J. Med. Sci.*, **239**, 120–126.

YARULLIN, KH. KH. (1963) Alterations in regional circulation in lesions of main blood vessels of the head. Plethysmography and rheoencephalography. *Klin. Med. (Moscow)*, **9**, 61–67.

YARULLIN, KH. KH. (1965 a) Rheoencephalography in diagnosis of vertebral artery pathology. In: *Symp. Acad. Med. Sci. USSR and Medical School Tartu*, Tartu, pp. 36–38.

YARULLIN, KH. KH. (1965 b) About the diagnosis of kinking by rheoencephalography. *Zh. Nevropatol. Psikhiat.*, **65**, 1476–1483.

YARULLIN, KH. KH. (1967) *Clinical Rheoencephalography*, Medizina, Leningrad.

YARULLIN, KH. KH. AND HADJIEV, D. (1968) Rheoencephalographic investigations on the pathogenesis of cerebral ischemic disturbances. In: MAXUDOV, G. A. (Ed.), *Symposium on Pathogenesis of Transient Ischemic Attacks and Cerebral Infarction*, Academy of Medical Sciences USSR, Moskow, pp. 345–353.

YARULLIN, H. AND HADJIEV, D. (1970) Rheoencephalographic investigations on the effect of Complamin in patients with ischemic disorders of the cerebral circulation. *Bull. Res. Inst. Neurol. and Psychiat. (Sofia)*, **14**, 29–33.

YOCHHEIM, K. A. (1962) Zur Therapie der Hirndurchblutungsstörungen. *Nervenarzt*, **1**, 32–34.

ZBINDEN, F. (1962) Rheographische Untersuchungen bei Patienten mit Migräne und vasomotorische Kopfschmerz. *Wien. Med. Wochschr.*, **112**, 211–213.

ZENOV, A. (1967) Versuch einer physiologischen Analyse der Veränderungen im Schädelrheogramm in Abhängigkeit von Veränderungen der Körperlage. *Psychiat. Neurol. Med. Psychol. (Lpz.)*, **19**, 387–391.

Regional Cerebral Blood Flow in Man

Establishment of "Normal" Control Values and Identification of the Abnormalities which Occur in "Stroke" Patients

IAIN M. S. WILKINSON*

The National Hospital, Queen Square, London W.C. 1 (U.K.)

The human cerebral hemisphere consists of two very distinct types of tissue, grey matter and white matter, which are perfused with blood at markedly different rates. The rate of perfusion of grey matter is approximately four times that of white matter in adult subjects under normal conditions of arterial P_{CO_2} and blood pressure. This has been ascertained by several workers (Ingvar et al., 1965; Høedt-Rasmussen, 1967; and Munck et al., 1968) by means of two-compartmental analysis of ^{133}Xenon clearance curves after injection of the isotope into the internal carotid artery. The use of multiple detectors situated on the lateral aspect of the patient's scalp has made it possible to estimate the rate of perfusion of grey and white matter simultaneously in many different regions of the cerebral hemisphere. It is this method which has been used to measure regional cerebral perfusion at the Institute of Neurology and National Hospital, Queen Square, London over the last three years. During this period data regarding regional perfusion of grey and white matter throughout the "normal" cerebral hemisphere have been produced, both in the conscious and in the anaesthetised subject. Furthermore the results obtained in the "normal" hemisphere have been used as controls for identification of abnormalities of regional cerebral perfusion in patients suffering from various forms of recent cerebral ischaemia.

METHOD

The details of methodology are stated in full elsewhere (Wilkinson et al., 1969). In essence, the blood flow studies were carried out immediately before diagnostic carotid angiography. A small bolus of ^{133}Xenon in saline solution was introduced into the upper cervical part of the internal carotid artery by means of a thin polythene catheter, and the ensuing clearance of the isotope from the cerebral hemisphere was monitored by 15 separate detectors situated on the lateral aspect of the patient's head (Fig. 1). Thus in each patient 15 clearance curves were obtained, each representing the clearance of ^{133}Xenon from a particular region of the cerebral hemisphere. Each clearance curve was plotted logarithmically against time and resolved by two-

---

* Iain M. S. Wilkinson, current address: Department of Neurology, Manchester Royal Infirmary. Manchester, 13 (U.K.)

References p. 103

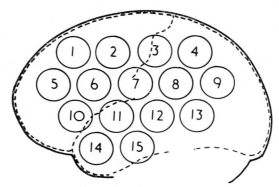

Fig. 1. Diagram to show the position of the 15 detectors on the lateral aspect of the patient's head.

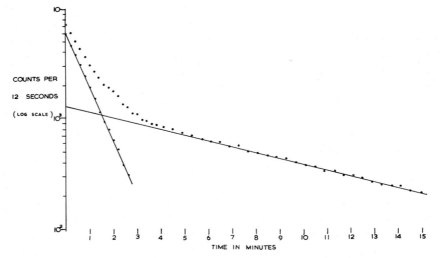

Fig. 2. A typical clearance curve, a logarithmic plot of count rate against time, represented by the upper series of dots. Two separate clearance exponentials are obtained from the original curve, represented by the two solid lines. The steep exponential represents the clearance of ^{133}Xenon from grey matter, and the shallow exponential represents its clearance from white matter.

compartmental analysis into two separate exponentials (Fig. 2). From the gradient of the steep exponential, the perfusion rate of grey matter (Fg) was calculated in millilitres blood/100 g grey matter/min. Similarly from the shallow exponential the perfusion rate of white matter (Fw) was calculated in millilitres blood/100 g white matter/min. Furthermore it was possible to calculate the percentage of the original clearance curve clearing at the fast rate and the percentage clearing at the slow rate; from this the relative weight of perfused grey matter (Wg) and the relative weight of perfused white matter (Ww) was calculated for the region of the cerebral tissue represented by each clearance curve. Thus for each region of the hemisphere the following three variables were estimated:

Fg = the rate of perfusion of grey matter.

Fw = the rate of perfusion of white matter.

Wg = the relative weight of perfused grey matter (for example: in a particular region of the hemisphere the perfused cerebral tissue consisted of x % grey matter and 100 − x % white matter).

A considerable amount of time and energy was devoted to making each of the detectors as regional as possible since this seemed to be axiomatic to the measurement of regional cerebral blood flow. The details of the modifications required for this are explained elsewhere (Wilkinson et al., 1969). The optimal setting of each detector was such that 77 % of the counts were recorded from the cylinder of cerebral tissue in front of the detector (Fig. 3), with 23 % of counts being derived from the brain tissue lying in front of adjacent detectors due to the Compton scatter effect.

Results in "normal" conscious subjects

Since regional cerebral blood flow studies were performed only at the time of diagnostic carotid angiography, none of the patients studied was strictly normal. The "normal" patients of this investigation were undergoing carotid angiography because of a suspected intracranial lesion. The criteria for "normality" were that there were no abnormal physical signs referable to the cerebral hemisphere and that the carotid angiogram subsequently proved to be normal. Frequently other investigations, including gamma scan of the brain and air encephalography, were performed in the patients, with normal results. The definitive diagnoses at the time of discharge from hospital in these patients were ipsilateral orbital pain, ipsilateral 3rd nerve palsy, pituitary adenoma, migraine (between attacks), contralateral optic nerve glioma, ipsilateral optic atrophy and epilepsy. No patient with the diagnosis of epilepsy was on treatment and none had suffered more than two attacks.

Ten conscious "normal" patients were studied. In each case 15 regional values for Fg, Fw, and Wg were obtained. In any one case, for each of the three variables, e.g. Fg, the mean value for the 15 regional values was calculated. This was called the mean value for the hemisphere for Fg in that patient. To make the regional results of one patient comparable with the rest, it was necessary to express the 15 regional values as a percentage of the mean value for the hemisphere. For each patient, therefore, there were six aspects to consider, first the mean values for the hemisphere of Fg, Fw and Wg, and secondly the regional patterns of Fg, Fw and Wg expressed in percentage terms.

The ten mean values for the hemisphere for each of the three variables were tabulated, and from them overall mean values for Fg, Fw and Wg were calculated,

TABLE 1

OVERALL MEAN RESULTS IN THE CONSCIOUS GROUP OF "NORMAL" PATIENTS

Number	Age (years)	AP_{CO_2} (mm Hg)	Mean B.P. (mm Hg)	Fg (ml/100 g/min)	Fw (ml/100 g/min)	Wg (%)
10	46 (18–64)	45 (40–50)	89 (72–115)	86.6 (± 17.1)	21.7 (± 3.7)	45.5 (± 4.8)

as shown in Table 1. These overall mean values are very similar to the values obtained for the whole hemisphere by other workers (Ingvar *et al.*, 1965; Høedt-Rasmussen, 1967; and Munck *et al.*, 1968). The grey matter perfusion rate is about four times higher than that of white matter, with values near to 80 and 20 ml/100 g/min respectively in conscious adult man at normal levels of arterial P_{CO_2} and blood pressure. The value for the relative weight of grey matter in the "normal" hemisphere, when measured in this way by laterally situated detectors, lies between 45 and 50% in all reported series.

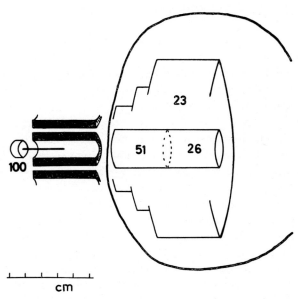

Fig. 3. A three-dimensional representation of the source of 100 counts registered by a modified detector such as was used in this investigation.

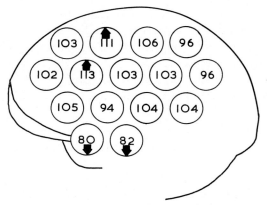

Fig. 4. Regional values for the perfusion rate in grey matter (Fg), expressed as percentages of the mean value for the hemisphere, in 10 conscious normocapnic "normal" subjects. Regions which are significantly above or below the mean value for the hemisphere at the $p < 0.001$ level are indicated by an arrow.

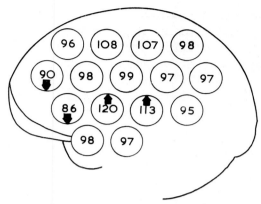

Fig. 5. Regional values for Fw in 10 conscious normocapnic "normal" subjects, (see legend of Fig 4).

The regional values, expressed in percentage terms, were accumulated into three composite diagrams (Figs. 4, 5 and 6) in the way described previously (Wilkinson *et al.*, 1969). In Figs. 4, 5 and 6 the regional patterns are shown at the $P < 0.001$ level of statistical significance, the regions which are significantly different from the mean value for the hemisphere at this statistical level being indicated by an arrow.

It can be seen in Fig. 4 that the grey matter in the temporal region was significantly less well perfused with blood than the rest of the hemisphere, whereas an area in the precentral region was significantly more highly perfused than the rest of the hemisphere. Ingvar *et al.* (1965) showed significantly lower cortical flow rates in the temporal region compared with the rest of the hemisphere, using a four-detector measuring unit. No artefactual explanation could be found to account for the observed regional pattern of perfusion of grey matter, and the low values in the temporal region are not due to the basal ganglia since the basal ganglia lie on the horizontal level of the insula, higher than the detectors covering the temporal lobe. It appears that the pattern shown in Fig. 4 represents the pattern of cortical perfusion rates throughout the "normal" cerebral hemisphere.

Fig. 5 shows the regional pattern for perfusion of white matter which was found in the ten conscious patients. The most notable feature was the significantly high perfusion rate of the white matter in the region of the internal capsule compared with the rest of the hemisphere. The explanation of this finding is not certain, but it may be that the white matter of the internal capsule has a richer capillary network than elsewhere in the hemisphere. From the work of Ross Russell (1963) there is no doubt that the white matter of the internal capsule has a greater abundance of small arteries between 100 and 400 μ in diameter than the white matter elsewhere, due to the numerous small perforating vessels which traverse the internal capsule from the putamen and globus pallidus to reach the thalamus and caudate nucleus. Whether this is associated with an increased capillary network is not established but Klosovskii (1963) has shown close inter-connections between the capillary network of the basal ganglia and that of adjacent white matter. There may thus be an anatomical basis for the finding of the high perfusion rate in the white matter of the internal capsule.

The low values for white matter perfusion which were found in the frontal regions may be partly or totally due to artefact. By means of its supraorbital, supratrochlear and meningeal branches the ophthalmic artery is the one main branch of the internal carotid artery to supply extracerebral structures which come within the field of measurement of the detectors used in this investigation. Slow clearance of ^{133}Xenon from the poorly perfused extracerebral structures may well tend to flatten the latter part of the clearance curves recorded in this region giving rise to falsely low values for white matter perfusion.

The pattern for the relative weight of perfused grey matter throughout the "normal" hemisphere is shown in Fig. 6. High values (equivalent to 55–60% grey matter) were

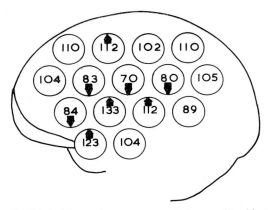

Fig. 6. Regional values for Wg in 10 conscious normocapnic "normal" subjects, (see legend of Fig. 4).

found over the insular region, extending forward and downwards over the anterior end of the temporal lobe. Low values (equivalent to 30–37% grey matter) were found in the regions of the corpus callosum and corona radiata, and intermediate values (equivalent to 50% grey matter) were found over the convexity of the hemisphere which was monitored tangentially by the detectors situated on the lateral aspect of the skull. Though this pattern seemed entirely reasonable on anatomical grounds, it was correlated with regional values of relative weight of grey matter throughout the hemisphere determined by post-mortem dissection of one cerebral hemisphere. The correlation was remarkably good both in terms of the similarity of pattern and actual numerical values. This anatomical correlation provided good confirmatory evidence of the validity of two-compartmental analysis as applied to the normal cerebral hemisphere.

In the conscious "normal" subject at normal levels of arterial P_{CO_2} and blood pressure there seems to be evidence of statistically significant regional variation of Fg, Fw and Wg throughout the cerebral hemisphere. This has become apparent in this study for two main reasons:

(i) two-compartmental analysis has been applied to multiple regional cerebral clearance curves,

(ii) the individual detectors have been modified with the single aim of making them as regional as possible, minimizing the amount of overlap between adjacent detector fields.

Results in "normal" anaesthetised subjects

Regional cerebral perfusion was studied in two groups of anaesthetised "normal" subjects. The same criteria of "normality" obtained in these two groups as was the case with the conscious "normal" subjects. The same method of blood flow measurement was employed and the results were expressed in the same way. Both groups of anaesthetised subjects were anaesthetised by the same technique which consisted of induction by short-acting barbiturate (methohexitone), followed by nitrous oxide–oxygen anaesthesia (at a constant ventilation rate of 15 litres/min) supplemented by neuroleptanalgesia in the form of droperidol and phenoperidine (full details of technique are reported by Wilkinson and Browne, 1970). This anaesthetic regime was deliberately chosen for two reasons. First it was one which, in the light of previous knowledge (Barker *et al.*, 1968; Fitch *et al.*, 1969), was likely to have little effect on cerebral blood flow in gross quantitative terms. Secondly this technique allowed the subjects to be studied at any desired level of arterial P_{CO_2} merely by regulating the amount of carbon dioxide in the inspired gas mixture.

The first group of anaesthetised patients were studied at an arterial P_{CO_2} level near to 45 mm Hg. This was to allow direct comparison of the results with the conscious group, whose overall mean arterial P_{CO_2} had been 45 mm Hg (Table 1). Six normocapnic patients were studied and their overall mean values for Fg, Fw and Wg are shown in Table 2.

TABLE 2

OVERALL MEAN RESULTS IN THE NORMOCAPNIC ANAESTHETISED GROUP OF "NORMAL" PATIENTS

Number	Age (years)	AP_{CO_2} (mm Hg)	Mean B.P. (mm Hg)	Fg (ml/100 g/min)	Fw (ml/100 g/min)	Wg (%)
6	34 (25–40)	45 (39–51)	82 (67–95)	77.3 ($\pm$ 16.9)	20.8 ($\pm$ 2.6)	51.5 ($\pm$ 3.6)

Comparison of these results with those obtained in the conscious group revealed that though Fg tended to be numerically lower in the anaesthetised group, there was no statistically significant difference in Fg, Fw or Wg between the two groups. This form of anaesthesia thus appears to have no gross quantitative effect on cerebral blood flow.

The regional patterns for Fg, Fw and Wg in the normocapnic anaesthetised patients were of interest. The patterns for Fw and Wg showed the same basic features as in the conscious group, so that a statistical comparison between anaesthetised and conscious groups revealed no significant differences whatsoever. The pattern of Fg in the anaesthetised group (Fig. 7) was significantly different from the pattern in conscious

References p. 103

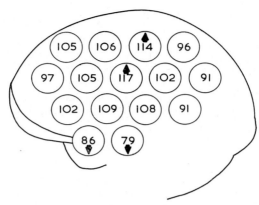

Fig. 7. Regional values for Fg in 6 anaesthetised normocapnic "normal" subjects, (see legend of Fig. 4).

patients, however. During anaesthesia the grey matter of the temporal region remained significantly less well perfused than elsewhere in the hemisphere, but a region of significantly high Fg was found over the region of the central sulcus. The essential difference between the pattern of Fg in the conscious and the anaesthetised patients lay in the location of the high flow area, being precentral in the conscious group, and over the central sulcus in the anaesthetised group. The explanation of this finding remains unanswered. It would be interesting to know whether the differing patterns of perfusion represent correspondingly different patterns of functional and metabolic activity of the cortex during the conscious and the anaesthetised state.

TABLE 3

OVERALL MEAN RESULTS IN THE HYPOCAPNIC ANAESTHETISED GROUP OF "NORMAL" PATIENTS

Number	Age (years)	AP_{CO_2} (mm Hg)	Mean B.P. (mm Hg)	Fg (ml/100 g/min)	Fw (ml/100 g/min)	Wg (%)
6	32 (20–40)	29 (25–32)	76 (63–87)	45.6 (± 6.5)	15.1 (± 2.1)	46.6 (± 4.9)

The second group of anaesthetised patients was studied during conditions of arterial hypocapnia, with arterial P_{CO_2} levels near to 30 mm Hg. The cerebral vasoconstrictive influence of arterial hypocapnia can be seen in Table 3, which contains the overall mean values for Fg, Fw and Wg in this group of six patients. Comparing these results with those obtained in the normocapnic subjects studied during the same anaesthetic technique, there was a highly significant ($p < 0.005$) difference in Fg and Fw, with no significant difference in Wg. This comparison showed that the anaesthetic regime of nitrous oxide supplemented by neuroleptanalgesia (droperidol and phenoperidine) left the cerebral circulation fully responsive to a reduction in arterial P_{CO_2}. A reduction in arterial P_{CO_2} from 45 to 29 mm Hg was accompanied by a 41 % reduction in Fg

and a 28% reduction in Fw. This reduction in perfusion rates during arterial hypocapnia was of the same order as was observed by Harper (1965) in animals and Wollman *et al.* (1968) in man. It is interesting to note that Fg appeared to be more
responsive to the change in arterial P_{CO_2} than Fw.

The regional patterns of Fw and Wg in the hypocapnic anaesthetised patients
showed no significant difference from their corresponding patterns in the normocapnic
anaesthetised and conscious patients. In all 3 groups the same basic pattern was
present for both these variables. It must be stated that one would not anticipate any
change in the pattern of Wg – the relative weight of perfused grey matter – since in the
normal hemisphere one would expect the whole hemisphere to remain perfused
with blood in the 3 circumstances in which it was studied in this investigation. The
stability of the pattern of perfusion of white matter is of interest, and is compatible
with the anatomical reason for the occurrence of high values for Fw in the region of
the internal capsule which was put forward earlier. The pattern of Fg in the hypocapnic anaesthetised patients (Fig. 8) was different from the corresponding pattern

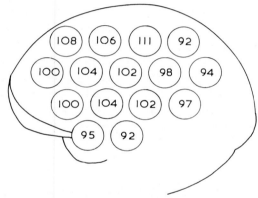

Fig. 8. Regional values for Fg in 6 anaesthetised hypocapnic "normal" subjects, (see legend of Fig. 4).
There were no values significantly above or below the mean value for the hemisphere at the $p < 0.001$
level.

in either of the other two groups of patients. In this group Fg was relatively homogeneous throughout the cerebral hemisphere so that no regional value was significantly
above or below the mean value for the hemisphere at the $p < 0.001$ level. The temporal
region no longer constituted a significantly low flow area, and no region of significantly
high values was found.

In this study of regional cerebral perfusion in the normal hemisphere Fg has been
observed to have been the most labile variable. Whereas the patterns of Fw and Wg
remained constant in all 3 groups of patients, Fg presented a different regional
pattern in each set of circumstances. Furthermore considerations of the flow values
in terms of mean values for the hemisphere (Tables 1, 2 and 3) showed that Fg
underwent a slight, but statistically insignificant, reduction comparing anaesthetised
and conscious patients at the same levels of arterial P_{CO_2} and blood pressure, and
that Fg showed a greater decrease than Fw when comparing hypocapnic with normo-

capnic patients studied during the same anaesthetic technique. Fg thus showed a greater capacity to change than Fw, and this is felt to be a reflection of the more direct correlation of cortical activity with the physiological circumstances of the patient.

Results in patients suffering from recent cerebral ischaemic events

Apart from their own intrinsic interest, the results obtained in the "normal" hemisphere constituted essential data for the investigation of disordered regional cerebral blood flow in "stroke" patients. The same method of regional cerebral blood flow measurement has been applied to patients who have suffered a recent cerebral ischaemic event either in the conscious state, or when anaesthetised by the technique used in the "normal" controls. The regional results for Fg, Fw and Wg which have been obtained in the "stroke" patients have been compared by statistical means with the appropriate accumulated pattern obtained in the "normal" hemisphere. Each regional value obtained in the "stroke" case has been compared with the corresponding regional value in the "normal" pattern, and it has been regarded as definitely abnormal if it has been different from the "normal" value at the $p < 0.001$ level of statistical significance. At this level one region in one thousand regions, *i.e.* 1 region in 60–65 patients (since 15 regions are measured in each patient) would be expected to appear abnormal by chance. A statistically reliable and comprehensive picture of the state of disordered cerebral perfusion has been disclosed by this method in these "stroke" patients studied to date. These patients have been of two broad categories, those who have suffered a completed stroke and those who have had previous transient ischaemic attacks.

(a) Patients with a completed stroke

Enough experience in patients with completed stroke has not yet accrued for any definitive general statement of our findings in this set of circumstances. There seems to be no doubt however that a detailed assessment of regional perfusion in these cases may be obtained by the method described above. Four illustrative cases will be presented here to indicate the sort of data which are currently accumulated in patients with completed strokes.

Case 1. A normotensive man of 53 who, 2 days prior to the blood flow study, suddenly became aphasic and developed a severe right hemiparesis associated with right-sided sensory loss and a right-sided homonomous hemianopia. By the time of the study the neurological deficit had recovered except for a dense motor dysphasia which was still present. There was no headache, loss of consciousness or neck stiffness. A left sided study was performed immediately prior to angiography.

The predominant abnormalities were in the regional pattern for Fg (Fig. 9). There was a region of low flow in the postero-inferior frontal region, and a larger region of high perfusion in the anterior parietal region. There was no disturbance of white matter perfusion but in the anterior frontal region there was a significantly low value for the relative weight of perfused grey matter. In the latter region the ratio of

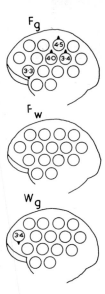

Fig. 9. Regional abnormalities in Fg, Fw and Wg in completed stroke case no. 1. Where the circle is left empty, the regional value in this patient was not significantly different from the normal value in that region. Where the circle is filled the value is the number of standard deviations by which the regional value in this patient varied from the normal regional value, and the arrow indicates the direction of the abnormality. Only regions which differed from the normal regional value by 3.3 standard deviations or more have been marked ($p < 0.001$), since this has been the statistical level of significance taken to indicate definite abnormality.

perfused grey matter to perfused white matter was low when compared with normal values. This finding is interpreted as follows. In this region there is an infarct, *i.e.* there is some cerebral tissue which is not being perfused at all. The infarcted tissue consists of more grey matter than white matter, so that the residual perfused tissue in this region has an abnormally low ratio of grey matter to white matter when compared with the normal value for that region of the cerebral hemisphere.

The accompanying carotid angiogram in this case showed an early filling vein in the parietal region, draining the region of grey matter hyperaemia into the superior longitudinal sinus.

This case is an example of a relatively extensive recent ischaemic event in the cerebral hemisphere. It should be emphasized that the area of low Fg was found in the region of the hemisphere concerned with motor speech, and that the region of post-ischaemic hyperaemia was present in a region of the hemisphere which may have been responsible for the severe hemiparesis and hemianaesthesia which lasted for 12 hours and completely recovered by the time of the blood flow study.

Case 2. A normotensive woman of 53 studied 8 days after the sudden onset of a right hemiparesis and moderate motor dysphasia. Satisfactory gradual recovery had occurred in the intervening 8 days, so that by the time of the study there was little if any disturbance of speech and only minimal residual right-sided weakness. There was no headache, loss of consciousness or neck stiffness. A left-sided study was carried out in association with carotid angiography.

References p. 103

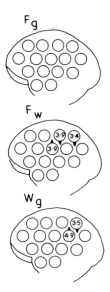

Fig. 10. Regional abnormalities in Fg, Fw and Wg in completed stroke, case no. 2 (see legend of Fig. 9).

In this patient there were no abnormalities in the rate of perfusion of grey matter (Fig. 10). There were marked abnormalities in Fw in the parietal region, with two regions of low flow and one region of hyperaemia. The relative weight of perfused grey matter to perfused white matter was disturbed in the parietal region also, which is interpreted as evidence of an infarct predominantly involving grey matter in one region and white matter in the other.

The accompanying carotid angiogram in this case showed no abnormality.

This case illustrates that regions of both high and low perfusion may be identified in the white matter of the cerebral hemisphere after a recent episode of ischaemia. In this case the Fw abnormalities were unaccompanied by any disturbance of grey matter perfusion but were associated with an infarct involving grey and white matter.

Case 3. A slightly hypertensive man of 47 studied 5 days after the abrupt onset of a left hemiparesis which was showing only slight improvement by the time of the blood flow study. There was no headache, loss of consciousness or neck stiffness. A right-sided blood flow study was performed immediately before carotid angiography.

There were no abnormalities whatsoever in the rate of perfusion of grey matter or white matter (Fig. 11). The only abnormality in this case was a disturbance of the ratio of perfused grey matter to perfused white matter in one region overlying the region of the internal capsule. A high value for the relative weight of perfused grey matter in the region is taken as evidence of the presence of an infarct in this region, involving white matter to a greater extent than grey matter. The predominant white matter in this region is the internal capsule. It appears that the only abnormality of regional cerebral perfusion which was present in this case was an area of non-perfusion, or infarct, predominantly affecting the white matter in the internal capsule. Such a

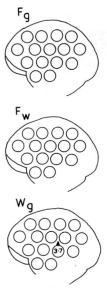

Fig. 11. Regional abnormalities in Fg, Fw and Wg in completed stroke, case no. 3 (see legend of Fig. 9).

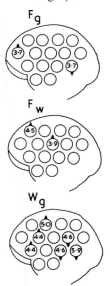

Fig. 12. Regional abnormalities in Fg, Fw and Wg in completed stroke, case no. 4 (see legend of Fig. 9).

case tends to confirm that a small strategically situated infarct in the region of the internal capsule can produce a relatively gross neurological deficit such as was found in this patient.

The accompanying carotid angiogram was normal.

Case 4. A normotensive man of 53 studied one day after the acute onset of dysphasia in association with a right-sided hemiparesis, hemianaesthesia and homo-

References p. 103

nomous hemianiopia, which had shown no improvement by the time of the blood flow study. There was no headache, loss of consciousness or neck stiffness. A left sided blood flow study was carried out in conjunction with carotid angiography.

The predominant regional abnormalities which were found in this case were in Wg (Fig. 12). There was a wide-spread disturbance of the relative weight of perfused grey matter to perfused white matter. These findings were taken to indicate the presence of a large infarct, mainly involving white matter anteriorly and grey matter posteriorly. There were accompanying abnormalities in the regional patterns of Fg and Fw, though these were less outstanding than those in Wg. There was a region of high Fg and another region of low Fg, and two regions of high Fw.

The accompanying carotid angiogram in this case showed a left-sided middle cerebral artery occlusion.

This case demonstrates quite well the detailed information regarding disturbed regional cerebral perfusion which may be obtained by this technique. The presence of an infarct is disclosed in association with middle cerebral artery occlusion. Regional abnormalities of actual tissue perfusion rates in grey and white matter, though present, are relatively minor features compared with the widespread evidence of brain tissue which is not being perfused at all.

This degree of insight into the state of disordered perfusion can only be obtained by two-compartmental analysis of the regional clearance curves. Other investigators are utilising indices of regional perfusion based on the gradient of the initial 2 minutes of clearance (F (initial)), and others are using regional weighted mean flow values indicating the total net flow through a region of cerebral tissue (using an assumed constant ratio of perfused grey matter to perfused white matter). Regional mean flow values and F (initial) values have also been estimated both in the "normal" and "stroke" patients of this investigation, but the results have proved much less informative, and only really comprehensible when compared with the regional results for Fg, Fw and Wg. Disturbances of white matter perfusion can only be identified by attention to the latter half of the clearance curves, and are not apparent in regional mean flow values or indices based on the initial two minutes of clearance. Grey matter perfusion rates cannot be correlated directly with regional mean flow values or F (initial) indices, since abnormalities in either of the latter two variables may be due to high or low values for Fg on the one hand or for Wg on the other. This is not to say that regional mean flow values of F (initial) indices have not been useful in the hands of other workers in increasing our knowledge regarding disturbances of regional perfusion. The F (initial) index has been particularly useful in the study of blood flow responses to short-lived physiological test situations, e.g. changes in arterial P_{CO_2} or blood pressure. In our own laboratory however, we consider the extra labour and statistical comparisons required to produce results as illustrated above are justified by the detailed information which is obtained by two-compartmental analysis of the clearance curves.

There are two main theoretical objections to performing two-compartmental analysis of regional cerebral clearance curves in stroke patients. The first is that the tissue:blood solubility coefficients of [133]Xenon for normal grey and white matter may not be applicable to the abnormal grey and white matter damaged by recent ischaemia. At the moment there is no sound answer to this criticism. It is a criticism which applies to all results for cerebral blood flow in abnormal brain tissue when measured by ^{133}Xenon clearance techniques, regardless of the method of calculation and the expressions of blood flow rates which are used.

The second objection is particular to two-compartmental analysis. Is it justifiable to resolve the regional clearance curves into two separate exponentials, when it seems likely on theoretical grounds that multiexponential clearance may occur in pathological circumstances? Our answer to this is a practical one. First the clearance curves which we have obtained in patients with "stroke" resolve themselves into two separate exponentials without difficulty. Secondly, pathological confirmation of blood flow results obtained in our laboratory by two-compartmental analysis has been obtained in three cases up to date. A paper is currently in preparation describing these in detail, but in essence regions of the brain which were identified as infarcts (*i.e.* regions of non-perfusion) by means of blood flow measurement in the way illustrated above, have later been confirmed as infarcts at post-mortem examination. The correlation between the findings of blood flow measurement and autopsy has been good both in terms of topography and in terms of the predominant tissue involved, *i.e.* whether grey matter or white matter was predominantly involved in the infarct. On the basis of this post-mortem evidence the method of two-compartmental analysis seems to be valid when applied to brains which are abnormal on account of acute vascular occlusive disease.

(b) Patients with transient ischaemic attacks

Rees *et al.* (1970) using the equipment and method of calculation described above, have studied a group of patients who have suffered previous transient ischaemic attacks. The patients were studied up to three months following the last clinically apparent episode of transient cerebral ischaemia. Localized abnormalities of either Fg, Fw or Wg were found in seven out of the ten patients when compared with the normal controls, whereas previous investigators (Skinhøj *et al.*, 1970) have been unable to detect any abnormalities of cerebral perfusion as measured by regional mean flow values and F (initial) values. Rees *et al.* pointed out that the reasons for their high incidence of focal abnormality probably lay in a greater sensitivity of technique, using highly regionalized detectors and two-compartmental analysis as the method of calculation. It is of great interest that lasting abnormalities of cerebral perfusion are present in such patients since the complete clinical recovery of the patient might suggest that this were not the case.

SUMMARY

(1) To collect good regional data regarding blood flow in different parts of the cerebral hemisphere, it is necessary to use multiple detectors which are specifically designed to minimize the amount of overlap between adjacent detector fields.

(2) Grey matter perfusion is not homogeneous throughout the "normal" hemisphere

in conscious patients. A definite regional pattern throughout the hemisphere exists. The temporal region is less well perfused than the rest of the hemisphere, and an area of high flow exists in the precentral region.

(3) Grey matter perfusion is not homogeneous throughout the "normal" cerebral hemisphere in patients anaesthetised by nitrous oxide and oxygen supplemented by neuroleptanalgesia (droperidol and phenoperidine). The regional pattern under these conditions is significantly different from the pattern found in conscious patients. During this anaesthetic regime the temporal region still constitutes a low flow area, but high values are found over the region of the central sulcus, rather than the pre-central region.

(4) Grey matter perfusion is relatively homogeneous throughout the "normal" cerebral hemisphere in patients anaesthetised by the same technique but studied during conditions of arterial hypocapnia. At the low levels of perfusion induced in this way the regional differences throughout the hemisphere are reduced.

(5) White matter perfusion is not homogeneous throughout the "normal" cerebral hemisphere. The region of the internal capsule is more highly perfused than elsewhere. The same regional pattern is found in conscious normocapnic patients, anaesthetised normocapnic patients and anaesthetised hypocapnic patients.

(6) The ratio of the weight of perfused grey matter to perfused white matter is by no means constant throughout the hemisphere. The relative weight of grey matter is high in the insular region, low over the corpus callosum and corona radiata, and intermediate or high over the convexity of the hemisphere. This pattern was found to be constant in the three groups of "normal" patients studied, and it correlated well with the pattern for the relative weight of grey matter obtained by post-mortem dissection on one normal hemisphere.

(7) Evidence is accumulating to confirm that two-compartmental analysis of regional ^{133}Xenon clearance curves provides a valid and detailed picture of the state of disordered perfusion which occurs in patients who have suffered various types of "stroke". Results in a small series of patients with a completed "stroke" are presented in this paper in whom regions of high and low perfusion of grey and white matter were found, and in whom regions of non-perfusion, i.e. infarcts, have been identified. Application of the same method has revealed focal abnormalities of the same type in patients with transient ischaemic attacks (Rees et al., 1970). The theoretical objections to performing two-compartmental analysis in patients with abnormal brains due to a recent "stroke" are discussed, and the evidence in favour of its validity presented.

ACKNOWLEDGEMENTS

This work was financed by the National Fund for Research into Crippling Diseases and was carried out in collaboration with Dr. J. W. D. Bull, Dr. G. H. du Boulay, Dr. John Marshall, Dr. J. E. Rees, Dr. R. W. Ross Russell and Mr. Lindsay Symon.

REFERENCES

BARKER, J., HARPER, A. M., MCDOWALL, D. G., FITCH, W. AND JENNETT, W. B. (1968) Cerebral blood flow, cerebrospinal fluid pressure, and E.E.G. activity during neuroleptanalgesia induced with dehydrobenzperidol and phenoperidine. *Brit. J. Anaesthesia*, **40**, 143–144.

FITCH, W., BARKER, J., JENNETT, W. B. AND MCDOWALL, D. G. (1969) The influence of neuro-leptanalgesic drugs on cerebrospinal fluid pressure. *Brit. J. Anaesthesia*, **41**, 800–806.

HARPER, A. M. (1965) The inter-relationship between arterial P_{CO_2} and blood pressure in the regulation of blood flow through the cerebral cortex. *Acta Neurol. Scand., Suppl.*, **14**, 94–103.

HØEDT-RASMUSSEN, K. (1967) *Regional cerebral blood flow. M. D. Thesis*, Munksgaard, Copenhagen.

INGVAR, D. H., CRONQVIST, S., EKBERG, R., RISBERG, J. AND HØEDT-RASMUSSEN, K. (1965) Normal values of regional cerebral blood flow in man, including flow and weight estimates of grey and white matter. *Acta Neurol. Scand., Suppl.*, **14**, 72–78.

KLOSOVSKII, B. N. (1963) *Blood Circulation in the Brain*, Monson, Jerusalem.

MUNCK, O., BARENHOLDT, O. AND BUSCH, H. (1968) Cerebral blood flow in organic dementia measured with the ^{133}Xenon desaturation method. *Scand. J. Clin. Lab. Invest.*, Suppl., **102**, XII: A.

REES, J. E., DU BOULAY, G. H., BULL, J. W. D., MARSHALL, J., ROSS RUSSELL, R. W. AND SYMON, L. (1970) Persistence of disturbances of regional cerebral blood flow after transient ischaemic attacks. Paper read September, 1970 at *Intern. Cerebral Blood Flow Symp.*, *London*, (Proceedings to be published by Pitmans, London).

ROSS RUSSELL, R. W. (1963) Observations on intracerebral aneurysms. *Brain*, **86**, 425–452.

SKINHØJ, E., HØEDT-RASMUSSEN, K., PAULSON, O. B. AND LASSEN, N. A. (1970) Regional cerebral blood flow and its autoregulation in patients with transient focal cerebral ischaemic attacks. *Neurology*, **20**, 487–493.

WILKINSON, I. M. S., BULL, J. W. D., DU BOULAY, G. H., MARSHALL, J., ROSS RUSSELL, R. W. AND SYMON, L. (1969) Regional blood flow in the normal cerebral hemisphere. *J. Neurol. Neurosurg. Psychiat.*, **32**, 367–378.

WILKINSON, I. M. S. AND BROWNE, D. R. G. (1970) The influence of anaesthesia and of arterial hypocapnia on regional blood flow in the normal human cerebral hemisphere. *Brit. J. Anaesthesia*, **42**, 472–482.

WOLLMAN, H., SMITH, T. C., STEPHEN, G., COLTON, E. T., GLEATON, H. E. AND ALEXANDER, S. C. (1968) Effects of extremes of respiratory and metabolic alkalosis on cerebral blood flow in man. *J. Appl. Physiol.*, **24**, 60–65.

Measurements in Man of Focal Intracerebral Blood Flow around Depth-Electrodes with Hydrogen Gas

CARL WILHELM SEM-JACOBSEN, OLE BERNHARD STYRI AND
ERIK MOHN

E.E.G. Research Laboratory, Gaustad Sykehus, Vinderen, Oslo 3 (Norway)

INTRODUCTION

In 1952, the author and his co-workers developed the depth-electrographic/neuro-surgical technique for diagnostic study and treatment of selected psychiatric and neurological disorders (Symposium, 1953). For the past 15 years the author has used this technique to systematically map the electrical activity as well as the response to electrical stimulation around 7200 indwelling electrodes in the brain of 220 patients.

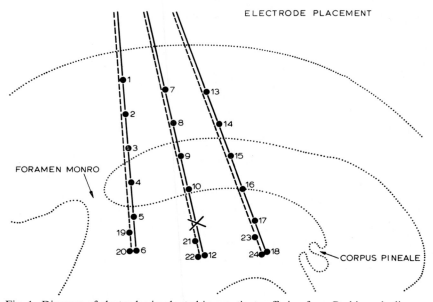

Fig. 1. Diagram of electrodes implanted in a patient suffering from Parkinson's disease.

C. W. Sem-Jacobsen, M. D., Medical Director, The EEG Research Laboratory, Gaustad Sykehus.
O. B. Styri, M. D., Medical Director, Department of Neurosurgery, Rikshospitalet.
E. Mohn, Statistician, Norwegian Computing Center.
The research reported herein has been sponsored in part by the United States Government, through the Department of the Army and the Atomic Commission.

References p. 113

(Sem-Jacobsen, 1968) The implanted electrodes (Fig. 1) have lately been made of platinum. In 1965, with Aukland, we demonstrated in four patients that it was possible to measure the focal blood flow around these electrodes with the hydrogen gas saturation/clearance technique (Aukland *et al.*, 1964; Sem-Jacobsen *et al.*, 1965).

In preliminary studies regional Cerebral Blood Flow (rCBF) were measured from 8–15 electrodes in 4 patients all suffering from Parkinson's disease. The patients aged 44–61 years, were studied while their electrodes were implanted for treatment. These patients were studied in 4–8 sessions with 2 measurements during each session. During this period adjustments were made to standardize the technique. The problems of drift and baseline determination were investigated. With co-workers at the Norwegian Computing Center a computer program for the analysis and handling of the data was developed.

Following the development of the program we have been able to handle in detail the data from patients studied so far, and preliminary results of 16 628 flow measurements have been analyzed (Sem-Jacobsen *et al.*, 1969). Further validation of our data with continuous gas analysis is planned.

MATERIAL

Following the preliminary development, rCBF measurements were made from 16 to 19 electrodes in each of 14 patients, 10 Parkinsonian and 4 others. Three patients were studied twice, first in one hemisphere and 6 to 12 months later in the other hemisphere in conjunction with an operation on that other side. The patients, aged 32 to 64, were studied while their electrodes were implanted for treatment in 1 to 22 sessions each, with 2 to 14 measurements during each session. Thus rCBF was determined from 2 to 152 times around each of the 285 electrodes – giving more than 16 628 flow values. 8314 flow values were based on saturation and 8314 on gas clearance measurements.

TECHNIQUE

During the preliminary studies the DY 2010B system was developed for instantaneous measurements and collection of H_2 gas saturation/clearance data on punch tape (Fig. 2). Information may be sampled from 1 to 25 electrodes at rates of up to 11 data sources per second. On line digital printing of data was used for monitoring.

Supplementary data on blood pressure, heart rate, and respiration were recorded.

The mathematical calculation is handled by a computer facilitating rapid print-out of blood flow around each electrode expressed in millilitres per min per 100 g of brain substance. A technique was developed and used for measurements of changes of short duration, such as during rest, flushing, physical and mental activity, as well as CO_2 breathing and sleep. By keeping the platinum hydrogen electrodes sufficiently negative, disturbances induced by oxygen were practically eliminated, and repeatable data were recorded several times a week over a period of several months.

In each session, after an initial stabilization period of 30 to 45 min, the patient

DY-2010 B GREY/WHITE MATTER LOCALIZING SYSTEM

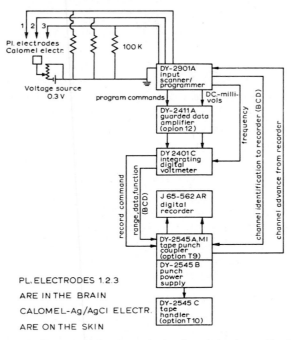

Fig. 2. Schematic diagram of the electrode circuit and the data collecting system.

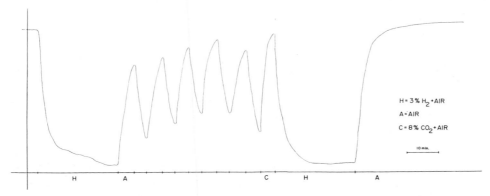

H = 3% H$_2$ + AIR

A = AIR

C = 8% CO$_2$ + AIR

10 min.

Fig. 3. Plotting of data collected during one session.

breathes air with 3% H$_2$ for 35 to 45 min to a saturation plateau. This is followed by several periods of clearance and resaturation of 4 to 5 min each (Fig. 3). During these short periods responses to physical activity, mental activity, CO$_2$,and so forth can be measured with control rest periods in between.

But is the whole brain resting just because we ask the patient to relax? It was found necessary to follow a strict protocol with comprehensive notes to be able to duplicate the observations. At the end of the sequence of short-time observations, we again recorded a saturation to plateau, followed by complete clearance back to the base line. In this way drifts in the system can be checked.

The flow calculation was based on the base line and the saturation plateau. The flow data in the chart were made on the basis of the first 20 measured points in the slope. Calculations were also made, based on the 10th to the 30th measurement.

For many electrodes the two calculations gave identical flow values. This suggests recording from a homogeneous gray or white matter. From other electrodes, such as the first electrode in Fig. 5, the second set of measurements constantly gave lower flow values indicating a fast and a slow component, and probably that records were being made from the border of gray and white substance.

STATISTICAL ANALYSIS

Consider a special session for a particular patient. The observations from one electrode are divided into $2m + 1$ phases, saturation (S)- or desaturation (D)-phases, according to whether the patient is inhaling H_2 or whether it is a clearance period. The observations are denoted by Y, time by t. Let $(t_{i1}, Y_{i1}), \ldots, (t_{in_i}, Y_{in_i})$ be the n_i pairs of observations in phase no. i. We suppose

$$Y_{ik} = \alpha^{(T_i)} + \beta^{(T_i)} t_{ik} + \gamma_i e^{-\lambda_i t_{ik}} + e_{ij}, \quad k = 1, \ldots, n_i, \; i = 1, \ldots, 2m + 1, \qquad (1)$$

where $\{e_{ik}\}$ are independent normally distributed errors with $E\,e_{ik} = 0$, var $e_{ik} = \sigma^2$ for all i, k. T_i equals S or D depending on the type of phase i. $\alpha^{(T_i)}$ is the *base*, $\beta^{(T_i)}$ the *drifting coefficient* of phase type T_i. The line $y = \alpha^{(T_i)} + \beta^{(T_i)}t$ is the base line. In the sequel, the index T_i will be dropped.

We will distinguish between 3 situations

(a) Both S and D are obtained in two phases. Then lower and upper baseline may be non-parallel, we may have $\beta^{(S)} \neq \beta^{(D)}$.

(b) D, but not S, is obtained in two phases. Then the two baselines are assumed to be parallel: $\beta^{(S)} = \beta^{(D)}$.

(c) Neither S nor D is obtained twice. Then we assume no drift: $\beta^{(S)} = \beta^{(D)} = 0$.

The reason for this partitioning is the great uncertainty in the estimation of the drifting coefficient when S and D is not obtained.

λ_i is the blood flow for phase i. The main object of the analysis is to estimate this parameter. Let $\tilde{\alpha}$ and $\tilde{\beta}$ be any two estimators of the base and drifting coefficient. Introduce new variables $\{Z_{ik}\}$ by $Z_{ik} = Y_{ik} - \tilde{\alpha} - \tilde{\beta}t_{ik}$. Then we estimate the blood flow in phase i by

$$\lambda_i = -\frac{1}{M} \sum_k{}' (t_{ik} - \bar{t}_i) \log (Y_{ik} - \tilde{\alpha} - \tilde{\beta}t_{ik}) \qquad (2)$$

where

$$M = \sum_k{}' (t_{ik} - \bar{t}_i)^2 \quad \text{and} \quad \bar{t}_i = \frac{1}{n_i} \sum{}' t_{ik}.$$

According to whether situation (a), (b) or (c) is fulfilled, we get different expressions for $\tilde{\alpha}$ and $\tilde{\beta}$.

Suppose S or D is obtained in phase j. We define *local* base for this phase by $\alpha_j = \alpha + \beta t_{jn_j}$. This local base is estimated by the mean of the h extreme observations in that phase:

$$\hat{\alpha}_j = \frac{1}{h} \sum_{k=1}^{h} X_{(k)},$$

where $X_{(1)}, \ldots, X_{(h)}$ are these extremes. Now, suppose S (or D) is obtained in both phase i and j. Then β and α are estimated by

$$\hat{\beta} = (\hat{\alpha}_j - \hat{\alpha}_i)/(t_{jn_j} - t_{in_i}), \quad \hat{\alpha} = \hat{\alpha}_i + \hat{\beta} t_{in_i} \tag{3}$$

This takes care of case (a) and the upper baseline in case (b). As for the other cases, when the baseline is not reached, we shall use a method suggested by C. S. Taylor (in Finney, 1958). In case (c) we have assumed the drift to be zero, which means that $Y_{ik} = \alpha + \gamma_i \exp(-\lambda_i t_{ik}) + e_{ik}$. The same model is obtained in case (b), lower baseline, after introducing new variables $Y'_{ik} = Y_{ik} - \hat{\beta}^{(D)} t_{ik}$. In this model Taylor's method results in

$$\alpha^* = \sum_i A_i^* \Big/ \sum_i (1 - \rho_i^*); \tag{4}$$

where

$$A_i^* = \bar{Y}_i^{(1)]} - \rho_i^* \bar{Y}_i^{(n)} \tag{5}$$

$$\rho_i^* = \sum_{k=2}^{n_i} (Y_{i,k-1} - \bar{Y}_i^{(n)}) (Y_{ik} - \bar{Y}_i^{(1)}) \Big/ \sum_{k=2}^{n_j} (Y_{i,k-1} - \bar{Y}_i^{(n)})^2 \tag{6}$$

where

$$\bar{Y}_i^{(1)} = \frac{1}{n_i - 1} \sum_{k=2}^{n_j} Y_{ik}, \quad \bar{Y}_i^{(n)} = \frac{1}{n_i - 1} \sum_{k=1}^{n_j - 1} Y_{ik}.$$

The method described above seems to give reasonable results. However, several things remain to be done, of which the more important are: testing the relevance of the model (1), study of the properties of the proposed estimation methods, and, if possible, obtaining confidence intervals for flow.

RESULTS

In the evaluation the recirculation of hydrogen from the body must be taken into account. For this purpose the continuous recording of the gas concentration in the inhaled air is important. Therefore we plan to set up a Mass Spectrometer for continuous sampling of the concentration of hydrogen, oxygen, nitrogen, and CO_2 from naso pharynx. Fig. 4 illustrates how, with the same strict protocol, observations may be duplicated.

Fig. 5 shows the complexity of the data obtained. The various blocks of measure-

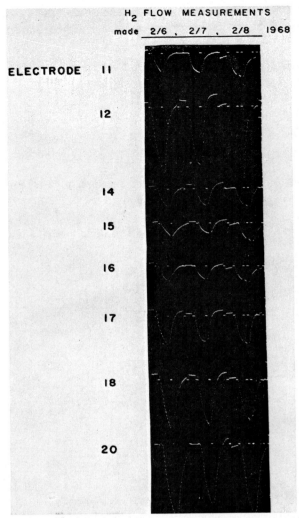

Fig. 4. Oscillograph tracings of data collected during 3 different sessions, from 8 different electrodes.

ments are made with intervals of days and weeks. For simplicity, data from only 3 electrodes in this patient are illustrated. They are taken from the diagram of data from 12 of the electrodes in this patient (Sem-Jacobsen *et al.*, 1969).

In comparing the two sessions M, during which motor activity was studied, and the two sessions CO_2, during which the response to CO_2 was measured, there is a marked difference between the M and the CO_2 sessions. Around most electrodes, however, there is agreement between the two M sessions. The same is also true for the two CO_2 sessions.

Fig. 5 illustrates that, even with an apparently strict protocol, it is hard to duplicate completely the changes in blood flow around *all electrodes* in two different sessions. When the simultaneous recordings from many electrodes from two such sessions are

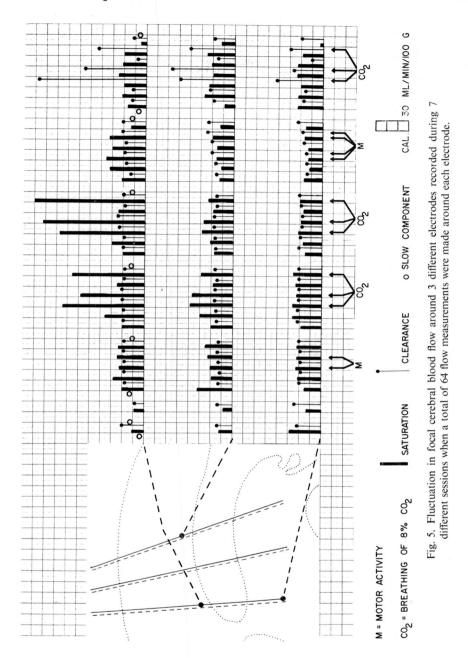

Fig. 5. Fluctuation in focal cerebral blood flow around 3 different electrodes recorded during 7 different sessions when a total of 64 flow measurements were made around each electrode.

compared in detail, the blood flow is often found to be altered around a few electrodes.

It is difficult, even observing the strictest protocol, to put the human brain in an identical situation at two different times. The slightest difference in mood or activity may cause alteration in the flow around one or more electrodes. The blood flow is measured at the same time around all electrodes in the patient. Therefore differences in the fluctuation of the blood flow are due to focal changes and not to systemic changes in blood pressure, heart rate, respiration or similar factors which one would have to consider if the measurements were made around one electrode at a time.

When studied in detail it is apparent how the response and the pattern in the response, vary from electrode to electrode. It is striking to see how CO_2 in the inspired or expired air elicits major changes in the blood flow in the area around certain electrodes, while hardly any change is found around other electrodes.

Motor movement and mental activity give rise to different changes in certain areas. It is evident from the data that the fluctuation in the blood flow can be extremely focal. The findings indicate the existence, in at least certain regions of the brain, of a well developed mechanism for increasing and reducing the blood flow. This is probably dependent on activity with increased or decreased need for blood supply in the various centers and systems.

Observations from one to two electrodes may be explained with simple models. When simultaneous measurements from more electrodes are studied, the explanation becomes increasingly difficult, and the complexity of the changes in the brain is evident.

For the past year, parallel with these studies, small solid state radiation sensors, 0.8 mm in diameter and 1.5 mm long, were adapted for introduction into the brain together with the platinum electrodes. When the problem of leakage in the insulation is solved, the solid state sensors will be used to monitor focal blood flow using Krypton-85 and Xenon-133.

CONCLUSION

Simultaneous measurements of focal cerebral blood flow were made around 16–19 electrodes during rest, physical activity, as well as during CO_2 breathing. Studies were carried out also during mental activity and sleep. A total of 16 628 rCBF determinations in ml/min/100 g were made. Increase, decrease, or no change were observed under a variety of conditions. The reproducible data give a picture of the complex, simultaneous focal changes in the blood flow in the various areas and systems of the brain. Gas analysis will be used in comprehensive tests to validate the data and to provide greater accuracy in their interpretation.

The data illustrate the complex focal changes in the blood flow in the brain. This information is useful in the treatment and understanding of head injuries and complications following brain surgery. The data may contribute to our understanding of the complex regulation of the cerebral blood flow in man.

SUMMARY

Intracerebral blood flow was measured from 16–19 electrodes in 14 patients, using the hydrogen technique. The patients were studied in 1 to 20 sessions with 2 to 14 measurements in each session. Thus rCBF was determined between 2 and 152 times around each of the 285 electrodes, giving 16 628 flow values during the past years.

Measurements were made during recovery from brain surgery, during sleep and wakefulness, as well as during physical and mental activity, etc. The data are reproducible from one session to another, each patient serving as his own control.

Marked focal fluctuations in blood flow were found in the subcortical structures. These fluctuations are probably due to physiological activity with corresponding increase or decrease in the need for blood supply in the brain centers and systems. CO_2 elicits major changes in the blood flow in certain areas, but no changes in others.

The information obtained contributes to our knowledge of cerebral blood flow, and is useful in the treatment of brain trauma as well as for neurosurgery in general.

REFERENCES

AUKLAND, K., BOWER, B. F. AND BERLINER, R. W. (1964) Measurement of local blood flow with hydrogen gas. *Circulation Res.*, **14**, 164.

FINNEY, D. J. (1958) The efficiencies of alternative estimators for an asymptotic regression equation. *Biometrika*, **45**, 374.

SEM-JACOBSEN, C. W. (1968) Depth-electrographic stimulation of the human brain and behavior. HORSLEY GANTT W. (Ed.), *14 Years of Studies and Treatment of Parkinson's Disease and Mental Disorders with Implanted Electrodes*, Charles C. Thomas, Springfield, Ill.

SEM-JACOBSEN, C. W., AUKLAND, K. AND AKRE, S. (1965) Attempts to localize gray and white matter around depth electrodes in human with hydrogen polarography. *Electroenceph. Clin. Neurophysiol.*, **19**, 617–618.

SEM-JACOBSEN, C. W., STYRI, O. B. AND MOHN, E. (1969) Simultaneous focal intracerebral blood flow measurements in man around 18 chronically implanted electrodes. In: BROCK, FIESCHI, INGVAR, LASSEN AND SCHÜRMANN (Eds.), *Cerebral Blood Flow, Clinical and Experimental Results*, Springer-Verlag, Heidelberg, pp. 44–46.

Symposium on intracerebral electrography (1953) *Proc. Staff Meetings Mayo Clinic*, **28**, 145–192.

The Measurement of Local Cerebral Blood Flow and the Effect of Amines

CLIVE ROSENDORFF

Department of Physiology, and Department of Medicine, University of the Witwatersrand, Johannesburg (South Africa)

Although the brain's great need for some component of the air was recognised by Hippocrates and incorporated into Galenical doctrine (Leake, 1962), it was not until 1783, more than a century after Harvey's description of the circulation of the blood, that serious attention was given to the cerebral circulation. Munro (1783), and later Kellie (1824), suggested that since the skull was rigid and its contents incompressible, no variation in either blood volume or circulation in the brain was possible. It was not until a century later that Hill (1896) proposed that the cerebral blood flow was in fact variable, but passively so, being determined by the systemic arterial and venous pressures. About the same time, Roy and Sherrington (1890), in a paper remarkable for its insight, had put forward the view that there was some intrinsic control of the cerebral circulation, based on local need and metabolic activity. It was not until the development of the pial window technique (Forbes and Cobb, 1938; Fog, 1939) that it was possible to investigate control mechanisms governing not only the total cerebral flow, but also regional variations.

Total cerebral flow

The "modern era" in cerebral blood flow measurement began in 1945, with the development by Kety and Schmidt (1945, 1948) of a method for the indirect measurement of *total* cerebral blood flow. The method utilises nitrous oxide (N_2O) as a freely diffusible tracer that is administered by inhalation for 10 minutes. During this period samples of arterial and jugular venous blood are collected at regular intervals, the N_2O saturation curves plotted, and the integrated arteriovenous difference in concentration computed. The mean cerebral blood flow over this ten-minute period is then calculated on the basis of the Fick principle (see Fig. 1).

Modifications of the Kety–Schmidt technique have included continuous integration of the arteriovenous difference of N_2O (Scheinberg and Stead, 1949; Fazekas *et al.* 1953), the substitution of Krypton-85 for N_2O as the indicator (Lassen and Munk, 1955), the use of the desaturation curve rather than the saturation curve (McHenry, 1964; Lassen and Klee, 1963) and the use of external scintillation counters to increase the accuracy of measurement of the numerator of the Fick equation (Lewis *et al.*,

References pp. 151–156

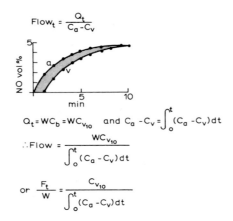

Fig. 1. A summary of the nitrous oxide saturation technique for the measurement of total cerebral
blood flow (Kety and Schmidt, 1945, 1948) – see text. Modified after Harper (1969).

Flow$_t$ = total cerebral blood flow.
Q_t = quantity of N₂O taken up by the brain from $t = 0$ up to time t
$C_a - C_v$ = $A - V$ difference in N₂O concentration between 0 and t minutes
W = Brain weight
C_b = N₂O concentration in brain at time t
C_{V10} = Venous blood concentration of N₂O at time $t = 10$.

1960; Lassen *et al.*, 1963). However, the method requires arterial and jugular venous
blood samples, and provides an estimate of total cerebral flow only.

Compartmental flow

An important development was the measurement of *compartmental* flow, *i.e.* flow
in grey and white matter, from the clearance of radio-active inert gases, such as ^{85}Kr
and ^{133}Xe, following intracarotid injection (Lassen *et al.*, 1963). These gases equilibrate rapidly between blood and brain tissue, and when the injection is stopped the
gas is cleared from the brain tissue by the perfusing blood. This rate of clearance can
be measured by means of an external scintillation counter. The curve of disappearance
of radioactivity, when plotted on semilogarithmic paper, can be analysed into two
components, a fast and a slow component, corresponding to flow through grey and
white matter respectively ("compartmental analysis") (Kety, 1965; Häggendal *et al.*,
1965; Harper and Jennett, 1967). Blood flows can then be calculated as:

$$F = \text{Blood flow (ml/100 g tissue/min)} = \frac{\lambda \cdot \log_e 2}{T\frac{1}{2}} \qquad \text{(i)}$$

where λ is the tissue:blood partition coefficient for grey or white matter, and $T\frac{1}{2}$
is the half-decay time for each exponential component (Fig. 2). The mathematical
derivation of this equation from the Fick principle has been described by Lassen
et al. (1963). Zierler (1965) has suggested the use of the formula, also derived from
the Fick equation:

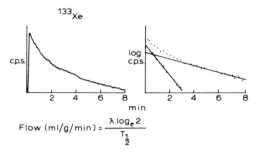

$$\text{Flow (ml/g/min)} = \frac{\lambda . \log_e 2}{T_{\frac{1}{2}}}$$

Fig. 2. The Inert Radioactive Gas clearance method for the measurement of blood through grey and white matter.
Advantages: no blood samples required; no arterial recirculation; compartmental analysis; "regional" flow.
Disadvantages: carotid puncture; inhomogeneity of flow; no local flow.

$$F = \frac{\lambda \cdot q_0}{\int_0^\infty q(t) \cdot dt} \qquad \text{(ii)}$$

where q_0 is the integrated area under the clearance curve, extrapolated to infinity. A more useful equation from the practical viewpoint is

$$F = \frac{\lambda \cdot (q_0 - q_{10})}{\int_0^{10} q(t) \cdot dt} \qquad \text{(iii)}$$

where q_{10} is the activity at 10 minutes, and the denominator is the integrated area under the curve from t_0 to t_{10}.

The best method of analysing clearance curves is still a subject of continuing fascination to those interested in cerebral blood flow. The "height over area" method (eqns. ii and iii) is easier and probably adequate under most circumstances, especially where the clearance curve is not a true exponential over its whole course. The value of compartmental analysis (eqn. i and Fig. 2) is the separate information it provides about blood flow through grey and white matter. It is true that cerebral grey matter is not completely homogeneous, and that, under certain circumstances, a multi-exponential clearance curve can be obtained from the cerebral cortex alone (Harper et al., 1961; Lassen, 1965; Fieschi et al., 1968). However, Harper and Jennett (1967) have compared simultaneous measurements of cortical blood flow (beta counting) and the fast component of the clearance of a gamma-emitting tracer in the monkey, and found a fairly good correlation. Also, the local cerebral cortical flow derived from the local injection of [133]Xenon in the rabbit, is of the same order of magnitude as that derived from the fast component of the binexponential clearance of an intra-carotid injection of the tracer in the same animal (Rosendorff and Cranston, 1969). Kety (1965) has stated "It may be that we are fortunate in working with the brain

References pp. 151–156

which has such a clear bimodal distribution of its population of perfusion rates, with practically no overlap between them, each distribution with a sharp peak and relatively small scatter".

Regional flow

A refinement of the above approach is the use of multiple external collimated counters, each looking at a "core" of brain tissue (Lassen et al., 1963; Ingvar et al., 1965). Ingvar et al. (1968) have used 8 scintillation detectors for simultaneous measurement of flow in eight regions, Lassen (1968) and Wilkinson et al. (1969) have used a 16-detector system, and Sveinsdottir et al. (1969) a 35-probe system. The same method of analysis, either "height over area" or "compartmental" may be used; in addition, the relative weights of grey and white matter within the counting area of each probe may be derived from the slopes of the two components of the clearance curve and their intercepts (Ingvar et al., 1965; Høldt-Rasmussen et al., 1966). Increasing the number and improving the geometry of the counters will improve the resolution of the system, but the localisation is still relatively crude, and it is impossible to distinguish between, say, cortical flow and non-cortical grey matter flow in the same counting field.

Local flow

Under certain circumstances this may be of importance, and during the course of studies on the hypothalamic control of thermoregulation in the rabbit (Cranston and Rosendorff, 1967 a and b, 1970; Cranston, Luff, Rawlins and Rosendorff, 1970; Cranston, Hellon, Luff, Rawlins and Rosendorff, 1970; Rawlins et al., 1970; Rosendorff and Mooney, 1970; Rosendorff et al., 1970) it became important to know the local blood flow in the hypothalamus under certain experimental situations.

For this purpose a technique was devised (Rosendorff, 1969; Rosendorff and Cranston, 1969, a and b; Cranston and Rosendorff, 1968 a and b, 1969) which involves the measurement of the rate of clearance of a small volume of ^{133}Xenon injected locally into the hypothalamus, or any other area chosen. Local injection methods have been described (Nillson, 1965; Espagno and Lazorthes 1965; Häggendal et al., 1965), but only for cortical and for subcortical white matter flow measurements. Nillson (1965) injected 1–5-μl volumes of a ^{85}Kr saline solution directly into the cerebral cortex, or into the subcortical white matter of anaesthetised craniotomised dogs. The values for flow through grey and white matter computed from these clearance curves corresponded fairly closely to the blood flow values obtained from the fast and slow components of the clearance of ^{85}Kr administered via a catheter in the internal carotid artery. He estimated that the injected ^{85}Kr did not diffuse more than 1–2 mm from the site of injection. Espagno and Lazorthes (1965) have performed similar experiments on man, and found a binexponential type of clearance of ^{133}Xe injected into the cerebral cortex. They suggest that this is due to diffusion of some of the Xenon into the subcortical white matter although this could also possibly be explained on the basis of lack of homogeneity of flow within circumscribed areas of the cortex. Häggendal and his colleagues (1965) found that microinjections of ^{85}Kr into the cortex of dogs gave rise to monoexponential clearance curves with the same flow values as those derived from the fast component of gamma or beta curves after intra-arterial ^{85}Kr injections in the same animal at the same arterial carbon dioxide tension. Similarly the rate of clearance of the tracer from a local injection into the subcortical white matter was very similar to that of the slow component of the curves derived from intra-arterial injections.

Other methods for the measurement of local cerebral blood flow have been developed. One, the heat clearance technique (Betz, 1965, 1968; Betz et al., 1966), depends upon the assumption that the temperature of a constantly heated point in a perfused tissue depends only upon the removal of heat by the blood. This method is obviously unsuitable for any studies on blood flow in the temperature-sensitive hypothalamus. Another technique involves the use of a hydrogen electrode in brain tissue to measure polarographically the rate at which desaturation of hydrogen occurs, after tissue saturation is achieved by H_2 gas inhalation (Aukland, 1965, 1968; Fieschi et al., 1965). With this method, no local injections are required; this is an advantage, since local tissue trauma will be less than the ^{133}Xe injection method. On the other hand, insertion of a needle may still be needed if one is to study the "micropharmacology" of local vessels, and the same needle can be utilised for ^{133}Xenon injections.

Another method for the measurement of local blood flow in experimental animals is the autoradiographic technique (Landau et al., 1955; Kety, 1960, 1965). The theoretical basis for this technique is as follows: a freely diffusible, unmetabolised tracer carried to a region by the blood will reach a concentration (C_i) in each small component (i) in time T, which depends upon the concentration in the arterial blood (C_a), during that period of time, and on local conditions of capillary blood flow per unit tissue mass (F_i/M_i), and the tissue–blood partition coefficient of the substance (λ_i);

$$C_i(T) = \lambda_i K_i e^{-K_i T} \cdot \int_0^T C_a \cdot e^{K_i t} \cdot dt \qquad \text{(iv)}$$

where

$$K_i = F_i/\lambda_i M_i \qquad \text{(v)}$$

Thus capillary blood flow through any small homogeneous segment of a region may be estimated from these equations, if the other quantities are known or can be measured. C_i is determined by autoradiography. The advantage of this method is the simultaneous measurement of blood flow in all parts of the brain, the disadvantage, which disqualifies it for the present study, is that only one estimate of flow can be made in any one area; serial measurement of flow or changes in flow are precluded. Further, it has been argued (Zierler, 1967, personal communication) that under the conditions in which autoradiography is usually performed, what is estimated is the relative volume of distribution of the infused tracer, and not the relative blood flow.

A variety of other techniques have been devised for the measurement of total, regional, and local cerebral blood flow. These include the ^{133}Xe inhalation technique (Mallett and Veall, 1963, 1965; Obrist *et al.*, 1967), mean transit time measurements following intracarotid injections of radio-iodinated serum albumin (Fieschi *et al.*, 1968), mode transit of times of [^{131}I]Hippuran (Oldendorf and Kitano, 1965; Taylor and Bell, 1968), impedance recording (Laitinen *et al.*, 1966), selective cannulation of cerebral veins (Foltz *et al.*, 1966), and flows through cerebral vessels using "square wave" electromagnetic flowmeters, thermovelocity (Herrmann, 1968) or thermodilution (Lowe and Dowsett, 1967) measurements in the internal jugular vein. The validity and usefulness of some of these methods in different experimental situations have been reviewed by McHenry (1966) and Harper (1967); none of them has been judged suitable for the present investigation.

The method used in the present study, namely the measurement of local flow derived from the rate of clearance of locally injected Xenon, has been subjected to careful study; the following section reports the results of experiments designed to explore the areas of usefulness, the validity, and perhaps most important of all, the limitations of this technique.

THE MEASUREMENT OF LOCAL CEREBRAL BLOOD FLOW IN THE CONSCIOUS RABBIT BY A ^{133}XENON INJECTION TECHNIQUE

All methods of measuring local blood flow in the brain are traumatic; it seems almost axiomatic that the more precisely blood flow is to be determined, the more traumatic is the technique that needs to be selected. The measurement of hypothalamic blood flow by the injection directly into brain tissue, via a cannula, of a radioactive gas dissolved in a volume of saline, could be assumed, a priori, to be so traumatic a technique that the changes induced by the measuring system would vitiate any understanding of the physiology or pharmacology of blood flow control in the area. Evidence that this is not so, that this technique is a useful approach to the problems of local flow control in the brain, is presented in this section.

All experiments were performed on adult chinchilla rabbits, weighing 2.5–3.00 kg.

The headplate used (Figs. 3 and 4) was an adaptation of that described by Monnier and Gangloff (1961), who had, in turn, adapted their technique from Hess (1932). Under pentobarbitone anaesthesia (30 mg/kg), the base-plate (C in Fig. 3) was screwed on to the skull. The base-plate had holes drilled $1\frac{1}{2}$ mm from the midline in the longitudinal axis, and at 3-mm intervals (aA, aB, aC, aD, aE and aF coordinates on each side); see Fig. 5. This base-plate was positioned on the skull so that the coronal suture was midway between the most anterior two pairs of holes, and the sagittal suture was midway between the two rows of holes. Bregma was then at midpoint of the square formed by the most anterior four holes. The base-plate was secured to the skull using short, stainless steel self-tapping screws. Holes were bored through the skull beneath those holes in the base-plate that were likely to be used, usually aA and aB on each side. The whole area was then sprayed with a polymyxin, bacitracin and neomycin aerosol (Swallowfield, Ltd.), and the skin closed around the edges of

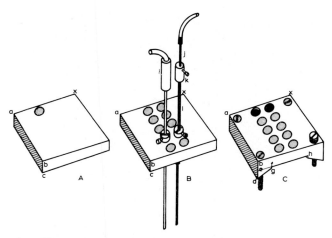

Fig. 3. The base-plate (C), carrier plate (B) and the araldite cover (A). Between experiments, A is used to cover C; at the time of each experiment, A is removed from C, and B is placed on C.

Legends:

i = Needle-mounted thermistor;
j = injection cannula;
k = adjustable sealing sleeve;
l = guide cannula;

ab = 15 mm	ax = 18 mm
bc = 3 mm	be = 3 mm
bd = 6 mm	ef = 3 mm
fg = 1 mm	dg = 4 mm

(Rosendorff and Mooney, 1971, Amer. J. Physiol., 220, 597–603)

the base-plate. An "Araldite" (Ciba) plate (A in Fig. 3), lubricated with sterile liquid paraffin, was screwed to the top of the base-plate to prevent upward growth of the skin over the base-plate, and the whole area sprayed with the transparent dressing "Nobecutaine" (Duncan, Flockhart and Evans Ltd.). The animal was then given an intramuscular injection of 100 000 units of benzylpenicillin and 0.1 g of streptomycin. At least one week elapsed before the animal was used for an experiment.

Cannulae and their insertion

A second rectangular steel plate (B in Fig. 3) 1.8 cm × 1.5 cm (the upper plate), was drilled with two rows of holes identical with those in the base-plate. Two cm lengths of stainless steel tubing (1) (Accles and Pollock Standard Hypodermic Tubing) were mounted in threaded collets in this plate, in the appropriate holes. These guide cannulae (1) protruded about 3–5 mm below the plate. A second cannula ("the injection cannula", j) was made with an adjustable sealing sleeve (k), (i.d. 0.22 mm, o.d. 0.44 mm), mounted in the end of a length of 00 nylon tubing, and inserted into the guide cannula (1), so that the injection cannula protruded a distance X cm, depending on the injection site, below the upper plate. The sealing sleeve (k) was then fixed on the injection cannula (j) at the top of the guide cannula (1), and the injection

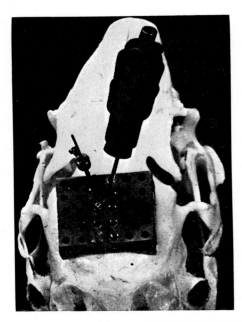

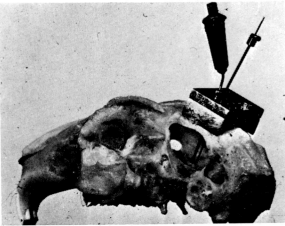

Fig. 4. The base-plate, carrier-plate, injection cannula, and a thermistor, shown *in situ* in a rabbit's skull. A "window" has been trephined in the calvarium; the tips of the cannula and thermistor can be seen.

cannula removed. The upper plate–guide cannula assembly was sterilised by boiling in distilled water for 10 min, cooled by brief immersion in sterile saline; the guide cannulae (l) were inserted through the appropriate holes in the base-plate (C), and the upper plate (B) carrying the guide cannulae was screwed to the base-plate (C). The injection cannulae (j) were flushed through with sterile, pyrogen-free saline solution, then with the solution to be injected, and finally placed in its guide cannula. Injections were made with a Hamilton micro syringe, graduated in microlitres,

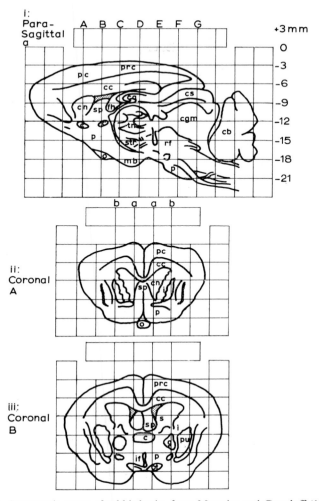

Fig. 5. Stereotaxic maps of rabbit brain, from Monnier and Gangloff (1961).
Legend:

c, ⎫ anterior   o, optic chiasma
ca, ⎭ commissure   ot, optic tract
cb, cerebellum   p, pre-optic area and hypothalamus
cc, corpus callosum   pc, precentral cortex
cgm, central grey matter   prc, paracentral cortex
cn, caudate nucleus   pu, putamen
cs, superior colliculus   rf, reticular formation
fh, fimbria hippocampus   s, corpus striatum
g, globus pallidus   sp, septum pellucidum
i, internal capsule   str, subthalamic region
if, infundibulum   tn, thalamic nuclei
mb, mamillary body   shaded area, lateral ventricle

mounted in a micrometer screw (Agla, Burroughs Wellcome Ltd). The position of the tip of an injection cannula in the hypothalamus was confirmed in some experiments by injecting 2–5 μl of a fine particulate carbon suspension, and the site of the injection determined by cutting serial sections of the brain. Fig. 6 shows the results of all rabbits injected. All of the sites of injection are within 1 mm of each other and within 1 mm of the stereotoxic coordinate aB – 16 mm.

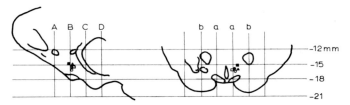

Fig. 6. Localisation of [133]Xenon injections in the anterior hypothalamus. These points were derived from the areas of maximum density of staining following the injection of 2.5–5.0 μl of carbon ink through the hypothalamic cannula.
Left: Parasagittal section through a. Right: Coronal section through B.
●T19   ○T22   ▲T28   ■T29   □T30

Since the counting geometry was required to be kept constant, the animals were restrained in conventional stocks, and the snout gently tied into a rubber ring which was securely fixed to the stocks. In this position the rabbit was unable to move its head, but had a free range of movement of trunk and limbs. This was the simplest way to ensure immobilisation of the head, and therefore of a constant distance between the head and the scintillation counter. The rabbits did not appear to be at all distressed by this enforced immobility. Before the experiments were carried out, each animal had been accustomed to this restraint by several exposures, and all those in which temperature was measured had shown no significant temperature change over 4–6 h.

All experiments were carried out in a temperature-controlled room at 22.0 ± 0.5 °C. Hypothalamic blood flow was measured at 15–30-min intervals by the clearance of small volumes of locally injected [133]Xenon dissolved in saline.

The [133]Xenon was supplied as 50 mC of the gas in equilibrium with 10 ml of sterile, pyrogen-free, normal saline, in a 10-ml vial. Since xenon comes out of solution very rapidly when exposed to air, the injection system was filled with the xenon solution taking great care to avoid a solution–air interface at any stage. The dead space in the vial was filled with sterile mercury. The injection cannula was introduced through the skull plate, positioned so that its tip was in the anterior hypothalamus (L a B or R a B, – 16 mm; see Figs. 5 and 6) and held in place with a grub screw.

The injection system is shown in Fig. 7, and the system for recording the γ-emission from the [133]Xenon solution is shown in Fig. 8. The counting system consists of a Thallium Activated Sodium Iodide crystal (Ekco, Type N609, $1\frac{3}{4}''$ diameter by $2''$ long), collimated by an adjustable brass collimator (3-mm thickness). The rest of the scintillation detection system consists of a photomultiplier tube and unity gain amplifier (Ecko M5401 A); this is connected to a counting system (Ecko M5050)

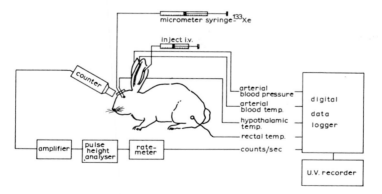

Fig. 7. Schematic diagram of the injection system for ^{133}Xe.
(Rosendorff, C. and Cranston, W. I. (1969) Measurement of hypothalamic blood flow in the conscious rabbit by a radioactive inert gas clearance technique. *5th Europ. Conf. Microcirculation, Gothenburg, 1968, Bibl. Anat.*, No. **10**, 292–297, Karger, Basel–New York.)

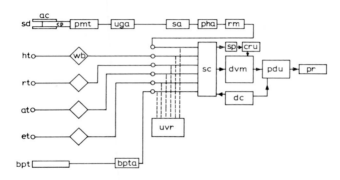

Fig. 8. Block diagram of the recording apparatus.

Legend:
ac, adjustable collimator
at, arterial blood thermistor
bpt, blood pressure transducer
bpta, blood pressure transducer amplifier
cp, crystal phosphor
cru, command range unit
dc, digital clock
dvm, digital voltmeter
et, environmental temperature
ht, hypothalamic thermistor

pdu, print drive unit
pha, pulse height analyser
pmt, photomultiplier tube
pr, printer
rm, ratemeter
rt, rectal thermistor
sa, wide band signal amplifier
sc, scanning unit
sd, scintillation detector
sp, system patchboard
uga, unity gain amplifier
uvr, ultra-violet recorder
wb, Wheatstone bridge circuit

consisting of a wide band signal amplifier, a single speed pulse height analyser, and a linear ratemeter. The time constant of the ratemeter used was either 3 sec for the first 30 sec of the clearance curve and 10 sec thereafter, or was 10 sec throughout. Since the half decay time for ^{133}Xenon clearance from the site of injection was rarely less than 1 min, and was usually of the order of 100 sec, $\tau = 0.1\ k$, where τ = the time constant value *RC* of the ratemeter assembly, and *k* is the time constant value for the exponential decay of activity during clearance (the input function). When this relationship holds, the observed rate of clearance, where $\tau = 10$ sec, is very close to the input function rate of clearance. This argument is expounded more fully in the Appendix and Fig. 25, which shows computer-derived curves of the alteration in observed exponential functions when the input function is modified by varying time constants.

The ratemeter was connected to the recording apparatus. This consisted of a 12-channel ultra-violet recorder (S.E.2005), which provided a continuous record of activity, and a digital data logging system (Solartron, Compact Logger, LY1470) with a print-out unit (Addo LX1652).

At least 5 min was allowed for stabilisation of the background, and then 2.5 to 10 μl of the ^{133}Xe-in-saline solution was injected through the cannula into the hypothalamus over a 1–3-sec period. The clearance curves were then followed for at least 5 min. Each curve was corrected by the subtraction of mean background activity, and re-plotted on semilogarithmic paper. The blood flows were calculated from the slope of the initial portion of the semilogarithmic plot of the clearance, using a value of λ (the hypothalamus: blood partition coefficient for ^{133}Xe) of 0.74. The derivation of this value, using a double-isotope technique, has been described in detail elsewhere (Rosendoff and Luff, 1970).

Control clearances

Clearance curves were mono-exponential (see Fig. 9) and the half-decay times varied

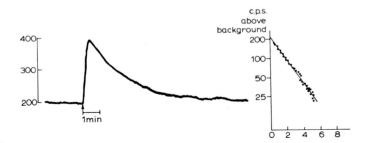

Fig. 9. ^{133}Xenon clearance curve. On the right is shown the semilogarithmic plot of the clearance, after the subtraction of mean background activities.
(Rosendorff, C. and Cranston, W. I. (1969) Measurement of hypothalamic blood flow in the conscious rabbit by a radioactive inert gas clearance technique. *5th Europ. Conf. Microcirculation, Gothenburg, 1968, Bibl. Anat.*, No. **10**, 292–297, Karger, Basel–New York.)

from 1.00 to 2.42 min in control animals. The half times were converted to nominal blood flow rates using the formula

$$\text{Blood flow (ml/g tissue/min)} = \frac{\lambda \cdot \log_e 2}{T_{\frac{1}{2}}},$$

where $\lambda = 0.74$, the tissue: blood partition coefficient for the rabbit hypothalamus

(Rosendorff and Luff, 1970) or $\lambda = 0.63$ for rabbit cerebrum (Andersen and Ladefoged, 1965). The mean background activity (H_b) was high, since the counter was "looking at" approximately 2 cm of the xenon-filled cannula. At the time of the injection of the xenon solution, the count rate increased to a maximum value which was within the range 200–1000 counts/sec, and was three times the background count rate. The subsequent clearance of the xenon by tissue perfusion was determined by subtracting a value for the mean background activity, and plotting the resulting curve on semi-logarithmic paper. $T\frac{1}{2}$ (the half-decay time, that is the time taken for activity to fall to half of the initial value) was plotted using the initial 1–2 min of the semilogarithmic plot of the clearance curve.

Control flows

In eight experiments on five rabbits, changes in hypothalamic blood flow were followed for 90–120 min. The mean control flow (at time = 0) for each experiment was calculated, and all subsequent flows in that experiment were expressed as a percentage of that control value.

The changes in blood flow over a 90–120-min period are shown in Fig. 10, and both

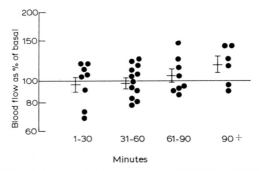

Fig. 10. Change in HBF with time. Ordinate: mean control H.B.F. is 100%, at time = 0. All subsequent H.B.F. values expressed as a percentage of the mean control H.B.F. All H.B.F. values are grouped in 30-min periods.

the blood flows and the blood flows expressed as a percentage of the control values, were grouped in 30-min intervals. The mean for each 30-min interval was then calculated, together with the range covered by one standard error on either side of the mean. There is no significant difference between the means of the "control period" and of the 0–30, 31–60, and 61–90-min groups. The 91–120-min mean is 119% of the control period, and this is significantly different (S.E.M. $\pm$ 9.0%, $t = 2.43$, $P < 0.05$) from the control flow.

The no-flow situation

In one experiment a large bore polythene catheter was inserted, via the femoral artery, with its tip in the aorta, under pentobarbitone anaesthesia. The animal was allowed to recover, and 2–3 hours later hypothalamic xenon clearance measured. The animal was then killed by rapid exsanguination, and the clearance of xenon was again assessed.

Fig. 11 shows the abolition of [133]Xenon clearance after cessation of hypothalamic perfusion.

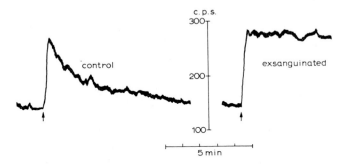

Fig. 11. Clearance of [133]Xenon injected into the hypothalamus in a control animal (left). On the right, the absence of clearance of [133]Xenon injected into the hypothalamus after exsanguination.

Autoregulation

Cerebrovascular autoregulation is the ability of the brain to maintain a constant blood flow despite changes in perfusion pressure. Autoregulation has been demonstrated in man and in various animals, but nearly all reported studies refer to total cerebral flow or cerebral cortical flow. Subcortical structures have received little attention, but in one study (Bozzao et al., 1968) autoregulation was demonstrated in the caudate nucleus and in subcortical white matter in the cat.

Cerebral autoregulation is easily abolished by tissue trauma, hypoxia, and hypercapnia. If autoregulation can be demonstrated by the local [133]Xenon technique, i.e. in spite of the presence of the hypothalamic cannula and in spite of the [133]Xenon-containing saline microinjections, then it may be concluded that the amount of tissue trauma, hypoxia or hypercapnia present locally is of little functional significance.

Changes in mean systemic arterial blood pressure were induced by bleeding and by angiotensin infusions. This method was adopted because it was simpler than techniques currently available for changing cerebrovascular perfusion pressure alone, and because, in the case of angiotensin, no direct action of this peptide on cerebral vessels has been reported.

Forty-eight measurements of hypothalamic blood flow were made, in seven adult male Chinchilla rabbits, weighing 2.5–3.5 kg. The rabbits were anaesthetised with pentobarbitone 30 mg/kg, supplemented when necessary during the experiment by further doses. The level of anaesthesia maintained was such that the corneal reflexes were intact. A tracheostomy was performed and the animals were respired by intermittent positive pressure ventilation, using a small animal respirator. The experimental set-up is shown in Fig. 12.

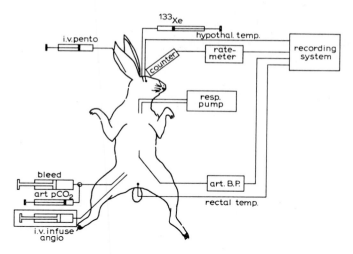

Fig. 12. Schematic representation of the experimental set-up for experiments on the autoregulation of hypothalamic blood flow.

The experiment was started with a slow infusion of sterile normal saline, using a Harvard infusion pump, and at least two hypothalamic blood flow measurements were made at the starting blood pressure. Angiotensin II amide ("Hypertensin", Ciba) infusions were used to produce a step-wise increment in mean arterial blood pressure, since angiotensin has been shown to have no direct effect on cerebrovascular resistance (Greenfield and Tindall, 1968), but raises the arterial blood pressure by a variety of mechanisms (Rosendorff *et al.*, 1970). After at least 15 min at each new blood pressure level, one or in some cases two blood flow measurements were made. The 15-min stabilisation period at each blood pressure level was adopted because of the demonstration, by Fog (1938), and Rapela and Green (1964), that following a sudden change in blood pressure, there is a time lag of 30 sec to 2 min before the onset of autoregulation. Later, 10–20-ml volumes of blood were withdrawn to produce a step-wise decrement in mean arterial pressure. At each blood pressure level at least one blood flow measurement was made.

At each blood pressure level 2 ml samples of arterial blood were withdrawn anaerobically, and P_{CO_2} was measured with a Severinghaus type CO_2 electrode and corrected to the animal's hypothalamic temperature using the data of Bradley *et al.* (1956).

Fig. 13 shows the results of a typical experiment in this series. In spite of marked changes in mean arterial blood pressure (MABP) the hypothalamic blood flow remained relatively constant. Only when the MABP fell below 60 mm Hg did auto-regulation fail, and the blood flow fell.

The results of these experiments were expressed as follows. The mean arterial blood pressure range of 81–100 mm Hg was taken as the "normal" blood pressure, and the mean blood flow for each rabbit at that blood pressure was ascribed a value of 1, and all other blood flows in that experiment at other blood pressure levels were

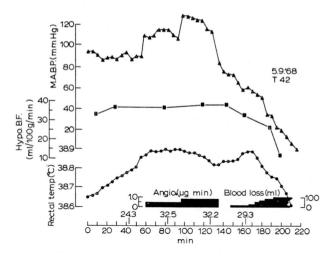

Fig. 13. Autoregulation of hypothalamic blood flow. Time course of one experiment. Traces are, from above down, mean arterial blood pressure in mm Hg, hypothalamic blood flow in ml/100 g/min, rectal temperature in °C, angiotensin infusion rate in μg/min, cumulative blood loss in ml. The abscissa is time in minutes, and values for arterial P_{CO_2}, in mm Hg, are also shown.

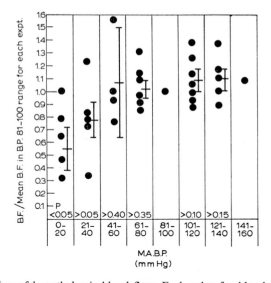

Fig. 14. Autoregulation of hypothalamic blood flow. Each value for blood flow is expressed as a ratio to the mean blood flow at a mean arterial blood pressure of 81–100 mm Hg in the same experiment (ordinate). The abscissa is the mean arterial blood pressure, in 20 mm Hg divisions. The means and standard errors of the means are shown, as well as the P values for significance of the difference of the means from 1.

expressed as a ratio to this value. This method of expressing the results allows for a comparison to be made between different animals, which vary considerably in their "normotensive" hypothalamic blood flows.

The results from all experiments, analysed in this way, are shown in Fig. 14, also with the means and standard errors of the mean for each group. None of the means of the flows in the blood pressure ranges from 21 to 140 mm Hg differ significantly from 1. It is only in the blood pressure range of 1–20 mm Hg that the mean flow differs significantly from 1 (mean 0.55 ± 0.17 SEM; $0.025 < P < 0.05$; $n = 5$). The conclusion is that probably within the range of mean arterial pressure of 21–140 mm Hg, and certainly in the range 41–140 mm Hg, autoregulation of hypothalamic blood flow has been demonstrated.

Local injection and carotid injection

A comparison was made in the pentobarbitone-anaesthetised rabbit between the blood flow derived from the clearance of locally injected xenon and that obtained from the clearance of xenon injected up the internal carotid artery. The fast component of the binexponential clearance of an intracarotid injection of ^{133}Xe represents flow through cerebral grey matter. This component was derived in an experiment in which a catheter was tied in the external carotid artery so that its tip lay at the origin of internal carotid artery. All branches of the external carotid were tied. Forty microlitres of [133]Xe (160 μC) was injected through the cannula and the clearance of the ^{133}Xe was recorded using the external counting system already described. The clearance curve, plotted on semilogarithmic paper, was analysed into its two components.

Blood flow in the cerebral cortex was then measured in the same animal by the local injection technique. The injection cannula was positioned with its tip in the cortex at L aB -2.5–3.0 mm (Fig. 5) and 2.5 μl (12.5 μC) ^{133}Xe injected. The clearance of the injected ^{133}Xe was also followed for about 10 min.

These traces are shown in Fig. 15. The clearance of ^{133}Xe from the brain following the intracarotid injection of a saline solution of the gas consists of two components,

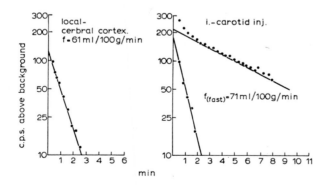

Fig. 15. Semilogarithmic plot of the clearance of ^{133}Xe injected into the cerebral cortex (left), and injected up the internal carotid artery (right). The latter clearance curve has been analysed into two components. The fast component of this compound curve is of the same order of magnitude as the rate of clearance of locally injected [133]Xe.
(Rosendorff, C. and Cranston, W. I. (1969) Brock, M. *et al.* (Eds.), *Cerebral Blood Flow*, Springer-Verlag, Berlin–Heidelberg, p. 37).

the faster of which is related to blood flow through grey matter. The value for grey matter flow derived from this slope (71 ml/100 g/min) is of the same order of magnitude as the blood flow in the cerebral cortex derived from the rate of clearance of locally injected ^{133}Xenon.

Histopathology

Twelve rabbit brains were removed, and subjected to histological examination. These were from rabbits which had had between one and five experiments performed on them, each experiment involving the insertion of one hypothalamic injection cannula and one thermistor. The brains were fixed in formol saline, and some were stained with haematoxylin and eosin, some with Luxol Fast Blue.

No gross disruption of hypothalamic tissue was seen in those animals which had had up to four experiments. In those brains which had been subjected to five or more experiments, severe oedema, inflammatory cell infiltrate and gliosis was seen, the severity of which increased with the number of experiments to which the animal had been subjected. Because of this finding no animals were subjected to more than four experiments.

DISCUSSION

The "signal to background" ratio for radioactivity was of the order of 3:1 after the injection of a 2.5 to 5-μl volume of injectate. This is a value which is of the same order of magnitude as that predicted on the basis of the following argument. Assuming that the counter is "looking at" 3 cm of the xenon-filled injection cannula, the volume of xenon contained in this length of cannula would be $\pi R^2 l = 3.14 (0.11)^2 30 = 1.14 \,\mu l$. After the injection, the counter is "looking at" this volume, 1.14 μl, plus the injected volume, 2.5 μl, giving a total of 3.64 μl. The ratio 3.64:1.14 = 3.19:1, which is of the same order of magnitude as the ratio of activity before and after the injection. The corollary of this argument is that one can calculate the length (l) of cannula within the counting field by using the relationship

$$\frac{\pi \cdot R^2 l}{\pi R^2 l + V_I} = \frac{Q_B}{Q_H},$$

where R is the radius of the lumen of the cannula (0.11 mm), V_I the volume injected, Q_B the background activity and Q_H the peak activity derived from extrapolating the clearance curve back to t_0, the time of injection.

The use of the initial slope of the clearance curve would seem to be theoretically valid, since this will give the fastest clearance rate, irrespective of diffusion, and is practically sound, because even if one could recognise a slow component, its activity would be so close to background levels that it would be very difficult to analyse on a compartmental or stochastic basis. There is no indication from these experiments what the diffusion distance for the injected xenon is, but it would appear to be limited to a single compartment, since only one component could be recognised in the clearance curves. The clearance curves after injections in grey matter are monoexponential (Fig. 9 and Häggendal *et al.*, 1965) giving values for cortical flow somewhat higher than hypothalamic flow, and so it is a reasonable assumption that the area of diffusion of xenon in the hypothalamus is uniformly perfused, and that this represents a region of subcortical grey matter in which flow is less than that in the cerebral cortex. It is now recognised that cerebral grey matter flow is not homogeneous, that is, it varies from one region to another, so it is not surprising that hypothalamic and cortical flow should differ, although this difference is reduced by anaesthesia.

The next question which arises is, given the probability that grey matter flow is non-homogeneous (Wilkinson *et al.*, 1969), how representative of cortical flow is that derived from one area of the cortex by local injection? The experiments in which local cortical flow was compared with flow derived from the fast component of the clearance of intracarotid xenon, were done under light barbiturate anaesthesia, which is reported to abolish differences in blood flow in different parts of the cortex (Sokoloff, 1959; Häggendal *et al.*, 1965) and also to increase uniformity of EEG activity (Gleichmann *et al.*, 1962). It is therefore likely that such differences in perfusion between one part of the cortex and the other as do exist, are small under conditions of barbiturate anaesthesia. (See also Fig. 16).

The effects of general anaesthetics are of interest. Barbiturate anaesthesia has been reported to lower (Schmidt *et al.*, 1945; Homberger *et al.*, 1946; Schieve and Wilson, 1953), increase (Wechsler *et al.*, 1951), or have no effect (Fazekas and Bessman, 1953; Wilson *et al.*, 1953) on cerebral blood flow. It has been suggested (Sokoloff, 1959), not unreasonably, that changes in cerebral circulation induced by barbiturates are secondary to some of their other effects, such as changes in arterial P_{O_2}, P_{CO_2} and pH, as well as cerebral metabolic rate or oxygen consumption. In the present experiments, cortical flow was approximately halved, while there was no significant change in

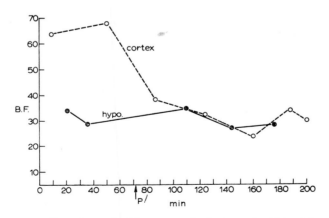

Fig. 16. Effect of pentobarbitone anaesthesia on cerebral blood flow.
Ordinate: blood flow in ml/100 g/min. Abscissa: Time in min. The open circles and the dotted lines represent blood flow in the cerebral cortex (aB – 3 mm) measured by the local injection technique. The closed circles and continuous lines are hypothalamic blood flow. *P* is the induction of anaesthesia with 30 mg pentobarbitone/kg body weight.

hypothalamic flow. This demonstrates a profound difference, not only in the blood flows in the control state, but also in the response to barbiturate anaesthesia, of two areas of grey matter.

The stability of hypothalamic blood flow over a 90-min period in the conscious rabbit, in spite of the physical restraint and the presence of the cannula tip in the hypothalamus, was an important finding. Any systematic change, or a very large variability, would have invalidated the technique. After 90 min there was a small increase in flow, of 19% of the control value. These experiments have not provided any evidence of the cause of this small rise of flow.

The findings from experiments in which the arterial pressure was altered by means of bleeding (Harper, a and b, 1965; Häggendal, 1965) indicate that the brain exhibits nearly perfect autoregulation in the mean arterial pressure range of 150 mm Hg down to 40–60 mm Hg. This autoregulation is dependent upon variations in overall cerebro-vascular resistance, which in turn will be influenced by other factors, such as P_{O_2} and P_{CO_2}. Thus, at arterial P_{CO_2} values higher than 70 mm Hg there is maximal vasodilation, and the CBF is passively related to pressure (Harper, 1966). Hypoxic states diminish auto-regulatory ability by a vasodilator action, resulting in a passive pressure–flow relationship at an arterial O_2 saturation level below 60%. Recent studies (Rapela and Green, 1968; Freeman, 1968; Freeman and Ingvar, 1968) have confirmed these observations. In the present experiments great care was taken to avoid hypoxia and hypercapnia by careful regulation of the respiratory minute volume.

Many authors have pointed out that cerebral autoregulation is easily abolished, e.g. by trauma, vascular perfusion procedures, periods of circulatory arrest, arterial and local tissue hypoxia, hypercapnia, and deep anaesthesia (Aiba et al., 1967; Freeman and Ingvar, 1968). According to some authorities (Skinhøj, 1966; Siesjö et al., 1968) extracellular acidosis may also affect CBF, and therefore autoregulation. The preservation of autoregulatory ability under the conditions of the present investigation would suggest that, if local tissue trauma, tissue hypoxia, hypercapnia or extracellular acidosis were induced by the presence of the hypothalamic cannula and by the serial injection of small volumes of ^{133}Xenon-containing saline, then they are of little functional significance.

THE ACTION OF INTRA-HYPOTHALAMIC NORADRENALINE ON HYPOTHALAMIC BLOOD FLOW

The effects of many drugs on the cerebral circulation are often very different from their effects on other vascular beds. According to Sokoloff (1959), "the physiological and pharmacological behaviour of the cerebral circulation is sufficiently unique that drug actions exerted on most other vascular beds can only rarely be assumed to be operating similarly in the brain". Although elsewhere in the body noradrenaline (NA) and 5-hydroxytryptamine (5-HT) have profound effects on blood vessels, their action on total cerebral blood flow is controversial, and their effect on hypothalamic flow unknown. The initial motivation to study the effects of amines on hypothalamic flow was that these drugs are known to affect thermoregulation in a variety of animals when injected into the lateral ventricles or directly into the hypothalamus (Cranston and Rosendorff, 1967 b), and it has been postulated (Cooper, 1966) that these compounds may affect body temperature via changes in hypothalamic perfusion.

Hypothalamic noradrenaline

Experiments were performed on 31 adult Chinchilla rabbits, involving 287 estimations of hypothalamic blood flow. Two fine injection cannulae, 0.4 mm o.d., were placed with their tips in identical positions in the anterior hypothalamus on either side of the midline (L and R aB–16 mm); each cannula was connected via a 2-metre length of 00 nylon tubing to a Hamilton 250-μl microsyringe, and the whole system was filled with ^{133}Xenon in sterile pyrogen-free normal saline solution (5 mC/ml) (Radiochemical Centre, Amersham, Bucks.). The tips of the injection cannulae were each 1.5 mm from the midline, and 3.0 mm from each other.

Micro-injections of 5–10 μl of the ^{133}Xe solution were made into each side of the hypothalamus alternately, allowing at least 15 min between injections. The clearance rates of the ^{133}Xe injectates were measured using the external counting system described above.

Equality of hypothalamic flow on either side of the hypothalamus

The first series of experiments (two rabbits) was designed to test the assumption that there is no systematic difference in hypothalamic blood flow on either side of the midline.

Fig. 17 shows the result of a typical control experiment. There was no difference

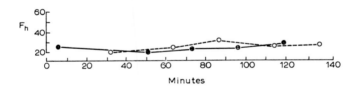

Fig. 17. Blood flow in the hypothalamus to the right (R) and left (L) of the midline (ml/100 g/min) ^{133}Xe–saline only injected on both sides.

in blood flow discernible between the two sides of the hypothalamus. Because of the tendency of hypothalamic blood flow to increase slightly but progressively with time (see Fig. 10), the following method of analysis of the results was adopted. The left side was designated the "control" side, and each "right side" blood flow value was expressed as a ratio (which could be called "the Activity ratio")

$$AR = \frac{F_R}{(F_{L1} + F_{L2})/2},$$

where F_R is the flow (ml/100 g/min) on the right side, F_{L1} and F_{L2} the flows on the left (control) side immediately preceding and following F_R. If, for example, a sequence of blood flows, with L = Left side (control) and R = Right side is: $L60$, $R25$, $L43$, $R23$, $L50$, $R27$, $L36$, then the ratios right side flow:mean preceding and following left side (control) flow would be

$$\frac{25}{(60 + 43)/2} = \frac{25}{51.5} = 0.49 \qquad \text{(i)}$$

$$\frac{23}{(43 + 50)/2} = \frac{23}{46.5} = 0.50 \qquad \text{(ii)}$$

$$\frac{27}{(50 + 36)/2} = \frac{27}{43} = 0.63 \qquad \text{(iii)}$$

This value was converted to a percentage (100 AR), and the arithmetic and geometric means, together with the standard errors of the means, were calculated. The application of the null hypothesis would then imply that these mean values should not differ significantly from 100%. Table 1 shows the results of all flows in experiments of this type, and use of Student's t test shows $0.475 < P < 0.4785$, $n = 8$, confirming the null hypothesis. This, therefore, confirms the impression derived from Fig. 10, namely that there is no significant difference in blood flow between the two sides of the anterior hypothalamus in the conscious rabbit.

TABLE 1

CONTROL EXPERIMENTS – XENON ONLY BOTH SIDES

No.	Left side (L) F	Right side (R) F	Mean L	$AR = R/\text{mean } L$	Log_{10} (10 R/mean L)
T51	50	54	46.5	1.16	1.064
	43	42	38.5	1.09	1.038
	34	37	34.5	1.07	1.030
	35	33	36.0	0.91	0.958
	37	37			
T55	27	22	25.0	0.88	0.946
	23	30	29.5	1.01	1.007
	36	25	30.5	0.82	0.912
	25	33	29.0	1.14	1.056
			Mean	1.01	1.001
				($\equiv$ 101%)	($\equiv$ 100.2%)
				(Arithmetic)	(Geometric)
			S.E.M.	0.014	0.019
			t	0.7142	0.065
			p	> 0.20	> 0.475

F = Hypothalamic Blood Flow (ml/100 g/min)
Mean L = Mean of two consecutive F on the left side.

Effect of intra-hypothalamic noradrenaline

The next series of experiments was evolved as follows. In each experiment one side of the hypothalamus was chosen at random and designated the control side. This side received [133]Xenon-in-saline injections only. The injection system on the opposite side was primed with the same [133]Xenon-in-saline solution to which *l*-noradrenaline (as the bitartrate) had been added, to make up a final concentration of 1 μg per injection (3 experiments), 2 μg (4 experiments), 10 μg (2 experiments), 20 μg (6 experiments), 40 μg (6 experiments), and 200 μg (2 experiments) per injection. In addition, in two experiments the effect of adding phenoxybenzamine, up to a final concentration of 50 μg per injection, to the 40 μg/injection noradrenaline–[133]Xe-saline solution, was determined; and in a further three experiments the effect of 50 μg/injection phenoxybenzamine alone was recorded. In another two experiments the effect of adding propranalol 20 μg per injection to the 1 μg/injection noradrenaline–[133]Xe-saline solution, was determined.

Arterial blood pressure (central ear artery) was measured using an ether pressure transducer.

The results of all experiments in which noradrenaline was added to the [133]Xenon-saline injectate are shown in Figs. 18–20. As in the control experiments described in the previous section, the "activity ratio"

$$AR = \frac{F_N}{(F_{C1} + F_{C2})/2}$$

was calculated. Here F_N is the hypothalamic blood flow (ml/100 g/min) on the noradrenaline side, and F_{C1} and F_{C2} the flows on the opposite (control) side immediately preceding and following F_N. Again, this ratio was expressed as a percentage,

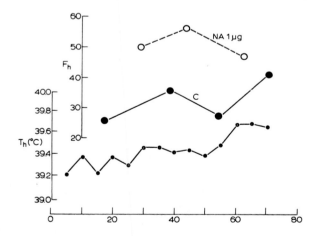

Fig. 18. A typical experiment, showing the effect on H.B.F. of NA (1 μg per injection) injected into the hypothalamus with the xenon (open circles, dotted lines), compared to H.B.F. values on the opposite side into which xenon only is injected (C = control; filled circles, continuous line). The lowest trace is hypothalamic temperature in °C.

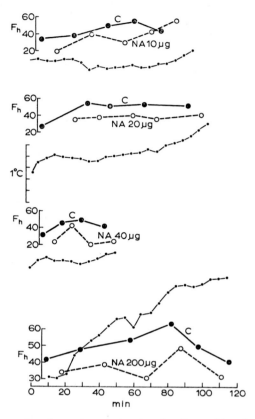

Fig. 19. Four typical examples of experiments showing the effects of intrahypothalamic NA, at four dose levels, on H.B.F. Closed circles and continuous lines are values for H.B.F. on the control side (C), and open circles and dotted lines are values for H.B.F. on the side into which NA was injected with the xenon, in doses of 10, 20, 40 and 200 μg per injection. Hypothalamic temperatures are also shown. Ordinate: H.B.F. in ml/100 g/min, and hypothalamic temperature, in °C. Abscissa: time in min.

and the geometric means calculated; the same test of significance as was used in the previous section was applied.

Fig. 18 shows, in one experiment, that noradrenaline, 1 μg/injection, increases hypothalamic blood flow; this is true of all the results using noradrenaline in this dose, the arithmetic mean value for 100 AR being 155.0 ± 12.7 (SEM), $P < 0.0005$, $N = 11$. The results for NA 2 μg/injection (Fig. 20) failed to show any significant effect on blood flow, mean $AR\%$ was 96.4 ± 23.9 (SEM), $P > 0.05$, $N = 18$. The results of experiments in which larger NA doses were used (10, 20, 40, 200 μg/injection) are shown in Figs. 19 and 20, and Table 2). At all of these dose levels hypothalamic flow on the treated side was significantly less than on the control side. The results of the tests of significance are shown in Table 2.

At all dosage levels NA produced a rise in the hypothalamic temperature (Figs. 19 and 20), but no significant change in systemic arterial pressure in those experiments

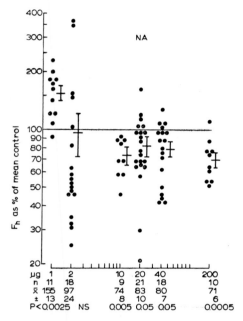

Fig. 20. Effect of intrahypothalamic NA on H.B.F. Ordinate: H.B.F. as a percentage of the mean control values (see text). Abscissa: dose of NA, in μg per injection. The means and S.E.M. for each dose are shown.

Legend: n = number of H.B.F. values in each group
x = mean
$\pm$ = S.E.M.
P = Significance value for difference of each mean from 100%.

TABLE 2

EFFECT OF ANTERIOR HYPOTHALAMIC INJECTION OF NORADRENALINE ON LOCAL FLOW

Drug	Dose ($\mu g/inj.$)	No. of injections	Mean AR%	P	Mean log$_{10}$ 10 AR	P
Control (saline)		8	101.0	N.S.	1.001	N.S.
NA	1	11	155.0	< 0.0025	1.175	< 0.0005
NA	2	18	96.4	N.S.	0.828	< 0.025
NA	10	9	73.5	< 0.005	0.854	< 0.005
NA	20	21	82.8	< 0.05	0.882	< 0.05
NA	40	18	79.5	< 0.05	0.874	< 0.0025
NA	200	10	70.9	< 0.0005	0.837	< 0.0025
Phenoxy	50	11	152.6	< 0.0025	1.168	< 0.0005
NA + phenoxy	40 } 50 }	7	137.4	< 0.005	1.166	< 0.0125
Propan	20	8	88.7	< 0.05	0.962	< 0.05
NA + propan	1 } 20 }	10	109.4	N.S.	1.027	N.S.

NA = Noradrenaline.
Phenoxy = Phenoxybenzamine.
Propran = Propranalol.
N.S. = Not significant.

in which B.P. was recorded. There was no change in arterial P_{CO_2} induced by the NA injections.

Effect of phenoxybenzamine

The addition of 50 μg of phenoxybenzamine to the NA 40 μg/injection, abolished the vasoconstrictor action of the NA. In fact the blood flow increased by 37% (Fig. 2 and Table 2). Phenoxybenzamine alone (50 μg/injection) increased hypothalamic blood flow by a mean of 52%.

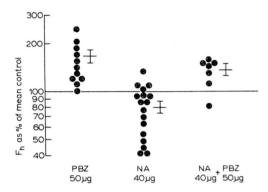

Fig. 21. Abolition of the vasoconstrictor effect of NA by phenoxybenzamine (PBZ). Ordinate: H.B.F. as a percentage of the mean control values (see text). The effects of 50 μg PBZ, 40 μg NA, and 40 μg NA plus 50 μg PBZ per injection are shown. Also shown are the means and S.E.M.

Effect of propranalol

The addition of 20 μg of propranalol to the NA 1 μg/injection, reduced the vasodilator effect of the NA from 55% above the control level to 9% above the control level (Table 2).

DISCUSSION

In 1959, Sokoloff wrote in his review of the pharmacology of cerebral blood flow: "Unlike the studies of epinephrine, those of *l*-norepinephrine have been few but clear and consistent". Häggendal (1965) demonstrated a "vasoconstricting effect" on cerebral vessels, of intravenously infused noradrenaline in the dog. In normotensive man, pressor doses of *l*-noradrenaline, whether administered intramuscularly (Sensenbach *et al.*, 1953) or by continuous intravenous infusion (King *et al.*, 1952; Moyer *et al.*, 1954; Fazekas *et al.*, 1960), produced either no change or a small fall in cerebral blood flow. The resulting increase in cerebrovascular resistance was interpreted at that time as indicating a cerebral vasopressor action of noradrenaline (Sokoloff, 1959). However, since we now recognise the existence of autoregulation, whereby the cerebral vessels have the capacity to regulate blood flow in response to changes in perfusion pressure, it is clear that an increased resistance can also occur in response to an elevated systemic arterial blood pressure. Thus the increase in cerebrovascular resistance following noradrenaline injection or infusion intravenously does not necessarily imply that the drug has a direct effect on the cerebral vasculature.

Green and Denison (1956), using an electromagnetic flowmeter to measure blood flow continuously in an isolated canine cerebral circulation preparation, showed that intracarotid injections of noradrenaline had no effect on the cerebral vascular bed. Greenfield and Tindall (1968) have investigated this problem in man. Continuous measurements of arterial blood pressure and flows in the internal and external carotid artery, using an electromagnetic flowmeter, were made during surgical exposure of these vessels. Intravenous administration of noradrenaline was accompanied by an increase in cerebrovascular resistance, injections of noradrenaline into the external carotid artery were accompanied by an immediate decrease in blood flow through that artery due to a direct action on the vascular bed supplied by the external carotid, while noradrenaline injections into the internal carotid artery had no immediate effect. It was concluded that noradrenaline had no direct action on the vascular bed, but that the increased cerebral vascular resistance following the intravenous administration of noradrenaline was due to autoregulation. Remarkably similar effects were observed after administration of adrenaline and angiotensin.

Whatever the role of a neural mechanism in the control of cerebral blood flow – and this is a question of considerable controversy (see Lassen, 1968; Scheinberg, 1968; James et al., 1969; for substantially opposing views) – there is no doubt that there is a rich adrenergic innervation of the cerebrosvascular system. The histochemical fluorescence method of Falck and Hillarp (see Falck and Owman, 1965) allows the direct demonstration of catecholamines in adrenergically innervated tissues. This technique has been applied to studies on the adrenergic innervation of the cerebral circulation system in rabbits, cats and dogs, and cerebral vessels have been found to have a rich adrenergic nerve supply (Nielsen and Owman, 1966; Falck et al., 1968) situated in nerve plexuses on the adventitial side of the media. The adrenergic ground plexus was less profuse in intra-parenchymal and pial arteries and arterioles in the brain than in the main arteries around in the circle of Willis. The isolated perfused rabbit ear artery is sensitive to noradrenaline applied via the lumen or via the medium bathing the adventitial surface of the artery, although the potency of intraluminal application is higher (De la Lande et al., 1966).

The subadventitial location of the adrenergic ground plexus, and the responsiveness of isolated blood vessels to externally applied drugs would suggest that parenchymal vessels in the brain might respond to externally applied drugs. Further, Baez (1969) has shown that, in the vessels of the rat mesentery, histamine and betahistine have prompter access to smooth muscle receptor cells when applied externally than when blood borne, and that these substances act on the same structures as do adrenaline and noradrenaline. It is therefore possible that the external administration of noradrenaline to blood vessels, that is through the adventitial side by intra-parenchymatous or intraventricular injections, is more appropriate to the study of adrenergic cerebral vascular control mechanisms than the use of the blood-borne route.

References pp. 151–156

Hypothalamic injections

The results of the present study suggest that there is a dose-dependent opposite effect of noradrenaline on hypothalamic blood flow in the conscious rabbit. Doses of 1 μg/injection produced an increase in local flow, and doses of 10 μg or more per injection reduce the hypothalamic blood flow, compared to the opposite (control) side. Changes of flow on the opposite (control) side are of interest. No change in control side was noted after injections of 1 μg and 2 μg NA. In the 10–200 μg NA/ injection range, however, there was an increase in control flow up to 60 min after the first NA injection, no net change in the 60–90-min period, and a reduction in flow after 90 min. Thus, in the first 60 min of the experiments the flows on the two sides changed in opposite directions, and in the period after 90 min, both sides showed a fall in flow.

These changes are explicable on the basis of a small dose of NA (1 μg/injection) causing a local vasodilatation, and a larger dose (10–200 μg/injection) a local vaso-constriction. The intermediate dose (2 μg/injection) produces no significant net change in cerebrovascular resistance. At the higher dose range (10–200 μg/injection) a small proportion of the injectate could diffuse the 3 mm across the midline to the control B.F. area. This fraction produces vasodilatation on the control side, as would the injection, directly into that side, of NA in 1 μg/injection doses. Repeated injections of the 10–200-μg dose will result, after 60 min, in an accumulation of NA on the control side equivalent to the local injection, on that side, of 2 μg/injection doses, with no net effect. Now, if the rate of diffusion of NA across the midline exceeds the rate of removal or inactivation of NA on the control side, then the concentration of NA will rise on that side. Therefore, the vasoconstrictor effects on the control side produced, after 90 min, by the further administration of 10–200 μg/injection doses, could be due to the accumulation, on that side, of concentrations of NA supra-threshold for vasoconstriction.

Other interpretations are possible; for example, that NA activates noradrenergic efferent neurones subserving reflex changes in blood flow distribution. Eliasson et al. (1951) and Hilton and his colleagues (see Hilton, 1966) have described hypothalamic areas, which when electrically stimulated, produce skin and intestinal constriction and muscle vasodilatation as part of a generalised defence reaction, and it is possible that these areas may be activated by noradrenaline. Little is known about the circu-lation in the brain following activation of these hypothalamic centres, but it is well known that electrical stimulation of those parts of the diencephalon and midbrain that integrate the defence reaction leads to a widespread activation of the brain, including the cerebral cortex (Starzl et al., 1951). There is, in turn, a high correlation between the frequency content of the EEG and the rate of cortical blood flow (Free-man and Ingvar, 1968), and a diffuse cerebral cortical vasodilatation might therefore be expected to occur in response to hypothalamic stimulation. In fact, it has been reported that 5-sec stimulation of the hypothalamus, just anterior and lateral to the mamillary bodies, can cause a 25–100% increase in cerebral blood flow lasting 5–6 min (Geiger and Sigg, 1955). The rise in arterial blood pressure will no doubt have contributed to the initial phase of this increase in flow, before autoregulation would normally be established, but the sustained increase in flow would suggest either abolition of the normal autoregulatory response to the rise in B.P. or else active neurogenic cerebral vasodilatation.

There are several problems associated with this latter hypothesis as an explanation of the local noradrenaline effect on ipsi- and contralateral hypothalamic blood flow. First, only increases in flow could be explained in this way. Secondly, the rabbits in the present experiments did not show the sympathetic activity characteristic of the defence reaction, namely pupillary dilatation, pilo-erection, pricking up of ears, etc.

Another possibility is that since noradrenaline injections into the hypothalamus cause an increase in body temperature, and since raising the body temperature by an increase in the environmental temperature produces a rise in hypothalamic blood flow (unpublished data), NA may increase hypothalamic flow via a non-specific effect on body temperature. That this is highly unlikely is suggested by the difference in response of the control and NA sides in the NA 1 μg/injection experiments. The control side showed no change in flow at a time when there was a significant increase in flow on the NA side; if there were an increase in cerebral flow as a result of NA-induced hyperthermia one might expect both sides to vasodilate *pari passu*. Further, in spite of the clear temperature-raising effect of NA in doses of 2 μg/injection, and in the range of 10–200 μg/injection, the former had no effect on hypothalamic blood flow, and the latter produced a fall in flow.

Effects of phenoxybenzamine and propranalol

The vasoconstrictor effect of 40 μg/injection of noradrenaline injected into the hypothalamus was antagonised, in fact reversed, by the addition of 50 μg of the alpha-receptor-blocking drug phenoxybenzamine. Phenoxybenzamine (50 μg/injection) alone increased blood flow. This is exactly analogous to the action of phenoxybenzamine in the human hand (Henning and Johnson, 1967), in which phenoxybenzamine infused intra-arterially produced a 30–40% increase in basal hand flow, and the vasoconstrictor action of noradrenaline was abolished. The vasodilator effect of 1 μg/injection of NA injected into the hypothalamus was antagonised by the addition of the beta-receptor-blocker propranalol.

These findings suggest that there are alpha and beta receptors in the resistance vessels of the hypothalamus, that beta receptors are activated by smaller doses of NA, and alpha receptors by larger doses. The net effect of the larger dose is an alpha-receptor-mediated vasoconstriction.

Adrenaline

Although not studied in the present series of experiments, a brief discussion of this catecholamine is relevant. Up to the late 1950's, it is probable that most studies of the cerebrovascular effects of adrenaline related to the natural adrenal medullary hormone.

This preparation, *e.g.* Adrenaline B.P. and Epinephrine U.S.P., contained appreciable amounts of (-)-noradrenaline (Auerbach and Angell, 1949; Goldenberg *et al.*, 1949) which has cerebral circulatory and metabolic effects which differ from that of pure adrenaline (King *et al.*, 1952; Sensenbach *et al.*, 1953).

Animal studies on the effects of adrenaline on the cerebral circulation have yielded conflicting results. Topical (brain surface) and intracarotid injections of adrenaline have been reported to produce vasoconstriction (Fog, 1939; Dumke and Schmidt, 1943; Faucon *et al.*, 1965) or vasodilatation (Forbes *et al.*, 1933; Norcross, 1938; Schmidt and Hendrix, 1937). Studies in man have failed to demonstrate any consistent action of adrenaline on cerebral blood flow (King *et al.*, 1952; Moyer *et al.*, 1954; Green and Denison, 1956; Greenfield and Tindall, 1968).

THE ACTION OF INTRA-HYPOTHALAMIC 5-HYDROXYTRYPTAMINE ON HYPOTHALAMIC BLOOD FLOW

The purpose of these experiments was to assess the effect on hypothalamic blood flow in the conscious rabbit, of 5-hydroxytryptamine (Serotonin, 5-HT) injected in doses which are known to affect the core temperature in the rabbit, 20, 40 and 80 μg as repeated injections directly into the hypothalamus. The same techniques and experimental design as were described in the last section for NA were used for 5-HT, and the results analysed in a similar manner.

Hypothalamic 5-HT

One hundred and twelve blood flow measurements were made in thirteen experiments on ten adult Chinchilla rabbits, weighing 2.5–3.0 kg. The rabbits were prepared, and the experiments carried out, in the same way as those described in the previous section. The injection system on the "test" side was primed with a ^{133}Xenon-in-saline solution (5 mC/ml) to which 5-hydroxytryptamine creatinine sulphate (May & Baker, Ltd.) had been added, to make up a final concentration (as 5-HT) of 20 μg (4 experiments), 40 μg (5 experiments) and 80 μg (4 experiments) per injection.

Rectal and hypothalamic temperatures and hypothalamic blood flow were recorded in all, and arterial blood pressure in some of the experiments. The experimental design was identical to that for the noradrenaline injection experiments described above.

Typical results are shown in Fig. 22. The same statistical analysis of the results was made as that described in the last section. Each blood flow measurement on the "test" side ($F_{5\text{-HT}}$) was expressed as a ratio (AR) to the mean of the control side flows immediately preceding and following it (F_{C1} and F_{C2}), thus:

$$AR = \frac{F_{5\text{-HT}}}{(F_{C1} + F_{C2})/2}$$

As in the case of the noradrenaline experiments, the arithmetic and geometric means

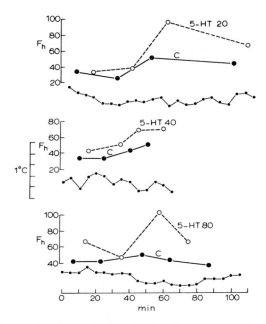

Fig. 22. Three typical examples of experiments showing the effects of intrahypothalamic 5-HT, at three dose levels, on H.B.F. Closed circles and continuous lines are values for H.B.F. on the control side, and open circles and dotted lines are values for H.B.F. on the side into which 5-HT was injected with the xenon, in doses of 20, 40 and 80 μg per injection. Hypothalamic temperatures are also shown.
Ordinate: H.B.F. in ml/100 g/min, and hypothalamic temperature, in °C. Abscissa: time in min.

expressed as percentages were derived, and tests of significance applied to these values with respect to 100%.

At all dose levels the hypothalamic blood flow was significantly greater on the 5-HT side than on the control side (Figs. 22 and 23). The arithmetic means were 124% (20 μg/injection), 154% (40 μg), and 169% (80 μg). No significant changes in blood flow with time were observed on the control side in these experiments. At all dose levels, 5-HT produced a small (0.05–0.2 °C) fall in hypothalamic and rectal temperature, which was transient lasting less than 10 min in all cases. No changes in arterial pressure were recorded following the 5-HT injections.

DISCUSSION

There is a large literature on the biosynthesis, distribution and possible biological significance of 5-hydroxytryptamine (see Page, 1958; Gyermek, 1961; Erspamer, 1963; Offermeier, 1965). Some aspects of 5-HT in thermoregulation have been reviewed (Cranston and Rosendorff, 1967 b) and this is the possible role of 5-HT in central nervous system activity that has preoccupied workers in the field in the past ten or so years. However, the early work on 5-HT was oriented around the cardiovascular effects, with often contradictory reports.

The effect of 5-HT on systemic blood pressure (B.P.) varies greatly according to

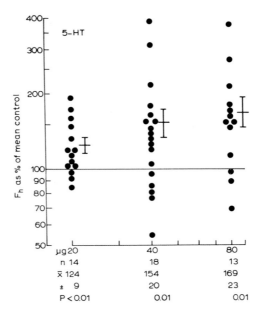

Fig. 23. Effect of intrahypothalamic 5-HT on H.B.F. Ordinate: H.B.F. as a percentage of the mean control values (see text). Abscissa: dose of 5-HT, in μg per injection. The means and S.E.M. for each dose are shown.

Legend: n = number of H.B.F. values for each group
x = mean
$\pm$ = S.E.M.
P = significance value for difference of each mean from 100%.

the animal species employed, the anaesthetic used, the route of administration, and the dose. For example, 5-HT causes vasoconstriction of most mammalian vessels – human forearm and umbilical vessels, rabbit ear artery and pulmonary vessels – and this is abolished by lysergic acid derivatives; according to Wurzel's (1966) recent work, however, 5-HT-induced contraction of the rabbit aorta is not inhibited by LSD, or by morphine, but is antagonised by another 5-HT inhibitor N-dimethyl-amino-N-benzyl-m-methoxycinnamamide (DBMC). On the other hand, the hypotensive effect of 5-HT in the rabbit, which has been suggested to be due to pulmonary vasoconstriction, is not altered by DBMC. Some vessels dilate in response to 5-HT, e.g. cutaneous vessels following intra-dermal or intra-arterial injection in man (Roddie et al., 1955), and others show a biphasic response ("amphibaric" in Page's terminology), or a dose-response relationship that, in some preparations, determines whether pressure will rise or fall (Page, 1958). In hypertensive patients the response to infused 5-HT was a small sustained rise of blood pressure, while in unanaesthetised neurogenic hypertensive dogs, it was a large fall (Page and McCubbin, 1956). Schmid et al. (1956) also found vasodilatation from slow infusion of 5-HT, but vasoconstriction when larger doses were given quickly. The possible mechanisms underlying these responses have been reviewed by Franchimont and Delwaide (1966).

There is surprisingly little information in the literature on the action of 5-HT on the vessels of the brain, an organ which contains a high concentration of the amine. This may be due to the prevalent opinion that 5-HT, being both lipid insoluble and ionised at physiological pH, does not readily pass the blood–brain barrier (Erspamer, 1961; Garattini and Valzelli, 1965; but see Bulat and Supek, 1967). However, interest in this field has been stimulated by the suggestion that 5-hydroxyindoles are involved in the pathogenesis of migraine (Curzon, 1968; Yahr, 1968; Anthony, 1968).

5-HT causes contraction of isolated segments of dog cerebral arteries (Bohr *et al.,* 1961), and local application of the drug to the middle cerebral artery of the cat causes prolonged spasm (Raynor *et al.,* 1961) as well as cerebral vasoconstriction in the monkey and baboon when injected into the internal carotid artery (Karlsberg *et al.,* 1963; Grimson *et al.,* 1969). On the other hand, Swank and Hissen (1964) have described an increase in cerebral blood flow in the dog. In man, it is suggested that 5-hydroxyindoles produce the small vessel vasodilatation that is one of the features of migraine, namely on the basis of the therapeutic effect in that condition of methysergide, a 5-HT antagonist (Sicuteri, 1959; Rooke *et al.,* 1962). Recent work has shown, however, that methysergide is inhibitory to a variety of vasoactive drugs, including kinins and histamine (Franchimont and Delawaide, 1966).

The present study has shown that 5-HT, when injected into the rabbit hypothalamus in doses of 20, 40 and 80 μg, causes a local vasodilatation. This cannot be due to a non-specific effect of body temperature change on hypothalamic blood flow, since an increase in skin and core temperature causes an increase in flow and vice versa. In the case of 5-HT, however, the increment of hypothalamic flow was associated with a small transient and variable fall in core temperature and cannot therefore be caused by it.

The absence of any significant effect on the control side would suggest that, unlike injected NA, any 5-HT which diffuses the 3 mm across the midline to the control side is insufficient to produce any effect on local flow.

On the other hand, intraventricular injection of 200 μg of 5-HT is followed by a sustained fall in hypothalamic flow (Rosendorff and Cranston, unpublished observations). Although this response is very variable, with a large scatter, this fall is statistically significant. The mechanism of this effect can only be speculated upon. It is reasonable to suppose that this action of 5-HT is a local vasomotor effect in the brain, and not the result of any change in systemic arterial pressure, since no such change was observed in those rabbits in which B.P. was measured. Also there is no reason to doubt that autoregulatory capacity was impaired in the 5-HT experiments, although this was not tested directly. This local effect could not have been due to the 200 μg 5-HT intraventricular injection producing, by diffusion, a hypothalamic 5-HT concentration equivalent to that produced by local injections of 20–80 μg of the drug, since these routes of administration and doses produced opposite effects. Therefore the effective local concentration of 5-HT achieved after the intraventricular injection must have been significantly greater or significantly less than that produced by the local 20–80-μg injections. There is a suggestion, in the dose-response curve shown in Fig. 22, that the greatest vasodilatation was caused by the largest local dose, and therefore progressively smaller doses, below 20 μg/injection, might be expected to produce progressively smaller vasodilator responses, until a dose is reached below which vasoconstriction is seen. A working hypothesis, therefore, is that the effective local concentration of 5-HT in the hypothalamus achieved after a single intraventricular injection of 200 μg of 5-HT, is considerably lower than that produced by repeated injections of 20 μg of 5-HT directly into the hypothalamus, and that this concentration has a vasoconstrictor effect. A dose-dependent, opposite, effect has been described with reference to the intravenous 5-HT action on arterial blood pressure (Page and McCubbin, 1956), and appears to apply to NA in the rabbit hypothalamus, so it is not inconceivable that a similar relationship exists in this situation. This hypothesis, unlike many others in the confusing and contradictory field of indole alkylamine pharmacology, is subject to relatively simple experimental testing.

SUMMARY

A method for measuring local cerebral blood flow in the conscious animal is described. The method depends upon the rate at which the physiologically inert, but freely diffusible isotope ^{133}Xenon, is cleared from its injection site in the brain tissue. A small volume (2.5 to 10 μl) of a ^{133}Xenon in saline solution is injected into the brain at the desired stereotoxic coordinate, via a fine stainless steel cannula. The rate of clearance is measured using an external scintillation counter, and the local flow (F) calculated as

$$F \text{ (ml/g tissue/min)} = \frac{\lambda \cdot \log_e 2}{T^{\frac{1}{2}}},$$

where $T^{\frac{1}{2}}$ is the half-decay time (min) of the clearance and λ is the tissue:blood partition co-efficient for ^{133}Xenon. λ is 0.74 in the rabbit hypothalamus.

Blood flow in the hypothalamus, a subcortical region of grey matter, is homogeneous within the area of diffusion of the tracer and within the limits of the technique. Pentobarbitone anaesthesia halves cortical flow; hypothalamic flow was unchanged. Autoregulation of local flow in the hypothalamus could be demonstrated within the mean arterial blood pressure range of 41–140 mm Hg.

One great advantage of this method is that it enables drugs to be added to the ^{133}Xenon–saline injectate, and therefore allows for an assessment of the effects of small doses applied locally to small vessels via their adventitial surface. Noradrenaline injected into the hypothalamus as 1 μg per injection caused an increase in local flow, while larger doses (10–200 μg per injection) were vasoconstrictor. The vasodilator effect of NA 1 μg, was blocked by propranalol, and the vasoconstrictor effect of NA 40 μg, was blocked by phenoxybenzamine.

5-Hydroxytryptamine was vasodilator at all doses studied.

The implications of these findings in terms of the possible neurogenic control of local cerebrosvascular tone are discussed.

APPENDIX

Correction to counting rate for ratemeter time constant

Symbols

RC – Ratemeter time constant; R – resistance; C – capacitance
K – biological decay constant; half-life $= \log_e 2/K$
N – activity of source at time t
N_0 – activity of source at time $t = 0$; $N = N_0 e^{-Kt}$
V_{out} – ratemeter reading at time t
I – current flowing through resistor (see essential ratemeter circuit, Fig. 24)

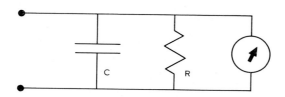

Fig. 24. Essential ratemeter circuit. (See text)

Q – charge on condenser at time t
q – charge delivered to condensor by each pulse from the detector.

The potential across the condenser is Q/C, therefore the current through the resistor, $I = Q/RC$.

The rate of charge on the condenser is the difference between the rate at which charge is supplied, and the rate at which charge is lost, *i.e.*

$$\frac{dQ}{dt} = N \cdot q - I$$

therefore

$$\frac{dQ}{dt} = N_0 \cdot q \cdot e^{-Kt} - \frac{Q}{RC}$$

or

$$\frac{dQ}{dt} + \frac{Q}{RC} = N_0 \cdot q \cdot e^{-Kt}$$

Solving this equation

$$Q\left(-K + \frac{1}{RC}\right) = N_0 \cdot q \cdot e^{-Kt} \qquad (a)$$

The complementary function is

$$Q = Q_0 \, e^{\frac{-t}{RC}} \qquad (b)$$

Combining (a) and (b)

$$Q = Q_0 \, e^{\frac{-t}{RC}} + \frac{N_0 \, q \cdot RC}{(1 - KRC)} \, e^{-Kt} \qquad\qquad \text{(c)}$$

If $Q = 0$ at $t = 0$, then

$$0 = Q_0 + \frac{N_0 \cdot q \cdot RC}{(1 - KRC)}$$

or

$$Q_0 = - \frac{N_0 \cdot q \cdot RC}{(1 - KRC)}$$

and the general solution (c) becomes

$$Q = \frac{N_0 \cdot q \cdot RC}{(1 - KRC)} (e^{-Kt} - e^{-\frac{t}{RC}})$$

The meter reading is proportional to the potential difference across the condenser and resistor which is Q/C, so the meter reading is:

$$V_{\text{out}} = \frac{A}{(1 - KRC)} (e^{-Kt} - e^{-\frac{t}{RC}})$$

where A is a constant of proportionality incorporating the constants N_0, q and R.
Re-arranging this equation:

$$V_{\text{out}} = \frac{A}{1 - KRC} \cdot (1 - e^{-\frac{t(1-KRC)}{RC}}) \cdot e^{-Kt}$$

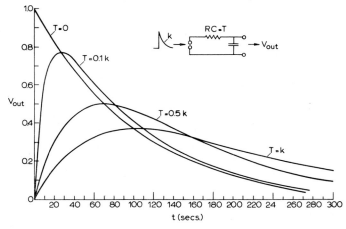

Fig. 25. Computer-derived curves showing the distortion produced in an exponential decay curve (k) by the recording system (*i.e.* ratemeter)tim e constant $RC = \tau$. The curve is unchanged only if $\tau = 0$. Curves for $\tau = 0.1\,k$, $0.5\,k$ and k are shown. For the derivation of these curves see *Appendix*.

Thus, for KRC of less than 1, the second term in brackets decreases as t increases, and eventually becomes negligibly small; so that M then falls exponentially with the decay constant K. Also this equation describes the relationship between the meter reading (V_{out}) and time (t), at various values of RC and K, from which the curves shown in Fig. 25 were derived.

ACKNOWLEDGEMENTS

Most of the experiments described in this paper were carried out in the Department of Medicine, St. Thomas' Hospital Medical School, London. Sections of the work were done in collaboration with the head of the department, Professor W. I. Cranston, to whom I am deeply grateful for advice, encouragement and support. I am also indebted to Dr. N. A. Lassen, Director of the Department of Clinical Physiology, Bispebjerg Hospital, Copenhagen, whose work first kindled in me an interest in cerebral blood flow, for his very helpful comments. Helpful advice and encouragement was received from Dr. S. S. Kety of Harvard University, Dr. K. Zierler, Johns Hopkins University, and Professor H. Barcroft, F.R.S., of St. Thomas' Hospital Medical School.

Financial support is acknowledged from the National Council for Research into Crippling Diseases, the British Heart Foundation, American Heart Association, the St. Thomas' Hospital Endowments Fund, Messrs. Roche Products Ltd., and Messrs. I.C.I. Ltd.

REFERENCES

AIBA, T., LANNER, L., STATTIN, S., WICKBOM, I. AND ZWETNOW, N. (1967) *Proc. VIII Symp. Neuroradiol, Paris.*

ANDERSEN, A. M. AND LADEFOGED, J. (1965) The relationship between haematocrit and solubility of Xenon-133 in blood. *J. Pharm. Sci.,* **54**, 1684.

ANTHONY, M. (1968) Plasma serotonin levels in migraine. *Advan. Pharmacol.,* **6B**, 203.

AUERBACH, M. E. AND ANGELL, E. (1949) The determination of arterenol in epinephrine. *Science,* **109**, 537–538.

AUKLAND, K. (1965) Hydrogen polarography in measurement of local blood flows; theoretical and empirical basis. *Acta Neurol. Scand.,* **41**, Suppl. **14**, 42–45.

AUKLAND, K. (1968) Measurement of local blood flow with hydrogen gas. In: BAIN, W. H. AND HARPER, A. M. (Eds.), *Blood Flow through Organs and Tissues,* E. and S. Livingstone, Ltd., London–Edinburgh.

BAEZ, S. (1968) Antagonistic effects of histamine and betahistine on the vasoconstrictor actions of catecholamines in mesentery microvessels. *Microcirculation, 5th Europ. Conf., Gothenburg, Bibl. Anat.,* **10**, Karger, Basel/New York, 1969, 292–297.

BETZ, E. (1968) Measurements of local blood flow by means of heat clearance. In: BAIN, W. H. AND HARPER, A. M. (Eds.), *Blood Flow through Organs and Tissues,* E. and S. Livingstone, London–Edinburgh, pp. 169–180.

BETZ, E., INGVAR, D. H., LASSEN, N. A. AND SCHMAHL, F. W. (1966) Regional blood flow in the cerebral cortex, measured simultaneously by heat and inert gas clearance. *Acta Physiol. Scand.,* **67**, 1–9.

BOHR, D. F., GOULET, P. L. AND TAQUINI, A. C. JR. (1961) Direct tension recording from smooth muscle of resistance vessels from various organs. *Angiology,* **12**, 478–485.

BOZZAO, L., FIESCHI, C., AGNOLI, A. AND NARDINI, M. (1968) Autoregulation of cerebral blood flow studied in the brain of cat. In: BAIN, W. H. AND HARPER, A. M. (Eds.), *Blood Flow through Organs and Tissues,* E. and S. Livingstone, London.

BRADLEY, A. F., STUPFEL, M. AND SEVERINGHAUS, J. W. (1956) Effect of temperature on P_{CO_2} and P_{O_2} of blood *in vitro*. *J. Appl. Physiol.*, **9**, 201–204.

BULAT, M. AND SUPEK, Z. (1967) The penetration of 5-hydroxytryptamine through the blood–brain barrier. *J. Neurochem.*, **14**, 265–271.

COOPER, K. E. (1966) Temperature regulation and the hypothalamus, *Brit. Med. Bull.*, **22**, 238–242.

CRANSTON, W. I., HELLON, R. F., LUFF, R. H., RAWLINS, M. D. AND ROSENDORFF, C. (1970) Observations on the mechanism of salicylate induced antipyresis. *J. Physiol.*, (in the press).

CRANSTON, W. I., LUFF, R. H., RAWLINS, M. D. AND ROSENDORFF, C. (1970) The effects of salicylate on temperature regulation in the rabbit. *J. Physiol.*, **208**, 251–259.

CRANSTON, W. I. AND ROSENDORFF, C. (1967 a) Monoamine oxidase inhibition and central temperature regulation in the conscious rabbit., *J. Physiol.*, **191**, 37–39.

CRANSTON, W. I. AND ROSENDORFF, C. (1967 b) Central temperature regulation in the conscious rabbit after monoamine oxidase inhibition. *J. Physiol.*, **193**, 359–373.

CRANSTON, W. I. AND ROSENDORFF, C. (1968 a) Local hypothalamic blood flow in the conscious rabbit. *J. Physiol.*, **204**, 25–26.

CRANSTON, W. I. AND ROSENDORFF, C. (1968 b) Hypothalamic blood flow in conscious rabbits; effects of monoamines and pyrogen., *Brit. J. Pharmacol. Chemotherap.*, **32**(2), 437.

CRANSTON, W. I. AND ROSENDORFF, C. (1969) The effect of noradrenaline and 5-hydroxytryptamine on local hypothalamic blood flow in the conscious rabbit. *J. Physiol.*, **204**, 108–109.

CRANSTON, W. I. AND ROSENDORFF, C. (1970) Acute effects of a monoamine oxidase inhibitor, tranylcypromine, on thermoregulation in the conscious rabbit. *Brit. J. Pharmacol.*, **38**, 530–536.

CURZON, G. (1968) 5-Hydroxyindoles and migraine. *Advan. Pharmacol.*, **6B**, 191–199.

DE LA LANDE, I. S., CANNELL, V. A. AND WATERSON, J. G. (1966) The interaction of serotonin and nor-adrenaline on the perfused artery. *Brit. J. Pharmacol. Chemotherap.*, **28**, 255–272.

DUMKE, P. R. AND SCHMIDT, C. F. (1943) Quantitative measurements of cerebral blood flow in the macaque monkey. *Amer. J. Physiol.*, **138**, 421–431.

ELIASSON, S., FOLKOW, B., LINDGREN, P. AND UVNAS, B. (1951) Activation of sympathetic vasodilator nerves to the skeletal muscles in the cat by hypothalamic stimulation. *Acta Physiol. Scand.*, **23**, 333–351.

ERSPAMER, V. (1961) Recent research in the field of 5-hydroxytryptamine and related indolealkylamines. *Fortschr. Artzneimittelforsch.*, **3**, 151–367.

ERSPAMER, V. (1963) In: U. S. VON EULER AND H. HELLER (Eds.), *Contemporary Endocrinology*, Academic Press, New York.

ESPAGNO, J. AND LAZORTHES, Y. (1965) Measurement of regional cerebral blood flow in man by local injections of Xenon[133]. *Acta Neurol. Scand.*, *Suppl.* **14** *ad* **21**, 58–62.

FALCK, B. AND OWMAN, C. (1965) A detailed methodological description of the flourescence method for the cellular demonstration of biogenic monoamines. *Acta Univ. Lundensis*, II (7), 1–23.

FALCK, B., NIELSEN, K. C. AND OWMAN, C. (1968) Adrenergic innervation of the pial circulation. *Scand. J. Lab. Clin. Invest.* Suppl. 102: VI, B.

FAUCON, G., DUCHÊNE-MARULLAZ, P., LAVARENNE, J., POTOCKI, B. AND FREDERICH, A. (1965) Effets circulatoires cérébraux de l'adrénaline et tonus vasomoteur cérébral. *Comptes Rend. Soc. Biol.*, **159**, 1703–1708.

FAZEKAS, J. F. AND BESSMAN, A. N. (1953) Coma mechanisms. *Amer. J. Med.*, **15**, 804–812.

FAZEKAS, J. F., BESSMAN, A. N., COTSONAS, J. J. JR. AND ALMAN, R. W. (1953) Cerebral haemodynamics in cerebral arteriosclerosis. *J. Gerontol.*, **8**, 137–145.

FAZEKAS, J. F., THOMAS, A., JOHNSON, J. V. V. AND YOUNG, W. K. (1960) Effect of arterenol (norepinephrine) and epinephrine on cerebral haemodynamics and metabolism. *A.M.A. Arch. Neurol.*, **2**, 435–438.

FIESCHI, C., AGNOLI, A. AND BATTISTINI, N. (1966) Mean transit time of a non-diffusible indicator as an index of regional cerebral blood flow. An experimental study in man with albumin I-131 and Krypton-85. *Trans. Amer. Neurol. Assoc.*, **91**, 224–226.

FIESCHI, C., BOZZAO, L. AND AGNOLI, A. (1965) Regional clearance of hydrogen as a measure of cerebral blood flow. *Acta Neurol. Scand.*, **41**, *Suppl.* **14**, 46–52.

FIESCHI, C., ISAACS, G. AND KETY, S. S. (1968) On the question of heterogeneity of the local blood flow in grey matter of the brain. In: BAIN, W. H. AND HARPER, A. M. (Eds.), *Blood Flow through Organs and Tissues*, E. and S. Livingstone, Ltd., London, 226–231.

FOG, M. (1938) The relationship between blood pressure and the tonic regulation of the pial arteries. *J. Neurol. Psychiat.*, **1**, 187–197.

FOG, M. (1939) Cerebral circulation I: Reaction of pial arteries to epinephrine by direct application and intravenous injection. *A.M.A. Arch. Neurol. Psychiat.*, **41**, 109–118.

FOG, M. (1939) Cerebral circulation II: Reaction of pial arteries to increase in blood pressure. *A.M.A. Arch. Neurol. Psychiat.*, **41**, 260–268.

FOLTZ, F. M., JOHNSON, D. C. AND NELSON, D. M. (1966) Methods for obtaining the venous outflow from the hypothalamus and hypophysis. *Proc. Soc. Biol. Med. Expt.*, **122**, 223–227.

FORBES, H. S. AND COBB, S. (1938) Vasomotor control of cerebral vessels. *A. Res. Nerv. Ment. Dis., Proc.*, **18**, 201.

FORBES, H. S., FINLEY, K. H. AND NASON, G. I. (1933) Cerebral circulation XXIV. A. – Action of epinephrine on pial vessels. B. – Action of pituitary and pitressin on pial vessels. C. – Vasomotor response in the pia and in the skin. *A.M.A. Arch. Neurol. Psychiat.*, **30**, 957–979.

FRANCHIMONT, P. AND DELWAIDE, P. J. (1966) Actions vasculaires de la serotonine chez l'homme. *Rev. Franc. Etudes Clin. Biol.*, **11**, 876–885.

FREEMAN, J. (1968) Elimination of brain cortical blood flow autoregulation following hypoxia. *Scand. J. Clin. Lab. Invest.*, *Suppl.*, **102**, V:E.

FREEMAN, J. AND INGVAR, D. H. (1968 a) Elimination by hypoxia of cerebral blood flow autoregulation and EEG relationship. *Exp. Brain Res.*, **5**, 61–71.

FREEMAN, J. AND INGVAR, D. H. (1968) Elimination of the cerebral blood flow EEG relationship and autoregulation by hypoxia. In: BAIN, W. H. AND HARPER, A. M. (Eds.), *Blood flow through organs and tissues*. E. and S. Livingstone, Ltd., London, pp. 258–259.

GARATTINI, S. AND VALZELLI, L. (1965) Serotonin, Elsevier, Amsterdam, p. 222.

GEIGER, A. AND SIGG, E. B. (1955) Significance of the hypothalamus in regulation of metabolism of brain. *Trans. Amer. Neurol. Assoc.*, 117–120.

GLEICHMANN, V. (1962) Regional cerebral cortical metabolic rate of oxygen and carbon dioxide related to the EEG in the anaesthetised dog. *Acta Physiol. Scand.*, **55**, 82–94.

GOLDENBERG, M., FABER, M., ALSTON, E. J. AND CHARGAFF, E. C. (1949) Evidence for occurrence of nor-epinephrine in adrenal medulla. *Science*, **109**, 534–535.

GREEN, H. D. AND DENISON, A. B. (1956) Absence of vasomotor responses to epinephrine and arterenol in isolated intracranial circulation. *Circulation Res.*, **4**, 565–573.

GREENFIELD, J. C. JR. AND TINDALL, G. T. (1968) Effect of norepinephrine, epinephrine and angiotensin on blood flow in the internal carotid artery of man. *J. Clin. Invest.*, **47**, 1672–1684.

GRIMSON, B. S., ROBINSON, C. S., DANFORD, E. T., TINDALL, G. T. AND GREENFIELD, J. C. (1969) Effect of serotonin on internal and external carotid artery blood flow in the baboon. *Amer. J. Physiol.*, **216**, 50–55.

GYERMEK, L. (1961) 5-Hydroxytryptamine antagonists. *Pharmacol. Rev.*, **13**, 399–439.

HÄGGENDAL, E. (1965) Effects of some vasoactive drugs on the vessels of the cerebral grey matter in the dog. *Acta. Physiol. Scand.*, **66**, *Suppl.* **258**, 55–79.

HÄGGENDAL, E., NILLSON, N. J. AND NORBACK, B. (1965) On the components of Kr^{85} clearance curves from the brain of the dog. *Acta Physiol. Scand.*, **66**, *Suppl.* **258**, 5–25.

HARPER, A. M. (1965 a) The inter-relationship between a P_{CO_2} and blood pressure in the regulation of blood flow through the cerebral cortex. *Acta Psychiat. Neurol. Scand.*, **41**, *Suppl.* **14**, 94.

HARPER, A. M. (1965 b) Physiology of cerebral bloodflow. *Brit. J. Anaesthesiol.*, **37**, 225–235.

HARPER, A. M. (1966) Autoregulation of cerebral blood flow: influence of the arterial blood pressure on the blood flow through the cerebral cortex. *J. Neurol. Neurosurg. Psychiat.*, **29**, 398–403.

HARPER, A. M. (1967) Measurement of cerebral blood flow in man. *Scot. Med. J.*, **12**, 349–360.

HARPER, A. M. (1969) Regulation of cerebral circulation. In: *Scientific Basis of Medicine Annual Reviews*, Univ. Lond. Athlone Press, pp. 60–81.

HARPER, A. M., GLASS, H. I. AND GLOVER, M. (1961) Measurement of blood flow in the cerebral cortex of dogs by the clearance of Krypton[85]. *Scot. Med. J.*, **6**, 12–17.

HARPER, A. M. AND JENNETT, W. B. (1967) Simultaneous measurement of beta and gamma clearance curves of radioactive inert gases from the monkey brain. In: BAIN, W. H. AND HARPER, A. M. (Eds.), *Blood Flow through Organs and Tissues*. Livingstone, London, pp. 214–225.

HENNING, M. AND JOHNSON, G. (1967) Interference of phenoxybenzamine and guanethidine with the vasoconstrictor responses of noradrenaline and angiotensin II in the hand. *Acta Pharmacol. Toxicol.*, **25**, 373–384.

HERMANN, E. (1968) Application of heat clearance method for measurements of cerebral blood flow in man. In: BAIN, W. H. AND HARPER, A. M. (Eds.), *Blood Flow through Organs and Tissues,* E. and M. Livingstone, London-Edinburgh, pp. 182–189.

HESS, W. R. (1932) *Die Methodik der lokalisierten Reizung und Ausschaltung subkortikalen Hirnabschnitte,* Georg Thieme Verlag, Leipzig.

HILL, L. (1896) *The Physiology and Pathology of the Cerebral Circulation; an Experimental Research,* Churchill, London.

HILTON, S. M. (1966) Hypothalamic regulation of the cardiovascular system. *Brit. Med. Bull.,* **22,** 243–248.

HØEDT-RASMUSSEN, K., SVEINSDOTTIR, E. AND LASSEN, N. A. (1966) Regional cerebral blood flow in man determined by intra-arterial injection of radioactive inert gas. *Circulation Res.,* **18,** 237–247.

HOMBERGER, E., HIMWICH, W. A., ETSTEIN, B., YORK, G., MARESCA, R. AND HIMWICH, H. E. (1946) Effect of pentothal anaesthesia on the cerebral cortex. *Amer. J. Physiol.,* **147,** 343–345.

INGVAR, D. H., CRONQUIST, S., EKBERG, R., RISBERG, J. AND HØEDT-RASMUSSEN, K. (1965) Normal values of regional cerebral blood flow in man, including flow and weight estimates of gray and white matter. *Acta Neurol. Scand.,* **41,** *Suppl.* **14,** 72–78.

INGVAR, D. H., LUNDMARK, T., RISBERG, J., VON SABSAY, E., BURKLINT, U. AND SUNDELIN, S. (1968) Recording of multiple clearance curves by means of a magnetic core memory. *Scand. J. Clin. Lab. Invest., Suppl.* **102,** XI H.

JAMES, I. M., MILLAR, R. A., PURVES, M. J. (1969) Observations on the extrinsic neural control of cerebral blood flow in the baboon. *Circulation Res.,* **25,** 77–93.

KARLSBERG, P., ELLIOTT, H. W. AND ADAMS, J. E. (1963) Effects of various pharmacologic agents on cerebral arteries. *Neurology,* **13,** 772–778.

KELLIE, G. (1824) On death from cold, and of congestions of the brain. *Trans. Med.-Chir. Soc.,* Edinburgh i, **84,** p. 123. Quoted by Hill, 1896.

KETY, S. S. (1960) Measurement of local blood flow by the exchange of an inert, diffusible substance. In: BRUNER, H. D. (Ed.), *Methods of Medical Research,* The Year Book Publ. Inc., Chicago, pp. 228–236.

KETY, S. S. (1965) Regional cerebral blood flow. *Acta Neurol. Scand.,* **41,** *Suppl.* **14,** 192–197.

KETY, S. S. (1965) Measurement of local circulation within the brain by means of inert diffusible tracers. *Acta Neurol. Scand.,* **41,** *Suppl.* **14,** 20–23.

KETY, S. S. (1965) Measurement of regional circulation in the brain and other organs by isotopic techniques. In: ROTH, L. J. (Ed.), *Isotopes in Experimental Pharmacology,* University of Chicago Press, Chicago, pp. 211–218.

KETY, S. S. and SCHMIDT, C. F. (1945) The determination of cerebral blood flow in man by the use of nitrous oxide in low concentrations. *Amer. J. Physiol.,* **143,** 53–66.

KETY, S. S. AND SCHMIDT, C. F. (1948) The nitrous oxide method for the quantitative determination of cerebral blood flow in man: theory, procedure and normal values. *J. Clin. Invest.,* **27,** 476–483.

KING, B. D., SOKOLOFF, L. AND WECHSLER, R. L. (1952) The effects of *l*-epinephrine and *l*-norepinephrine upon cerebral circulation and metabolism in man. *J. Clin. Invest.,* **31,** 273–279.

LAITINEN, L., JOHANSSON, G. G. AND SIPPONEN, P. (1966) Recording of regional cerebral circulation by an impedance method. A preliminary report. *Brain Res.,* **2,** 184–187.

LANDAU, W. M., FREYGANG, W. H., ROWLAND, L. P., SOKOLOFF, L. AND KETY, S. S. (1955) Local circulation of living brain: values in unanaesthetised and anaesthetised cat. *Trans. Amer. Neurol. Assoc.,* **80,** 125–129.

LASSEN, N. A. (1965) Blood flow of the cerebral cortex calculated from [85]Krypton beta clearance recorded over the exposed surface; evidence of inhomogeneity of flow. *Acta Neurol. Scand.,* **41,** *Suppl.* **14,** 24–28.

LASSEN, N. A. (1968) Preliminary experience with oscilloscope and Polaroid camera as recorder unit in a multichannel scintillation detector instrument. *Scand. J. Clin. Lab. Invest., Suppl.* **102,** XI: I.

LASSEN, N. A. (1968) Neurogenic control of CBF. *Scand. J. Clin. Lab. Invest., Suppl.* **102,** VI: F.

LASSEN, N. A., HØEDT-RASMUSSEN, K., SORENSEN, S. C., SKINHOJ, E., CRONQUIST, S., BODFORSS, B. AND INGVAR, D. H. (1963) Regional cerebral blood flow in man determined by a radio-active inert gas (Krypton-85). *Neurology,* **13,** 719–727.

LASSEN, N. A. AND KLEE, A. (1965) Cerebral blood flow determination by saturation and desaturation with Krypton-85 and evaluation of the validity of the inert gas method of Kety and Schmidt. *Circulation Res.,* **16,** 26–32.

LASSEN, N. A. AND MUNCK, O. (1955) The cerebral blood flow in man determined by the use of radioactive Krypton. *Acta Physiol. Scand.,* **33,** 30–49.

LEAKE, C. D. (1962) The historical development of cardiovascular physiology. In: *Handbook of Physiology, Circulation*, Vol. 1, 11–22.

LEWIS, B. M., SOKOLOFF, L., WECHSLER, R. L., WENTZ, W. B. AND KETY, S. S. (1960) A method for the continuous measurement of cerebral blood flow in man by means of radioactive Krypton (Kr[97]). *J. Clin. Invest.*, **39**, 707–716.

LOWE, R. D. AND DOWSETT, D. J. (1967) A catheter probe for measurement of jugular venous blood flow in man by thermal dilution. *J. Appl. Physiol.*, **23**, 1001–1003.

MCHENRY, L. C. JR. (1964) Quantitative cerebral blood flow determination, application of Krypton-85 desaturation technique in man. *Neurology*, **14**, 785–793.

MCHENRY, L. C. JR. (1966) Cerebral blood flow. *New Engl. J. Med.*, **274**, 82–91.

MALLETT, B. L. AND VEALL, N. (1963) Investigation of cerebral blood flow in hypertension, using radioactive-xenon inhalation and extracranial recording. *Lancet*, **i**, 1081–1082.

MALLETT, B. L. AND VEALL, N. (1965) Measurement of regional cerebral clearance rates in man using Xenon-133 inhalation and extracranial recording. *Clin. Sci.*, **29**, 179.

MONNIER, M. AND GANGLOFF, H. (1961) Atlas for stereotaxic brain research on the conscious rabbit. *Rabbit Brain Research*, Vol. **1**, Elsevier, Amsterdam.

MOYER, J. H., MORRIS, G. AND SNYDER, H. (1954) A comparison of the cerebral haemodynamic responses to aramine and norepinephrine in the normotensive and hypotensive subject. *Circulation*, **10**, 265–270.

MUNRO, A. (1783) Observations on the structure and functions of the nervous system. Creech, Edinburgh. Quoted by Hill, 1896.

NIELSEN, K. C. AND OWMAN, C. (1966) Control of ventricular fibrillation by a beta-adrenergic blocking agent (INPEA) during induced hypothermia in cats. *Life Sci.*, **5**, 1611–1623.

NILLSON, N. J. (1965) Observations on the clearance rate of beta radiation from Krypton-85 dissolved in saline and injected in microlitre amounts into the grey and white matter of the brain. *Acta. Neurol. Scand.*, **41**, *Suppl.* **14**, 53–57.

NORCROSS, N. C. (1938) Intracerebral blood flow: an experimental study. *A.M.A. Arch. Neurol. Psychiat.*, **40**, 291–299.

OBRIST, W. D., THOMPSON, H. K. JR., KING, C. H. AND WANG, H. S. (1967) Determination of regional cerebral blood flow by inhalation of [133]Xenon. *Circulation Res.*, **20**, 124–135.

OFFERMEIER, J. (1965) *Serotonin and its Derivatives. A study on Structure–Activity Relations*, Thoben Nijmegen, pp. 9–133.

OLDENDORF, W. H. AND KITANO, M. (1965) Isotope study of brain blood turnover in vascular disease. *Arch. Neurol.*, **12**, 30.

PAGE, I. H. (1958) Serotonin (5-hydroxytryptamine); the last four years. *Physiol. Rev.*, **38**, 277–335.

PAGE, I. H. AND MCCUBBIN, J. W. (1956) Arterial pressure response to infused serotonin in normotensive dogs, cats, hypertensive dogs and man. *Amer. J. Physiol.*, **184**, 265–270.

RAPELA, C. E. AND GREEN, H. D. (1964) Autoregulation of cerebral blood flow. *Circulation Res.*, **15**, *Suppl.* **1**, 205–211.

RAPELA, C. E. AND GREEN, H. D. (1968) Autoregulation of cerebral blood flow during hypercarbia and during hypercarbia and controlled (H+). *Scand. J. Clin. Lab. Invest.*, *Suppl.* **102**, V.C.

RAWLINS, M. D., ROSENDORFF, C. AND CRANSTON, W. I. (1970) The mechanism of action of antipyretics. In: *Pyrogen and Fever*, Ciba Foundation Symposium, in the press.

RAYNOR, R. B., MACMURTY, J. G. AND POOL, J. L. (1961) Cerebrovascular effects of topically applied serotonin in the cat. *Neurology*, **11**, 190–195.

RODDIE, I. C., SHEPHERD, J. T. AND WHELAN, R. F. (1955) The action of 5-hydroxytryptamine on the blood vessels of the human hand and forearm. *Brit. J. Pharmacol.*, **10**, 445–450.

ROOKE, E. D., RUSHTON, J. C. AND PETERS, G. A. (1962) Vasodilating headache: a suggested classification and results of prophylactic treatment with UML 491 (methysergide). *Proc. Mayo Clin.*, **37**, 433–43.

ROSENDORFF, C. (1969) Studies on hypothalamic blood flow and control of thermoregulation in the rabbit. *Ph. D. Thesis*, University of London.

ROSENDORFF, C. AND CRANSTON, W. I. (1969 a) Measurement of hypothalamic blood flow in the conscious rabbit by a radioactive inert gas clearance technique. 5th Europ. Conf. Microcirculation, Gothenburg, 1968. *Bibl. Anat.*, *10*, Karger, Basel–New York, pp. 292–297.

ROSENDORFF, C. AND CRANSTON, W. I. (1969 b) Application of the [133]Xenon clearance method to the measurement of local blood flow in the conscious animal. In: BROCK *et al.* (Eds.), *Cerebral Blood Flow – Clinical and Experimental Results*, Springer-Verlag, Berlin–Heidelberg–New York, pp. 36–38.

ROSENDORFF, C., LOWE, R. D., LAVERY, HELEN AND CRANSTON, W. I. (1969) Cardiovascular effects of angiotensin mediated by the central nervous system of the rabbit. *Cardiovasc. Res.*, **4(1)**, 36–43.

ROSENDORFF, C. AND LUFF, R. H. (1970) An indirect method for the determination of the tissue-blood partition coefficient for ^{133}Xenon. *J. Appl. Physiol.*, **29**, 713–716.

ROSENDORFF, C. AND MOONEY, J. J. (1971) Central nervous system sites of action of a purified leucocyte pyrogen. *Amer. J. Physiol.*, **220**, 597–603.

ROSENDORFF, C. AND MOONEY, J. J. AND LONG, C. N. H. (1970) Sites of action of leucocyte pyrogen in the genesis of fever in the conscious rabbit. *Federation Proc.*, **29(2)**, 1547.

ROY, C. S. AND SHERRINGTON, C. S. (1890) On the regulation of the blood supply to the brain. *J. Physiol.*, **11**, 85–108.

SCHEINBERG, P. (1968) Evidence for a brain centre regulating CBF. *Scand. J. Clin. Lab. Invest.*, *Suppl.* **102**, Vl: C.

SCHEINBERG, P. AND STEAD, E. A. JR. (1949) Cerebral blood flow in male subjects as measured by nitrous oxide technique: normal values for blood flow, oxygen utilisation, glucose utilisation, and peripheral resistance with observations on effect of tilting and anxiety. *J. Clin. Invest.*, **28**, 1163–1171.

SCHIEVE, J. F. and WILSON, W. P. (1953) The influence of age, anaesthesia and cerebral arteriosclerosis on cerebral vascular activity to carbon dioxide. *Amer. J. Med.*, **15**, 171–174.

SCHMID, E., WALTZ, H. AND FREUND, G. (1956) Zur Kreislauf- und Atmungs-wirkung von Serotonin (5-Hydroxytryptamin) am Wachen Hund. *Arch. Exp. Pathol. Pharmacol.*, **228**, 307–313.

SCHMIDT, C. F. AND HENDRIX, J. P. (1937) The action of chemical substances on cerebral blood vessels. *Res. Publ. Ass. Nervous Mental Disease*, **18**, 229–276.

SCHMIDT, C. F., KETY, S. S. AND PENNES, H. H. (1945) Gaseous metabolism of the brain of the monkey. *Amer. J. Physiol.*, **143**, 33–52.

SENSENBACH, W., MADISON, L. AND OCHS, L. (1953) A comparison of the effects of *l*-nor-epinephrine, synthetic *l*-epinephrine, and U.S.P. epinephrine upon cerebral blood flow and metabolism in man. *J. Clin. Invest.*, **32**, 226–232.

SICUTERI, F. (1959) Prophylactic and therapeutic properties of L-methyl-lysergic acid butanolamide in migraine. *Intern. Arch. Allergy*, **15**, 300–307.

SIESJÖ, B. K., KJÄLLQUIST, Å., PONTÉN, U. AND ZWETNOW, N. (1968) Extracellular pH in the brain and cerebral blood flow. In: LUYENDIJK, W. (Ed.), *Cerebral Circulation, Progress in Brain Research*, Vol. 30, Elsevier, Amsterdam, pp. 93–98.

SKINHØJ, E. (1966) Regulation of cerebral blood flow as a single function of the interstitial pH in the brain. *Acta Neurol. Scand.*, **42**, 604–607.

SOKOLOFF, L. (1959) The action of drugs on the cerebral circulation. *Pharmacol. Rev.*, **11**, 1–85.

STARZL, T. E., TAYLOR, C. W. AND MAGOUN, H. W. (1951) Collateral afferent excitation of the reticular formation of the brain stem. *J. Neurophysiol.*, **14**, 479–496.

SVEINSDOTTIR, E., LASSEN, N. A., RISBERG, J. AND INGVAR, D. (1969) Regional cerebral blood flow measured by multiple probes: digital computer and oscilloscope systems for rapid data retrieval. In: BROCK, M. *et al.* (Eds.), *Cerebral Blood Flow – Clinical and Experimental Results*, Springer-Verlag, Berlin–Heidelberg–New York, pp. 27–28.

SWANK, R. L., HISSEN, W. AND FELLMAN, J. H. (1964) 5-Hydroxytryptamine (serotonin) in acute hypotensive shock. *Amer. J. Physiol.*, **207**, 215–22.

TAYLOR, A. R. AND BELL, T. D. (1968) An intravenous isotope technique for estimating cerebral blood flow. Uses in the management of intracranial hypertension. In: BAIN, W. H. AND HARPER, A. M. (Eds.), *Blood Flow through Organs and Tissues*, E. and S. Livingstone, Ltd., London–Edinburgh, pp. 314–325.

WECHSLER, R. L., DRIPPS, R. D. AND KETY, S. S. (1951) Blood flow and oxygen consumption of the human brain during anaesthesia produced by thiopental. *Anaesthesiology*, **12**, 308–314.

WILKINSON, I. M. S., BULL, J. W. D., DU BOULAY, G. H., MARSHALL, J., ROSS RUSSELL, R. W. AND SYMON, L. (1969) Heterogeneity of blood flow throughout the normal cerebral hemisphere. In: BROCK, M. *et al.* (Eds.), *Cerebral Blood Flow*, Springer-Verlag, Berlin–Heidelberg, pp. 18–19.

WILSON, W. P., ODOM, G. L. AND SCHIEVE, J. F. (1953) The effect of carbon dioxide on cerebral blood flow, spinal fluid pressure, and brain volume during pentothal sodium anaesthesia. *Current Res. Anesthesiol.* **32**, 268–273.

WURZEL, M. (1966) Serotonin receptor in rabbit artery. *Amer. J. Physiol.*, **211**, 1424–1428.

YAHR, M. D. (1968) Discussion of 5-hydroxyindoles and migraine. *Advan. Pharmacol.*, **6B**, 201–202.

ZIERLER, K. (1965) Equations for measuring blood flow by external monitoring of radio-isotopes. *Circulation Res.*, **16**, 309–321.

Rapid Assessment of Cerebral Hemodynamics*

JOHN C. KENNADY

Laboratory of Nuclear Medicine and Radiation Biology and the Department of Surgery/Neurosurgery, UCLA School of Medicine, Los Angeles, California 90024 (U.S.A.)

INTRODUCTION

There is no question that the more information the physician has available to him regarding a particular intracranial problem, the more accurate and successful will be his assessment and treatment of the disease process. A carefully recorded history and neurological examination still ranks primary in importance inasmuch as the results from all of the diagnostic procedures have to elucidate and correlate with the clinical symptoms and signs.

The assessment of cerebral hemodynamics has involved the use of diffusible indicators based on the Fick principle (Kety and Schmidt, 1945, 1948; Lassen and Ingvar, 1961; and Glass and Harper, 1963), non-diffusible indicators (Nylin *et al.*, 1960; Oldendorf, 1962 and Kennady *et al.*, 1963) and the application of flowmeters on the carotid arteries (Hardesty *et al.*, 1961; Tindall *et al.*, 1963 and Greenfield and Tindall, 1968). Initially, total cerebral blood flow was calculated. Subsequently, it became apparent that significant changes could occur in regional blood flow without alteration of total cerebral blood flow. This prompted several investigators to use multiple small detectors, rather than a single large detector, for regional monitoring of the radioisotope tracer passage. Recording data from each source directly onto magnetic tape prior to graphic readout as a clearance curve increased quantity and progressively improved the quality of the results. Mathematical analysis of the temporal and spatial relationships between these multiple curves requires considerable time in order to determine whether a region of altered blood flow exists within the hemisphere (Zierler, 1965). The time factor has been improved with the use of a programmed computer (Sveinsdottir *et al.*, 1969). The accuracy of such calculations is dependent upon adequate detector collimation and minimum overlap of adjacent regions.

This paper is a review of our results using the image intensifier videocamera (Magnacamera®) and non-diffusible radiopharmaceuticals in the assessment of 175 patients with various types (*i.e.* acute and chronic vascular disease, vascular and avascular tumors, arteriovenous malformations, idiopathic seizures and trauma) of

* The studies reviewed were supported by Contract AT(04-1) GEN 12 between the Atomic Energy Commission and the University of California.

References pp. 188–189

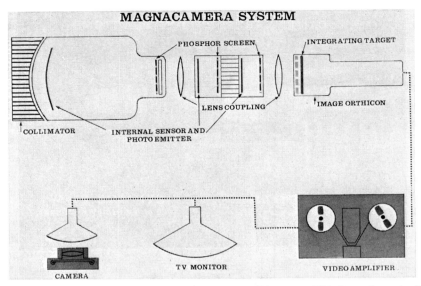

Fig. 2. The image intensifier videocamera (Magnacamera R) system. This is a schematic diagram showing the essential components. Not shown is the quantifier that couples between the videoamplifier and the television monitor described in the text.

TEST AGENTS AND INJECTION TECHNIQUE

The radiopharmaceutical of choice in these studies is [99m]Technetium-labeled human serum albumin microaggregates ([99m]TcAA), 1–8 microns in diameter. This test agent is made in the following manner: 6 to 10 ml [99m]TcO$_4$ is placed in a beaker with a magnetic stirring bar and heated at 55 °C. The solution is lowered to pH 1.5 with 2 N HCl. Then 0.05 ml ferric chloride (48.4 mg/ml) is added and let set 1 min. Next 15 mg ascorbic acid (100 mg/ml) is added without preservative followed by raising to pH 8.5–9.5 with 2 N NaOH. Then 5 mg human serum albumin is added and the pH is lowered to 1.0. The solution is stirred for 2 min and the pH slowly raised to 5.5–5.7. This solution is passed through a resin column and 5 % final volume/pH 5.6 acetate buffer is added through a 0.22-micron millipore filter. The resultant 8 to 12 ml is put in a 50-ml vial and placed in a large heated ultrasound bath for 8 min at 97 °C, then cooled. The particle size is checked under the microscope on a hemocytometer chamber. Usually the particle suspension has to be then placed in a cold ultrasound bath for about 5 min for correct particle size of less than 10 microns.

Initially the dose used was 5 mC and 1.0 ml, but with a recent increase in sensitivity of the videocamera system the dosage has been reduced to 2.5 mC and 0.2–0.4 ml. Similar amounts of [99m]Technetium pertechnetate have also been given when the aggregates are not available. The microparticles are similar in size to erythrocytes; they drift toward the anode in electrolysis and cinephotomicroscopic studies show that they do not clump together or with blood elements nor adhere to the vessel intima (Kennady and Taplin, 1965). Hence, there is one definite advantage in using

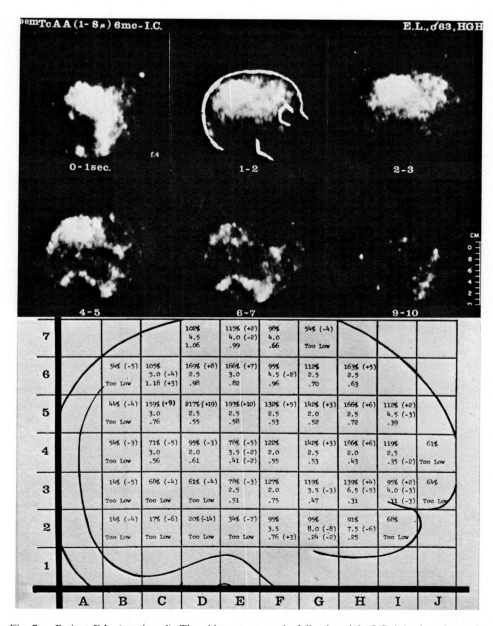

Fig. 7 a. Patient E.L. (continued). The videocamera study following right I.C. injection shows the tumor well in 1–2 sec and it retains the test agent longer than in adjacent brain. The quantifier results show a very high percent mean maximum ^{99m}Tc concentration in the tumor region compared to very low percentages and flow rates in the posterior and inferior regions.

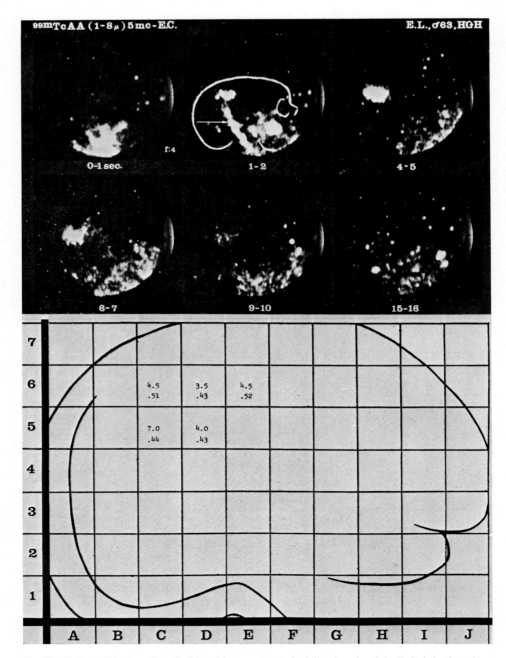

Fig. 7 b. Patient E.L. (continued). The videocamera study following the right E.C. injection shows the specific meningeal artery (arrow) supplying the tumor which appears smaller than in Fig. 7 a. The ⁹⁹ᵐTcAA does not appear to leave the tumor as rapidly; confirmed by comparing the inverse $T \frac{1}{2}$ values for respective 1.5-cm² areas.

region(s) of the hemisphere as clearly delineated areas of decreased radiodensity following injection of the radiopharmaceutical (Kennady, 1969 a).

Patient F.L., age 54 years, had adenocarcinoma of the lung with metastasis to his left hemisphere. Following his angiogram which showed a depression in the pericallosal branch of the anterior cerebral artery and no tumor "stain", the videocamera studies were performed (Fig. 8). In the superior frontoparietal region, an area of decreased radiodensity (arrows) is readily observed within 2 sec and does not show any evidence of additional test agent in later pictures.

The percent mean maximum ^{99m}TcAA concentration is significantly reduced at the vertex and in the anterior frontal areas on quantification (Fig. 8). This, along with marked reduction in the inverse T $\frac{1}{2}$ values, suggests impairment of blood flow through the anterior cerebral artery. By comparison, the inverse T $\frac{1}{2}$ values are significantly lower in the central parietal area but the concentration of the test agent is equivalent to the control group percentages. This would indicate impedance of blood flow in the middle cerebral artery bed caused by increased venous pressure resulting from early increase in intracranial pressure secondary to rapid tumor growth.

At operation, the dura was tense, the tumor area was quite necrotic for the most part and the total region involved corresponded in size and location to that seen in the camera picture. A subtotal removal was accomplished. The patient was subsequently given radiation therapy.

Cystic tumors

Patients with cystic tumors are not unlike those studied in the avascular group. They are often distinguished from the latter by demonstration of the vascular nodule within an avascular area by radiocontrast studies.

Both carotid and vertebral artery angiograms were done on patient L.L., 33 years, who complained of headaches and a visual field disturbance. The left internal carotid angiogram showed some elevation of terminal branches of the angular and posterior parietal arteries. The left vertebral angiogram demonstrated an avascular tumor with a small area of very fine blood vessels located posteriorly in the parieto-occipital region.

The videocamera study was done with the catheter in the vertebral artery (Fig. 9). It is well established that in the vertebral system the pressure gradient is lower and the blood flow volume is less than in the carotid system. Therefore unlike the carotid injection studies, a high concentration of the test agent is seen in the pictures taken during the first 6 sec following injection. In the 11–12-sec picture the nodule (arrow) is seen. The prolonged retention of the test agent is probably due, in part, to using ^{99m}Tc pertechnetate which has entered the extravascular space through an altered blood–brain (nodule) barrier after 15–20 sec. However, the dose given is approximately six times less than that used in routine brain scanning and there is a significant dilution factor.

Only the inverse T $\frac{1}{2}$ values are given in the lower half of Fig. 9 inasmuch as our series has no control patients with normal vertebral studies. It would appear that the superior and posterior portions of the nodule area have a slower flow than the anterior and inferior regions. Admittedly, these values are of questionable significance because

References pp. 188–189

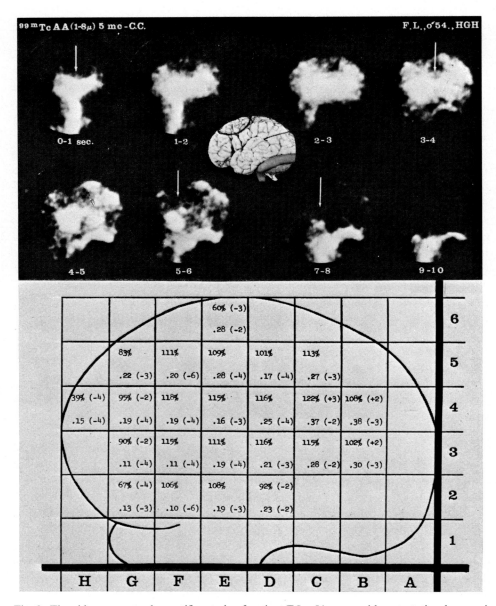

Fig. 8. The videocamera and quantifier study of patient F.L., 54 years, with metastatic adenocarcinoma in the left frontoparietal region. The avascular area is seen early and persists (arrows). Percent mean maximum ^{99m}Tc concentrations are low in this region with widespread decrease in the inverse $T\frac{1}{2}$ values.

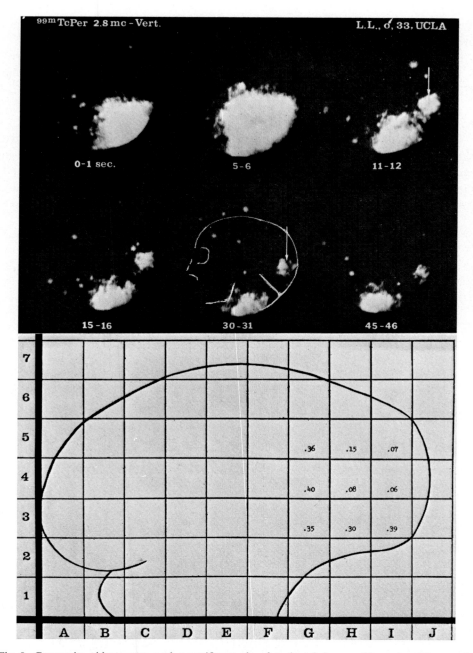

Fig. 9. Composite videocamera and quantifier study of patient L.L., age 33 years, with a cystic astrocytoma in the left occipital lobe. Following vertebral artery injection the cyst nodule appears later (arrow) and the inverse $T \frac{1}{2}$ values are very low in this region.

of the extravasating test agent. However, a recent patient given ^{99m}TcAA also shows low inverse $T\ \frac{1}{2}$ values in the region of her nodule.

This patient was operated upon successfully and a large cystic cavity was encountered in the parieto-occipital area with a well vascularized posteriorly placed nodule. Histologic diagnosis: Cystic astrocytoma gr ii.

Arteriovenous malformations

This is the most dramatic group of patients in the series in terms of rapid events. With the rapid drop in the blood pressure gradient between large arteries and large veins without an intervening capillary bed, blood volume and flow is increased and rapid imaging is paramount for the study of any details of the anomaly (Kennady *et al.*, 1968).

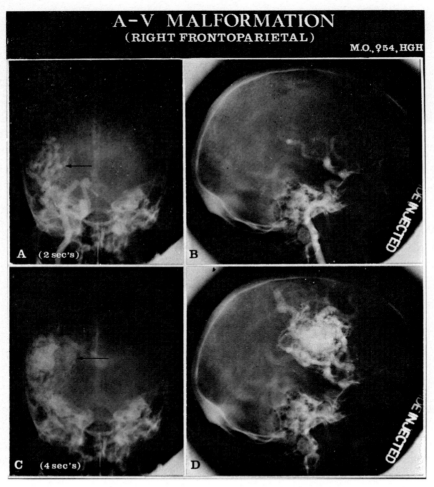

Fig. 10. Arteriovenous malformation. The right internal carotid angiogram of patient M.O., 54 years with a large frontoparietal A–V malformation. Note the early filling (2 sec) of markedly enlarged arteries (arrows); the racemose and two large draining veins are seen within 4 sec.

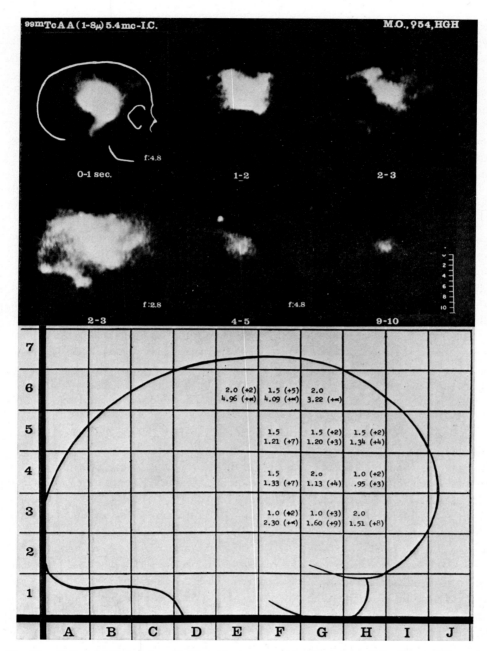

Fig. 10 a. Patient M.O. (continued). The videocamera study shows immediate filling of the malformation; the two draining veins in 1–2 sec and most of the ^{99m}TcAA out within 4–5 sec. The 2–3-sec picture is taken again at F : 2.8 to show minimal test agent in the adjacent cortex. Fast arterial–capillary times and very high inverse $T\ \frac{1}{2}$ values are seen in the racemose region.

Patient M.O., 54 years, was admitted to the hospital because of a syncopal attack. Her neurological examination was within normal limits except for a bruit over her right hemicranium. The angiographic study (Fig. 10) shows a large frontoparietal arteriovenous (A–V) malformation with the large arteries filling within 2 sec, the racemose and large veins in 4 sec. The right anterior cerebral artery and other branches are not visualized. The anomaly also received blood from the left side. The video-camera study (Fig. 10 a) shows the A–V malformation filling within 1 sec with little or no test agent entering the surrounding vasculature. The two veins seen draining the racemose in the angiogram are also demonstrated in the 1–2-sec picture. The major portion of the ^{99m}TcAA has passed through within 4–5 sec.

Only in the region of the A–V malformation is the concentration of the test agent high enough to be statistically significant to allow quantification. The arterial–capillary times are significantly fast in the majority of the areas and the inverse $T \frac{1}{2}$ values are the fastest flows recorded in this series (1.13 to 4.96 ml/mg/ml). In view of these results it is surprising that this patient did not have any significant neuro-logical abnormalities. Her syncope was undoubtedly precipitated by a stress situation that she has now been told to avoid. No operative procedure has been proposed at this time because of high risk of neurological impairment and she is being followed in the outpatient clinic.

Patient P.J., 27 years, exemplifies the more frequent history obtained in this group: headaches and the sudden onset of cephalgia with evidence of meningeal irritation and a cranial bruit. Lumbar puncture indicated slow subarachnoid bleeding. His angiogram demonstrated an A–V malformation in the right parieto-occipital region with a large draining vein into the lateral sinus. The anterior cerebral and all the middle cerebral artery branches were visualized.

In Fig. 11, his videocamera study shows one branch of the middle cerebral artery (probably the posterior parietal) primarily supplying the malformation in the 0–0.5-sec picture. The large vein draining toward the lateral sinus is seen after one second and the test agent passes through the racemose by 3.5–4 sec. There is little evidence of ^{99m}TcAA in other regions of the hemisphere and this is verified by the significantly low (−2 to 6 S.D.) percent mean maximum concentrations of the test agent seen on quantification. Only in the region of the malformation are the percentages higher than in the control group (+3 to 7 S.D.) whereas the arterial–capillary times and the inverse $T \frac{1}{2}$ values are similar. This may be explained on the basis of the test agent entering the subadjacent cortical tissue as well – adding to the maximum concentration of ^{99m}TcAA but prolonging the flow values. However, a more tenable explanation is the negating effect of the many points taken along the lower portion of the recorded downslope on the three sample times along the steep upper part of this slope when using the least squares method to determine the monoexponential fit. This situation did not arise in the first patient because of the close proximity of the malformation to the markedly dilated middle cerebral artery trifurcation branches with a perfusion pressure probably similar to that in the carotid syphon and a large blood volume. Together, this would produce the high peaks, fast arterial–capillary times and the very rapid ml/mg/ml flow rates recorded.

KENNADY, J. C. AND TAPLIN, G. V. (1965) Albumin macroaggregates for brain scanning. Experimental basis and safety in primates. *J. Nuclear Med.*, **6**, 566–581.

KENNADY, J. C. AND TAPLIN, G. V. (1967 a) Investigations of brain hemisphere scanning with radio-albumin macroaggregates. In: HIDALGO, J. U. (Ed.), *Symposium on Computers and Scanning*, Society of Nuclear Medicine, New York, p. 198.

KENNADY, J. C. AND TAPLIN, G. V. (1967 b) Shunting in cerebral microcirculation, *Amer. Surgeon*, **33**, 763–771.

KENNADY, J. C. AND TAPLIN, G. V. (1968) Regional cortical blood flow studies with radioalbumin macroaggregates. In: BAIN, W. H. AND HARPER, A. M. (Eds.), *Blood Flow through Organs and Tissues*, Livingstone, Edinburgh, p. 239.

KENNADY, J. C., TAPLIN, G. V. AND GRISWOLD, M. L. (1965) Arteriolar blockade studies with radio-albumin macroaggregates. *Reprint of Scientific Exhibit*, Presented at the American College of Surgeons Meeting, Atlantic City, N.J., Oct., 1965.

KETY, S. S. AND SCHMIDT, C. F. (1945) The determination of cerebral blood flow in man by the use of nitrous oxide in low concentrations, *Amer. J. Physiol.*, **143**, 53–66.

KETY, S. S. and SCHMIDT, C. F. (1948) The nitrous oxide method for the quantitative determination of cerebral blood flow in man: theory, procedure and normal values. *J. Clin. Invest.*, **27**, 476–492.

KING, E. G., WOOD, D. E. AND MORLEY, T. P. (1966) The use of macroaggregates of radioiodinated human serum albumin in brain scanning, *Canad. Med. Assoc. J.*, **95**, 381–389.

LASSEN, N. A. AND INGVAR, D. H. (1961) The blood flow of the cerebral cortex determined by radio-active Krypton[85], *Experientia*, **17**, 42–43.

MEIER, P. AND ZIERLER, K. L. (1954) On the theory of the indicator-dilution method for measurement of blood flow and volume. *J. Appl. Physiol.*, **6**, 731–733.

NYLIN, G., SILFVERSKIOLD, B. P., LOFSTEDT, S., REGNSTROM, O. AND HEDLUND, S. (1960) Studies on cerebral blood flow in man, using radioactive labelled erythrocytes. *Brain*, **83**, 293–335.

OLDENDORF, W. H. (1962) Measurement of mean transit time of cerebral circulation by external detection of an intravenously injected radioisotope. *J. Nuclear Med.*, **3**, 382–398.

ROSENTHALL, L. (1965) Human brain scanning with radioiodinated macroaggregates of human serum albumin. *Radiology*, **85**, 110–114.

SVEINSDOTTIR, E., LASSEN, N. A., RISBERG, J. AND INGVAR, D. H. (1969) Regional cerebral blood flow measured by multiple probes: An oscilloscope and a digital computer system for rapid data pro-cessing. In: BROCK, M., FIESHI, C., INGVAR, D. H., LASSEN, N. A. AND SCHÜRMANN, K. (Eds.), *Cerebral Blood Flow*, Springer-Verlag, Berlin, p. 27.

TINDALL, G. T., ODOM, G. L., DILLON, M. L., CUPP, H. B., JR., MAHLEY, M. S., JR. AND GREENFIELD, J. C., JR. (1963) Direction of blood flow in the internal and external carotid arteries following occlusion of the ipsilateral common carotid artery. *J. Neurosurg.*, **20**, 985–994.

YAMADA, H., JOHNSON, D. E., GRISWOLD, M. L. AND TAPLIN, G. V. (1969) Radioalbumin micro-aggregates for reticuloendothelial organ scanning and function assessment. *J. Nuclear Med.*, **10**, 453–454.

ZIERLER, K. L. (1965) Equations for measuring blood flow by external monitoring of radioisotopes. *Circulation Res.*, **16**, 309–321.

Regional Cerebral Blood Flow in Physiologic and Pathophysiologic States

MARTIN REIVICH*

Cerebrovascular Physiology Laboratory of the Department of Neurology, University of Pennsylvania, Philadelphia, Penna. 19104 (U.S.A.)

Because of the heterogeneity of perfusion rates in the brain and the focal nature of changes in various physiologic and pathologic states, it is important to be able to accurately measure changes in regional cerebral blood flow. Qualitative methods for measuring changes in regional cerebral perfusion consisting of observation of the superficial vasculature of a limited area of the exposed cortex (Forbes, 1928) or of the use of temperature-sensing devices on the cortex (Schmidt and Hendrix, 1937) were the only techniques available until the theoretical work of Kety in 1951. This work was the basis of the first quantitative technique for measuring regional cerebral blood flow (rCBF) developed by Landau *et al.* in 1955.

More recently methods for measuring regional cerebral blood flow have been developed which make use of detectors to measure radioactivity from small regions of the brain (Lassen and Ingvar, 1961; and Ingvar *et al.*, 1965). These methods enable repeated flow determinations to be made in the same animal and are applicable to man, advantages which the autoradiographic technique developed by Landau *et al.* does not have. However, they are not truly regional in the sense of being able to determine the flow in a discrete anatomic structure in the brain. They measure average flow in a cone of tissue which is "seen" by the probe. The autoradiographic technique remains the only truly regional method for measuring cerebral blood flow throughout the entire brain simultaneously.

AUTORADIOGRAPHIC METHOD FOR MEASURING REGIONAL CEREBRAL BLOOD FLOW

There are certain limitations to the original technique which utilized $[^{131}I]$trifluoro-iodomethane ($[^{131}I]CF_3$). This gas is not commercially available and must be synthesized for each experiment. Possible errors may be introduced by volatilization of the gas from the surface of the frozen brain sections. This was minimized by using thick sections, however, it was then difficult to prepare adjacent sections for histological comparison. The relatively high energy of the beta radiations (0.608 MeV)

* Associate Professor of Neurology, Department of Neurology, Hospital of University of Pennsylvania. Recipient of Career Research Development Award K3-HE-11, 896-05.

References pp. 225–228

of the ^{131}I label and its gamma emission lowers the resolution of the autoradiographs, and the short half-life of the isotope producers timing problems. Finally, the solubility of $[^{131}I]CF_3$ in blood varies with hematocrit. The partition coefficients between the various tissues and blood, therefore, vary from animal to animal. It is, thus, necessary to determine them in each animal. For these reasons and because of certain advantages to be pointed out, a modification of this technique was developed using ^{14}C anti-pyrine (Reivich et al., 1969).

Antipyrine is freely diffusable in total body water and its distribution in the body is proportional to the water content of various tissues (Brodie and Axelrod, 1950). This suggested that the brain–blood partition coefficient might be similar for all regions of the brain. The compound is very slowly metabolized in the liver (6% per hour) so that a possible error from this source would be negligible in the 1-min duration of the studies. The use of a ^{14}C label has several advantages. It is a pure beta emitter of low energy (0.155 MeV) and therefore produces autoradiograms of better resolution than ^{131}I. Furthermore, the long half-life of ^{14}C enables permanent standards to be made and allows a smaller dose of isotope to be used since longer exposure times are possible. The use of a non-gaseous tracer obviated its possible loss from the surface of the sections thus making it possible to use sections only 20 microns thick. This allows serial sections to be obtained so that histological studies can be undertaken along with the autoradiographic studies. Since the tracer is not gaseous, the autoradiograms can be made at room temperature instead of $-70\,^\circ$C.

This method is based upon the principles of inert gas exchange and in particular is an application of the Fick principle (Fick, 1871). This principle for a biologically inert, freely diffusable tracer substance may be stated as follows: The time rate of change of the amount of tracer substance within the tissue is equal to the difference between the rates at which the substance is brought to the tissue in the arterial blood and removed from it in the venous blood. It can be shown (Kety, 1960) that for a region of brain homogeneous with regard to flow this can be expressed mathematically as follows:

$$C_i(T) = \lambda_i k_i \int_0^T C_a(t)\, e^{-k_i(T-t)}\, dt \tag{1}$$

where $C_i(T)$ is the concentration of the tracer substance in that region of the brain at time T, λ_i is the tissue–blood partition coefficient of the tracer for that region, k_i is the flow per unit volume of tissue weighted by the reciprocal of λ_i, and $C_a(t)$ is the time course of change of arterial concentration of tracer material.

The assumptions upon which this technique is based are: (1) the region considered is homogeneous with respect to flow and solubility of the tracer material used, (2) no arterial–venous shunts are present, (3) there is instantaneous equilibrium achieved between the tracer material in blood and tissue, (4) the tracer is not metabolized by the tissue.

If the region being studied is not homogeneous with respect to flow or the tissue–blood partition coefficient, the venous blood from that tissue will not be representative of the tissue concentration of tracer even though diffusion equilibrium is present. This is because the average tissue concentration is influenced by the weights of the component areas while the average venous concentration is in addition weighted by the flows to the component areas. There is some evidence suggesting that the cerebral cortex and other gray matter structures are heterogeneous as regards flow even within areas 1 to 2 mm² (Lassen and Ingvar, 1961; and Fieschi, 1964). The error introduced by heterogeneity of flow within a region during the 1-min. duration of tracer material infusion, can be estimated as follows. The tissue concentration of tracer at 1 min in each component can be calculated using equation (1) and an appropriate value for k_i and λ_i. The mean tissue concentration, $\bar{C}_i(T)$, would then be given by:

$$\bar{C}_i(T) = W_1 C_1(T) + W_2 C_2(T) \tag{2}$$

where the subscripts refer to the two components. The mean flow predicted by this mean tissue concentration could then be calculated from equation (1), and compared to the true mean flow which for a two-component system is given by the expression: as shown by Ingvar and Lassen, 1962.

$$\bar{f} = W_1 k_1 \lambda_1 + W_2 k_2 \lambda_2 \tag{3}$$

Fieschi (1964) has found two components in the caudate nucleus, thalamus, and geniculate bodies with k_i's of 1.0 and 0.2 respectively. Assuming two components with these perfusion rates and weights of 60% and 40% respectively, the true mean flow would be underestimated by 10%. If the ratio of the weights of these components was 5 to 1 the error would be only 6%. Whether this degree of heterogeneity actually exists is open to question. Kety (1965) has presented some data on regional flow determinations performed at 1 and 2 min in a series of cats which suggests that the error introduced into the autoradiographic technique due to heterogeneity is not great.

The question as to the presence of arteriovenous shunts in the brain is more difficult to answer. The majority of studies of the angioarchitecture of the brain both in man and in experimental animals have failed to reveal any arteriovenous anastomoses in the cerebral vascular system with the exception of the leptomeningeal circulation (Campbell, 1938; Scharrer, 1940). Precapillary arteriovenous anastomoses have been observed in the pial circulatory system of man (Rowbotham and Little, 1965) but not in the brain parenchyma.

Particles up to 60 microns in diameter have been injected into the carotid arteries of dogs and have been observed to appear in the cerebral veins (Swank and Hain, 1952; and Benda and Brownell, 1960). This has been taken as indirect evidence for the existence of arteriovenous shunts. More recently precapillary channels joining arterioles with venules which measure 8 to 12 microns in diameter have been described in human brains (Hasegawa et al., 1967). Similar channels 6 to 8 microns in diameter were seen in dog brains. These channels were described as being present in abundance in the brain parenchyma. The physiologic significance of these anastomoses remains unknown and their effect, if any, on the measurement of regional cerebral blood flow is unclear.

References pp. 225–228

How well the requirement for instantaneous diffusion is met can be approached from several points of view. Copperman (1951) has calculated on the basis of the intercapillary distances present in gray and white matter that diffusion equilibrium should be virtually complete in less than one second. There are also experimental data available which support this theoretical prediction. Fieschi (1964) has measured blood flow in the white matter of the cat using H_2 electrodes and finds a value which is almost identical to that found by Landau *et al.* (1955) using $[^{131}I]CF_3$. The molecular weights of these gases have a ratio of $1:100$ which together with the larger intercapillary distances present in white matter should maximize any error due to diffusion limitation. The failure to find a discrepancy in calculated flow values supports the assumption that diffusion equilibrium occurs very rapidly.

The tracer material used in this technique, $[^{14}C]$antipyrine, is neither metabolized nor produced by the brain.

Thus, the assumptions upon which this technique are based appear to be fairly well fulfilled. In order to calculate the blood flow to a given homogeneous region it can be seen from equation (1) that one must know: (a) the tissue–blood partition coefficient of the tracer substance for that region of the brain, (b) the concentration of tracer substance in that region of the brain at some time, T, which has been chosen as 1 min, and (c) the time course of change of arterial concentration of tracer material from the beginning of its infusion to time T.

Since antipyrine is both excreted unchanged in the urine and metabolized in the liver (Brodie and Axelrod, 1950) in order to obtain a steady state for the determination of the tissue–blood partition coefficient the blood supply to the liver and the kidneys was occluded by ligatures in a series of rats prior to the intravenous injection of the $[^{14}C]$antipyrine. At the end of 1 hour a blood sample was obtained by cardiac puncture and the brain frozen and cut in half sagittally. From one half of the brain autoradiograms were prepared while from the other half, samples of white and grey matter were obtained and the concentration of $[^{14}C]$antipyrine in them determined. In 17 such determinations the tissue–blood partition coefficients for grey and white matter were found to be 1.00 ± 0.026 and 0.97 ± 0.026 respectively. There was no significant difference between these values so that the average value of 0.99 was accepted as the brain–blood partition coefficient for antipyrine. There was no difference for the value of the partition coefficient among various white or grey structures throughout the entire brain as demonstrated by the autoradiograms which showed a homogeneous density throughout.

The second factor which must be determined in order to calculate regional cerebral blood flow is the arterial concentration of tracer material during the 1-min period of infusion of this substance. A sampling system was used which enabled 0.04 ml blood samples to be collected every second. This system consisted of a Harvard peristaltic finger pump ($\#1201$) and a paper drive. The samples were collected as spots of blood on $\#3$ Whatman filter paper. Each spot was cut out and placed in a counting vial containing naphthalene dioxane phosphor solution and 1 ml of water, and counted in a liquid scintillation counter.

The correction for smearing in this sampling system was obtained by introducing

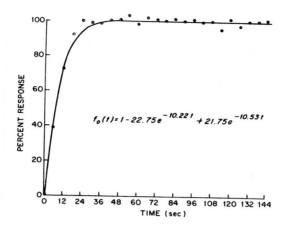

Fig. 1. Response of arterial sampling system to a step function input. Response can be described by an equation of the form illustrated, *i.e.*, the difference of two exponentials.

a step function change in $[^{14}C]$antipyrine concentration in the catheter system. The results of such an experiment are shown in Fig. 1. Such a smearing determination is done after each study with the animal's own blood before the catheter is removed from the pump. In this way any effects of changes in pump setting or blood viscosity are eliminated. The response of the system to a step function change in tracer concentration was found empirically to be adequately described by an equation of the form:

$$f_0(t) = 1 - A_1 e^{-r1t} + A_2 e^{-r2t} \qquad (4)$$

where $f_0(t)$ represents the concentration of $[^{14}C]$antipyrine at any time t, A_1 and A_2 are the relative sizes of the exponentials and r_1 and r_2 are their rate constants. Knowing the response, $f_0(t)$, of the sampling system to a step function change in concentration of isotope, the behavior of the system in response to any type of change in isotope concentration is defined. Using equation (4) and Laplace transforms, it can be shown that the relationship in operational notation between the true arterial curve, $C_a(t)$, and that after it has been smeared through the sampling system, $C'_a(t)$ is:

$$C_a(t) = \left[\frac{1}{r_1 r_2} D^2 + \frac{r_1 + r_2}{r_1 r_2} D + 1 \right] C'_a(t) \qquad (5)$$

where r_1 and r_2 are defined above and D^2 and D respectively are second and first derivative operators. Substituting equation (5) into equation (1) produces:

$$C_1(T) = \frac{\lambda_i k_i (k_i - r_1)(k_i - r_2)}{r_1 r_2} \int_0^T C'_a(t) e^{-k_i(T-t)} \, dt - \frac{\lambda_i k_i (k_i - r_1 - r_2)}{r_1 r_2} C'_a(T) +$$

$$\frac{\lambda_i k_i}{r_1 r_2} \cdot \frac{dC'_a(T)}{dt} \qquad (6)$$

thus defining k_i in terms of measurable variables. (See *appendix* for complete derivation of equations (5) and (6.)

Since equation (6) cannot be solved explicitly for k_i a computer program was written to make the computation of $C_i(T)$ by means of the trapezoid rule for various values of k_i.

Finally the tissue concentration of the tracer material must be determined. This is done by preparing autoradiograms from sections of the animal's brain. At time T which is usually 1 min after the start of administration of the radioactive tracer material the circulation to the brain is rapidly stopped by an intravenous injection of saturated KCl and the brain frozen. Effective cerebral perfusion is stopped by this method usually within 5 sec. In studies that have been performed in monkey fetuses (Reivich *et al.*, 1970 a) the whole animal has been dropped into isopentane cooled in liquid nitrogen.

The frozen brain is then cut into 20-μ sections in a cryostat which are picked up with a coverslip and immediately placed on a hotplate at 60 °C. The sections dry within 2 to 3 sec. Studies comparing the autoradiograms obtained by this method with those obtained from sections which were kept frozen at all times revealed no apparent loss of resolution with the quick drying technique. These sections were then placed on medical x-ray film with a set of standards containing known concentrations of [^{14}C]antipyrine. Thus, a calibration curve is obtained for each film relating optical density to isotope concentration. The calibration curve corrects for differences in exposure and developing that occurs between films.

Originally the standards which were used consisted of sections from the brains of rats which had been prepared as described above for the determination of the brain–blood partition coefficient. Standards prepared in this manner are good for only a limited period of time since being unfixed tissue they begin to deteriorate and changes in the [^{14}C]antipyrine concentration occur. Therefore, permanent standards have been made consisting of plastic containing [^{14}C]antipyrine which have been calibrated against freshly prepared rat brain tissue. This calibration also corrects for the fact that the plastic standards are of infinite thickness whereas the brain standards and tissue sections are 20 microns thick.

The tissue concentration of isotope in the various cerebral structures seen on the autoradiograms is determined quantitatively by measuring the optical density of the film and converting this value into isotope concentration by means of the calibration curve obtained for each film from the standards. The densitometer used in these measurements permits a resolution of approximately 1 mm^2.

Autoradiograms have been made after the injection of ^{131}I-labeled serum albumin which does not leave the vascular space (Landau *et al.*, 1955; Sokoloff, 1961). These studies demonstrated that the autoradiograms obtained with the use of freely diffusible tracers are not measurably affected by the quantity of isotope remaining in the blood in the various tissues but represent almost exclusively the concentrations of the tracer in the extravascular tissue. Thus tissue blood flow and not tissue blood volume is being measured by this technique, *i.e.* the contribution to the optical density from intravascular isotope is negligibly small.

TABLE 1

REGIONAL CEREBRAL BLOOD FLOW IN AWAKE CATS

	Landau et al. (1955) 10 Cats	Reivich et al. (1969) 6 Cats	P Value
Superficial cerebral structures			
Cortex			
Sensory motor	1.38 ± 0.12	1.09 ± 0.04	
Auditory	1.30 ± 0.05	1.22 ± 0.11	
Visual	1.25 ± 0.06	1.17 ± 0.04	
Miscellaneous association	0.88 ± 0.04	0.81 ± 0.05	
Olfactory	0.77 ± 0.06	0.74 ± 0.05	
White matter	0.23 ± 0.02	0.21 ± 0.01	
Deep cerebral structures			
Medial geniculate body	1.22 ± 0.04	1.43 ± 0.11	
Lateral geniculate body	1.21 ± 0.08	1.64 ± 0.14*	< 0.02
Caudate nucleus	1.10 ± 0.08	1.02 ± 0.07	
Thalamus	1.03 ± 0.05	1.06 ± 0.06	
Hypothalamus	0.84 ± 0.05	0.68 ± 0.06	
Basal ganglia and amygdala	0.75 ± 0.03		
Amygdala		0.54 ± 0.03	
Hippocampus	0.61 ± 0.03	0.62 ± 0.04	
Optic tract	0.27 ± 0.02	0.20 ± 0.01*	< 0.05
Midbrain and pons			
Inferior colliculus	1.80 ± 0.11	1.74 ± 0.08	
Superior olive	1.17 ± 0.13	1.08 ± 0.07	
Superior colliculus	1.15 ± 0.07	1.10 ± 0.16	
Inferior olive		0.75 ± 0.03	
Reticular formation	0.59 ± 0.05	0.65 ± 0.03	
Cerebellum and medulla			
Cerebellum			
Nuclei	0.79 ± 0.05	0.84 ± 0.03	
Cortex	0.69 ± 0.04	0.83 ± 0.03*	< 0.05
White matter	0.24 ± 0.01	0.24 ± 0.01	
Medulla			
Vestibular nuclei	0.91 ± 0.04	0.92 ± 0.03	
Cochlear nuclei	0.87 ± 0.07	0.95 ± 0.11	
Pyramid	0.26 ± 0.02	0.22 ± 0.02	

Values are means ± SE, given in ml/g per min. * Significant differences. All other pairs of values not significantly different.

Several factors may contribute to errors in the determination of the tissue concentration of tracer material from the autoradiograms. Since the sections are less than infinite thickness, any variation in the thickness of the 20-micron sections will produce apparent changes in [^{14}C]antipyrine concentration. Another possible error is the variability in the duplicate readings of the optical density of the autoradiograms. The magnitude of the error from these two sources was determined by making multiple readings on a set of 16 serial sections cut from a rat brain equilibrated with [^{14}C] antipyrine for 1 hour. The variation within sections was 1.9% of the mean optical density while the variation between sections was 5.6%. The variation within sections is probably due mainly to errors in making duplicate optical density measurements. The variation between sections includes this error plus the errors due to variations in the section thickness. Variability in replicate samples of the plastic standards is another source of error. This was reduced by exposing all the standards on x-ray film and reading their optical density. The most divergent standards in each group were discarded so that the resulting standard deviation of each mean value was no greater than 1.1% of that value.

The results obtained with the original and modified techniques agree remarkably well. In Table 1, twenty-three regions are compared in two series of awake cats in which regional cerebral blood flow was measured by these techniques. In only 3 regions was there a significant difference between the flows obtained with these two methods. At the 0.05 level of significance one would expect between one and two significant differences to occur by chance alone when this many comparisons are made. Therefore, there appears to be excellent agreement between these two autoradiographic techniques for measuring regional cerebral blood flow.

This technique for estimating regional cerebral blood flow has been used to study cerebral hemodynamics in a number of physiological and pathological conditions.

REGIONAL CEREBRAL BLOOD FLOW DURING SLEEP

In addition to the studies mentioned above in awake animals, measurements of rCBF have been performed during sleep with electroencephalographic slow waves (S-SW) and sleep with rapid eye movements (S-REM) (Reivich et al., 1968). There is evidence that S-REM, in contrast to S-SW, is a period of marked central nervous system activity. Evarts (1962) demonstrated a marked increase in single unit activity in the occipital cortex of the cat during S-REM. It was also shown (Evarts, 1964) that discharge frequencies of pyramidal tract neurons are about twice as great during S-REM as during S-SW. A marked increase in spontaneous unit discharge during S-REM was also recorded in the mesencephalic reticular formation (Huttenlocker, 1961) and in the lateral geniculate body and vestibular nuclei (Bizzi, 1965; and Bizzi et al., 1964). An increase in metabolic activity might be anticipated in association with this increased neuronal activity during S-REM. A consequent increase in cerebral blood flow might be expected as there is now a large body of evidence relating the metabolic activity of the brain and cerebral blood flow.

By means of thermal techniques, a relative increase in blood flow in the cortex and in the rhombencephalic reticular formation has been found while a relative decrease in flow in the mesencephalic reticular formation has been noted in cats during S-REM (Kanzow *et al.*, 1962; Baust, 1967). In addition, Kawamura and Sawyer (1965) measured increases in the temperature of the forebrain and hypothalamus during S-REM in cats.

However, quantitative studies of either total cerebral blood flow or regional flow during S-REM have not yet been performed. An attempt was, therefore, made to obtain such information.

Studies were performed in unrestrained, unanesthetized adult cats. The method of Scheatz (1965) was used for the chronic implantation of electrodes to record electrocorticogram (ECG), electromyogram (EMG) from posterior neck muscles, and the electro-oculogram (EOG). Catheters were placed in the femoral artery and vein. All operative procedures were completed at least 4 days prior to the experiment. Each animal designated for a sleep study was sleep-deprived for a period of 24–48 hours just before the experiment to encourage the occurrence of REM sleep and slow wave sleep. The animals designated for awake studies underwent no sleep curtailment.

Immediately before the regional blood flow measurement, an arterial blood sample was obtained and analysed for pH, P_{CO_2}, P_{O_2}, and haematocrit.

Six studies were done in awake cats, five in cats during S-SW and six in cats during S-REM. The criteria for S-REM were a low voltage fast ECG, silent EMG, and the presence of irregular rapid eye movements. In addition, observation of the animal regularly revealed twitching movements of the vibrissa and the extremities. During S-SW, the ECG showed high voltage slow waves, the EMG showed activity (although reduced in amplitude from the awake period) and rapid eye movements were absent (Fig. 2). There was no significant difference in the values for haematocrit, P_{CO_2}, P_{O_2}, or pH among the three groups (Table 2). Fig. 3 shows some representative autoradiograms from these studies.

There was a significant increase in flow in every one of the twenty-five regions measured during S-REM. This increase varied from 62% in the cerebellar white matter and sensory motor cortex to 173% in the cochlear nuclei. During S-SW, a significant increase in flow occurred in only ten of the twenty-five regions, and these

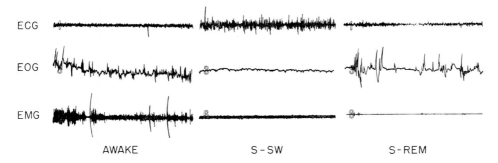

Fig. 2. Electrocorticogram (ECG), electro-oculogram (EOG) and electromyogram (EMG) recorded from an awake animal, an animal during S-SW and an animal during S-REM demonstrating the characteristic patterns seen.

References pp. 225–228

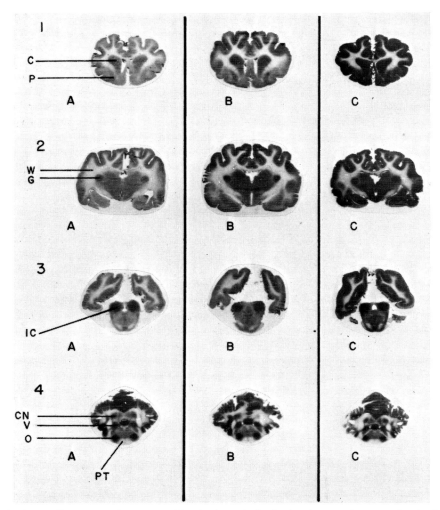

Fig. 3. Autoradiograms at four coronal levels through the brain of an awake control animal (A), an animal during S-SW (B), and an animal during S-REM (C). The structures labelled are (C) caudate nucleus, (P) putamen, (W) cerebral white matter, (G) lateral geniculate body, (IC) inferior colliculus, (CN) cerebellar nuclei, (V) vestibular nuclei, (O) inferior olive, and (PT) pyramidal tract.

TABLE 2

ARTERIAL BLOOD CONSTITUENTS

	P_{CO_2} mm Hg	P_{O_2} mm Hg	pH	Haematocrit %
Awake controls	34 ± 2.9	102 ± 8.4	7.44 ± 0.01	29 ± 6.6
S-SW	31 ± 1.8	84 ± 0.7	7.43 ± 0.02	22 ± 3.1
S-REM	32 ± 1.2	85 ± 1.3	7.44 ± 0.02	26 ± 1.1

Values are means ± S.E.

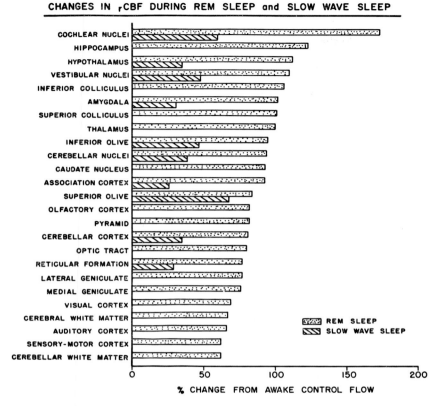

Fig. 4. Those regions of the brain showing a significant change in flow during S-SW and S-REM are plotted as a percentage change from the awake control flow.

changes were smaller in magnitude, varying from 26% in the association cortex to 68% in the superior olive.

Fig. 4 shows these structures arranged in order of decreasing change of flow during S-REM. Most of the structures with more than 100% increase in flow are located in the brain stem and diencephalon, while the least change in flow occurred in areas of the cortex subserving sensory and motor modalities, and in white matter.

The marked increases in regional blood flow found during S-REM substantiate the suggestion that the temperature increases measured in the brain during S-REM may be due to increases in blood flow (Kawamura and Sawyer, 1965; Wurtz, 1967).

Relative changes in cortical blood flow measured by a heat clearance technique demonstrated a 30–50% increase in flow during S-REM as compared to S-SW. The quantitative measurements of perfusion rates in the present study were in close agreement revealing an increase of 45–82% in the cortex during S-REM as compared to S-SW. The only other measurement of blood flow by heat clearance techniques (Baust, 1967) demonstrated an increased flow during S-REM in the rhombencephalic reticular formation and a decreased flow in the mesencephalic reticular formation.

References pp. 225–228

The magnitude of these changes was not reported. We found a 77% increase in flow in the rhombencephalic reticular formation during S-REM compared to the awake controls. The flow in the mesencephalic reticular formation was not measured.

The generalized increases in regional cerebral blood flow during S-REM support the possibility that this is a period of increased cerebral metabolism and activity. This hypothesis is further supported by the observations on the spontaneous activity of single neurons in the mesencephalic reticular formation, superior colliculi, visual cortex, pyramidal tract, and vestibular nuclei, which all show bursts of rapid discharges during S-REM. In contradistinction, during S-SW very little change from the quiet waking control was seen in the discharge rate of these neurons.

No direct studies of cerebral metabolism during S-REM have been performed. Brebbia and Altshuler (1965) measured total body oxygen utilization in man during sleep and found that it was greatest during S-REM and least during stages III and IV of S-SW. During S-SW Hyden and Lange (1965) showed that there is a two- to three-fold increase in succinate oxidase activity in cells of the reticular formation. This enzyme plays an important role in the aerobic metabolism of glucose and in the energy production of the brain. However, Mangold et al. (1955) found no significant change in the overall cerebral metabolic rate for oxygen during S-SW in man. They did, however, find a significant increase in total cerebral blood flow of the order of 10%. If the twenty-five regions investigated in the present study are weighted according to their relative sizes, an increase of about 15% in total cerebral blood flow would be expected during S-SW. A similar calculation shows that approximately an 80% increase in total cerebral blood flow would occur during S-REM.

No direct evidence concerning the method of production of the large blood flow changes seen during S-REM is provided by this study. It cannot be attributed to changes in arterial P_{O_2}, P_{CO_2}, or pH. A decrease in neurogenic vasoconstrictor tone must be considered but there is little evidence to support such an hypothesis. Blood pressure changes were not monitored during these studies. However, it is not likely that they could account for the flow changes seen during S-REM since, although blood pressure becomes erratic, it does not show large and consistent increases (Snyder et al., 1964). Furthermore, one would also have to postulate a loss of auto-regulation during S-REM in order to incriminate changes in blood pressure as causing flow changes. Thus the most likely hypothesis is that local increases in cerebral metabolism may be the important factor in producing the regional changes in blood flow demonstrated. The performance of cerebral metabolic studies during S-REM may shed further light on the method of production and significance of these large increases in flow that have been found.

REGIONAL CEREBRAL BLOOD FLOW FOLLOWING TRAUMA

The effects of cerebral trauma on regional changes in the control of cerebral blood flow have been investigated (Reivich et al., 1970 b). Duret, as early as 1878 postulated that cerebral vasomotor paralysis with consequent production of cerebral edema resulted from cerebral trauma. Similar suggestions have been made by others (Evans and Scheinker, 1945; Courville, 1942; Rand and Courville, 1931; Langfitt *et al.*, 1968). The latter have shown that blunt non-necrotizing trauma to the exposed cortex followed by arterial hypertension caused acute brain swelling. It was postulated that cerebral autoregulation had been abolished or diminished by the trauma and that the subsequent increase in arterial pressure was transmitted to the capillaries and veins producing an increased hydrostatic gradient across the capillary membrane with resultant cerebral edema. Fog (1968) has stated that in his studies on the vasomotor reactions of pial arteries, autoregulation was abolished in those animals in whom trauma to the brain had occurred during preparation.

Although cerebral blood flow has been studied after acute head injury in experimental animals (Denny-Brown and Russell, 1941; Brown and Brown, 1954; German *et al.*, 1947; Meyer and Denny-Brown, 1955; Meyer *et al.*, 1969) and man (Taylor and Bell, 1966; Taylor, 1969; Baldy-Moulinier and Frerebeau, 1969) no systematic attempt has been made to directly investigate the autoregulatory response of the cerebral vessels in this condition. Experiments were, therefore, undertaken to investigate the changes in vasomotor tone and the autoregulatory ability of the brain following mechanical trauma to the cerebral cortex.

A series of cats was studied in which a bilateral craniotomy was performed under light anesthesia with 70% nitrous oxide and 30% oxygen after an induction with thiopental. The animals were paralyzed with gallamine and artificially respired. End tidal P_{CO_2} was continuously monitored and intermittent arterial samples were obtained for P_{CO_2}, P_{O_2} and pH. Arterial blood pressure and sagittal sinus pressure were recorded.

In order to avoid damage to the underlying brain during the craniotomy, fluid was withdrawn from the cisterna magna allowing the brain to fall away from the overlying skull. The dura was opened and reflected and the brain covered with a thin polyethylene sheet in order to prevent drying or the escape of Krypton-85 from the brain during the blood flow studies. When the preparation was complete, 1 ml/kg body weight of a 3% solution of Evans blue dye in saline was injected intravenously. After an interval of 30 min the brain was inspected to see whether there was any blue staining. If this was present, it was presumed that the brain had been traumatized during preparation and the animal was discarded.

Regional cerebral blood flow was measured by two techniques. Two end window Geiger–Mueller tubes 0.5 inches in diameter were placed over homologous areas of the exposed cortex. Krypton-85 dissolved in saline was infused via a catheter placed in each common carotid artery and its cortical clearance was monitored from both hemispheres before and after mechanical trauma to the cerebral cortex at various levels of mean arterial pressure. Regional cerebral blood flow was also measured after cerebral trauma by the autoradiographic technique.

Arterial pressure was lowered by slowly bleeding the animal into an heparinized syringe and then raised by reinjecting the blood.

After control measurements were obtained one hemisphere was traumatized by means of a jet of compressed nitrogen at 50 lbs/square inch delivered from a fixed distance of 2 cm from the surface of the brain. The duration of the blast and the

interval between blasts was controlled. The normal square wave form of the release
of gas was modified to that of a sine wave in order to prevent sudden displacement
of the whole brain and tearing of bridging veins. The brain was depressed approximately 4 mm with each impulse. The duration of each blast was $\frac{1}{2}$ sec and the interval
between blasts was 2 sec. Twelve such blasts were administered.

During the control studies the mean $\pm$ standard error arterial P_{CO_2} was 29.3 $\pm$
0.6 mm Hg while during the post-trauma measurements the value was 28.9 $\pm$ 0.9 mm
Hg. The mean $\pm$ S.E. arterial P_{O_2} was 123 $\pm$ 3.8 mm Hg during the control phase
and 126 $\pm$ 4.9 mm Hg following trauma. The mean $\pm$ S.E. arterial pH was 7.378 $\pm$
0.025 and 7.370 $\pm$ 0.032 in the control and post-trauma studies respectively. There were
no significant differences between any of these measurements. During the control
studies the autoregulatory ability of the cortex was demonstrated to be intact. Mean
arterial pressure was changed from 75 to 187 mm Hg without any significant effect
on cortical blood flow. Following cerebral trauma mean arterial pressure was varied
from 65 to 215 mm Hg. Cortical blood flow passively followed the changes in mean
arterial pressure indicating a loss of autoregulation. The regression lines and 95%
confidence limits for the control and post-trauma data are shown in Fig. 5. There is a

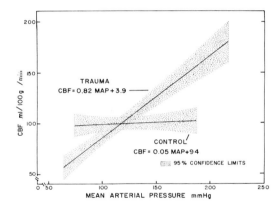

Fig. 5. The regression lines relating cortical blood flow (CBF) and mean arterial pressure (MAP)
for the control and post-trauma data are shown with their 95% confidence limits. There is a highly
significant difference between the slopes of the two lines ($p < 0.001$). The slope of the control data is
not significantly different from zero.

highly significant difference between the slopes of these two lines ($p < 0.001$). The
slope of the control data is not significantly different from zero. If the cortical blood
flow data in the region of normal mean arterial pressure in these animals, i.e. about
120 mm Hg, are examined, no significant difference is seen between the control and
trauma studies. This suggests that a primary vasodilation does not occur after trauma
under these conditions.

A loss of autoregulation was also demonstrated by the autoradiographic regional
cerebral blood flow studies. In addition these studies provided information regarding
the distribution of these changes in autoregulation. Usually the loss of autoregulation

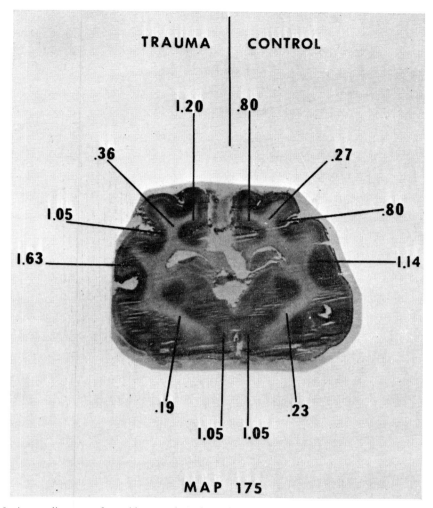

Fig. 6. Autoradiogram of a mid-coronal section of the brain in an animal whose mean arterial pressure (MAP) was elevated to 175 mm Hg. In the traumatized hemisphere the flows in the cortex and subcortical white matter are higher than in the control hemisphere. The deep midline structures do not show this difference in flow. The numbers are flow values in ml/g/min.

was confined to the traumatized hemisphere but did extend to areas in that hemisphere not directly traumatized. These changes were most marked in the cortex and underlying white matter while more deeply placed structures such as the thalamus, hypothalamus and the basal ganglia did not show much change in flow. Structures in the posterior fossa also were unaffected. In one of the animals studied, loss of autoregulation was also seen in parts of the opposite non-traumatized hemisphere. Fig. 6, 7, and 8 show autoradiograms from animals whose mean arterial pressure was 175, 100 and 75 mm Hg respectively. The areas of loss of autoregulation in the cortex and underlying white matter of the traumatized hemisphere are clearly seen.

References pp. 225–228

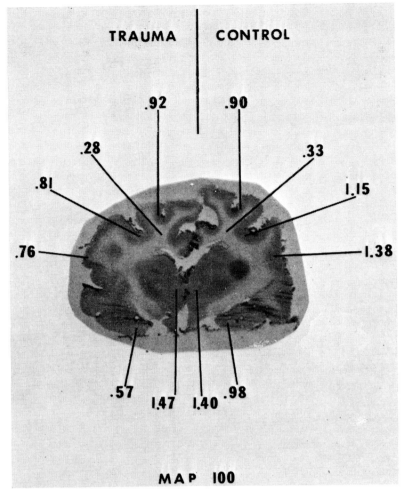

Fig. 7. Autoradiogram of a mid-coronal section of the brain in an animal whose mean arterial pressure (MAP) was reduced to 100 mm Hg. Reductions in flow are present in the cortex and white matter of the traumatized hemisphere. These changes are also present in regions not directly traumatized in the same hemisphere. The deep midline structures do not show these changes. The numbers are flow values in ml/g/min.

Cerebrosvascular resistance was calculated from these data and plotted against mean arterial pressure as shown in Fig. 9. There is a highly significant difference ($p < 0.001$) between the slopes of the regression lines relating cerebrovascular resistance and mean arterial pressure for the control and post-trauma data. The slope of the post-trauma data is not significantly different from zero. These data demonstrate that the reactivity of the cerebral vessels is abolished after trauma and that a constant value of cerebrovascular resistance is maintained. This value is not significantly different from the normotensive control value. Thus, lack of vasomotor reactivity or vasomotor paralysis is present without vasodilation following mechanical trauma

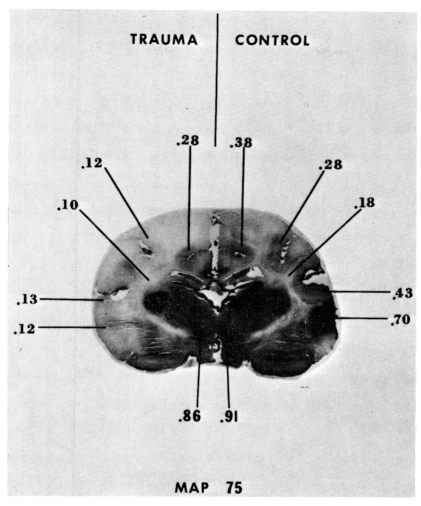

Fig. 8. Autoradiogram of a mid-coronal section of the brain in an animal whose mean arterial pressure (MAP) was reduced to 75 mm Hg. Marked reductions in flow are present in the cortex and white matter of the traumatized hemisphere. These changes are also present in regions not directly traumatized in the same and contralateral hemispheres. The deep midline structures do not show these changes. The numbers are flow values in ml/g/min.

to the cortex. This lack of vasodilation was found to be present over the entire range of mean arterial pressures studied in these experiments.

Almost one hundred years ago, Duret (1878) postulated that the loss of vasomotor control plays a role in the production of cerebral edema and the clinical manifestations of head injury. Courtney in 1899 suggested that vasoparalysis and accompanying vasodilation was followed by passage of water into the brain parenchyma. Evans and Scheinker in 1945 hypothesized that trauma caused vasoparalysis of the capillaries and venules with slowing of blood flow. The latter then produced hypoxia and an

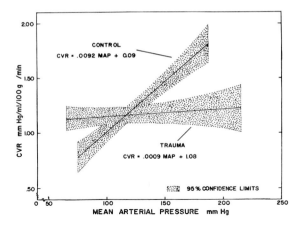

Fig. 9. The regression lines relating cerebrovascular resistance (CVR) and mean arterial pressure (MAP) for the control and post-trauma data are shown with their 95% confidence limits. There is a highly significant difference between the slopes of the two lines ($p < 0.001$). The slope of the trauma data is not significantly different from zero.

accumulation of CO_2 with further vasodilation and increased permeability of vessel walls.

Langfitt *et al.* (1968) have shown that trauma to the exposed cortex followed by hypertension results in immediate brain swelling accompanied by marked elevation of sagittal sinus pressure. The swelling occurs within seconds of the rise in blood pressure and is produced without any change in the permeability of the blood–brain barrier to albumin as evidenced by a lack of staining of the brain by intravenously injected Evans blue. Electron-microscopic examination of these brains (Schutta *et al.*, 1968) revealed an enlargement of the extracellular space in the cortex and white matter which at times contained a fluffy precipitate thought to be extravasated protein. Usually, however, the swollen brain showed no increased permeability of the blood–brain barrier to plasma protein and the accumulated fluid was therefore thought to be a plasma ultrafiltrate. It was postulated that the edema fluid was produced by an increased hydrostatic gradient across the capillary membrane resulting from a loss of autoregulation with the transmission of the subsequent increase in arterial pressure to the capillaries and veins.

In studies in cats in which cerebral concussion was produced with the skull intact (Langfitt *et al.*, 1966) it was found that after an initial transient rise in intracranial pressure coincident with the blow there was a secondary rise. It was hypothesized that the secondary rise was due to cerebrovascular dilation produced by the concussive blow with a consequent increase in brain blood volume, *i.e.* that cerebral vascular resistance was reduced.

From the data available in the literature, it is not clear whether a primary vaso-dilation occurs in the traumatized region. It may be that merely a failure to vaso-constrict occurs so that in the presence of hypertension, the velocity of flow is increased but not the intracranial blood volume. The concomitant rise in intracranial pressure that occurs has been interpreted as evidence for cerebrovascular dilation (Langfitt et al., 1966) however, this could as well be due to edema formation.

Several investigators have tried to determine whether cerebral blood volume changes following cerebral concussion. White et al. (1943) found no change in the blood content of the brain in cats after accelerative concussion. Langfitt et al. (1968) were able to demonstrate a two-fold increase in cerebral blood volume following cerebral trauma, however, the technique used did not distinguish between intra- and extra-vascular blood. Since there was always some intracranial hemorrhage present and the change in blood volume measured was 0.5 ml, it could not be demonstrated conclusively that there was actually an increase in intravascular blood volume. Lewis et al. (1968) found that the intracranial blood volume in cats subjected to head injury increased markedly at about 30 min after trauma to more than 7 ml or approximately 50% of the volume of the cranial cavity. However, again the method used to measure cerebral blood volume did not discriminate between intra- and extravascular blood. Since the mortality from the blow delivered in these studies was about 40%, this constituted a severe injury and there probably was a significant amount of intracranial bleeding.

Since respiratory embarrassment is a frequent concomitant of cerebral concussion (Meyer and Denny-Brown, 1955) any vasodilation that does occur could very easily be secondary to hypercarbia rather than a primary effect of the blow itself. In fact, it may be that only the non-traumatized vessels retain their CO_2 responsiveness and it is these that respond to hypercapnia and not the vessels in the traumatized region.

Several investigations of cerebral circulation following head injury have been performed. Brown and Brown (1954) demonstrated that internal carotid blood flow in monkeys subjected to cerebral concussion decreased during the first three seconds following a blow to 24% below control levels followed by an increase reaching a peak of about 250% of control at 30 sec with a gradual return to control levels by 6 min. Similar changes were found in arterial blood pressure. Since they had previously found a maximal decrease in femoral artery flow at the time of maximal elevation of arterial pressure (Brown et al., 1952) they postulated that the blow produces an intense excitation of the nervous system resulting in a maximal peripheral vaso-constriction and consequent elevation of blood pressure. Cerebral blood flow then passively follows this change in pressure. Thus, they imply a loss of cerebral auto-regulation. Meyer and Denny-Brown (1955) also found in cats and monkeys an increase in cortical blood flow which occurred with a latency of 10 to 20 sec after a concussive blow. This change in flow was uninfluenced by cervical sympathectomy or vagotomy and could occur independent of any rise in blood pressure. In more recent studies (Meyer et al., 1969) it was found that mild concussion in baboons produced a 4% increase in CBF and a 7% increase in cerebral metabolic rate for oxygen ($CMRO_2$) lasting about 1 min. Severe concussion, on the other hand, produced a 12% reduction in cerebral blood flow and a 10% reduction in $CMRO_2$. German et al. (1947) studied cerebral concussion in dogs and found an 86% increase in CBF and a 42% increase in $CMRO_2$ with a decrease in cerebrovascular resistance. The dissociation between CBF and $CMRO_2$ in these latter studies suggest the presence of a luxury perfusion syndrome. The authors hypothesized that the trauma inhibited a tonic neural vascular control mechanism. Thus, animal studies have fairly consistently shown an increase in cerebral blood flow following cerebral concussion.

Two studies have been performed in man. Taylor and Bell (1966) found a 15% increase in the mean cerebral circulation time in patients with concussional head injury. They postulated that this was due to increased vasomotor tone. Baldy-Moulinier and Frerebeau (1969) found that in six comatose patients following head injury, without evidence of a hematoma, that average rCBF was fairly normal (43 ml/100 g/min). Loss of autoregulation was demonstrated to be present in the one case in which it was tested.

The present studies support the concept that cerebral trauma produces a loss of autoregulation. They fail to confirm the hypothesis that a primary cerebral vasodilation occurs and suggest that this is not the case if oxygenation is maintained and hypercarbia prevented.

REGIONAL CEREBRAL BLOOD FLOW DURING FETAL HYPOXIA

There have been reported two distinct pathological patterns of brain damage following asphyxia in the term monkey fetus. With complete interruption of gas exchange between the fetus and mother for periods lasting $4\frac{1}{2}$ to 16 min the pathological changes are largely restricted to the thalamus and brain stem (Ranck and Windle, 1959; Windle et al., 1962; Myers, 1968). No evidence of brain swelling has been found associated with this insult (Myers, 1968). The second pattern of pathological change is seen with a more prolonged but partial impairment of gas exchange between mother and fetus. Here there is major involvement of the cortex, the underlying white matter, and the basal ganglia (Myers, 1967 a, b). In addition, brain swelling is often present (Myers et al., 1969). This latter pattern of pathological change is much more often seen than the former in perinatal brain damage in the term human infant (Towbin, 1970). In an attempt to further elucidate the underlying factors producing these pathological changes, studies of rCBF were performed in term monkey fetuses subjected to prolonged partial asphyxia (Reivich et al., 1970 a).

A series of eight pregnant rhesus monkeys between the 155th and 163rd day of gestation (the average length of pregnancy in this species is 168 days) was studied. They were anesthetized with pentobarbital, 35 mg/kg parenterally, intubated and artificially respired. A catheter was placed in the maternal femoral artery to monitor blood pressure and to obtain blood samples for pH, P_{CO_2} and P_{O_2} throughout the procedure.

Under sterile conditions, the gravid uterus was exposed and the uterine wall and amniotic sac were incised well away from the placental disks. The right arm of the fetus was then delivered through the incision and catheters were placed in the fetal brachial artery and vein. The arm was then replaced into the uterus and the incision in the uterus and abdominal wall closed with the fetal catheters leading out for collection of blood samples, monitoring of blood pressure and infusion of [^{14}C]-antipyrine for rCBF determination.

Four of the fetuses were maintained in as optimal a condition as possible and used for control measurements of regional cerebral blood flow. In the other four, fetal hypoxia was produced for periods of time varying from 1.6 to 3.7 hours, by reducing the maternal inspired oxygen concentration to 12–14%.

In the control animals mean arterial P_{O_2} and standard error were 28.8 ± 1.3 mm Hg, P_{CO_2} was 48.3 ± 3.5 mm Hg and pH was 7.30 ± 0.02. The time course of change of these parameters in an experimental animal is illustrated in Fig. 10. Oxygen tension fell from an initial value of 36 mm Hg to 16 mm Hg over a period of 4 h and 40 min. Carbon dioxide tension rose from an initial value of 43 mm Hg to 85 mm Hg and pH fell from 7.38 to 6.83 during that time. The values of these parameters for all animals are summarized in Table 3. The duration of acidosis in each fetus at pH levels

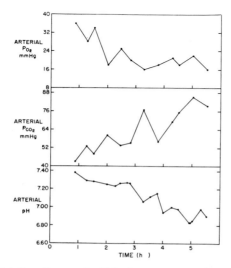

Fig. 10. Changes in arterial P_{O_2}, P_{CO_2} and pH in fetus no. 1494 following reduction of maternal inspired oxygen to 12–14%. Over a period of 4.67 h, P_{O_2} fell from 36 to 16 mm Hg, P_{CO_2} rose from 43 to 85 mm Hg and pH fell from 7.38 to 6.83.

TABLE 3

ARTERIAL BLOOD VALUES

No.	Duration of acidosis (h)			Duration of hypercarbia (h) $P_{CO_2} > 55$ mm Hg	Duration of hypoxia (h) $P_{O_2} < 18$ mm Hg
	$pH \leqslant 7.20$	$pH \leqslant 7.00$	$pH \leqslant 6.90$		
1496	0	0	0	0	0
1498	0	0	0	0	0
1489	0	0	0	0	0
1491	0	0	0	0.5	0
1497	1.3	1.0	0.1	1.3	1.3
1488	1.2	0.4	0	1.2	0.8
1494	2.4	1.6	0.4	3.2	0.9
1492	2.6	1.1	0.5	2.4	2.1

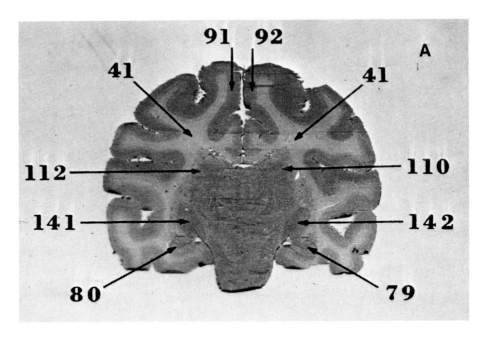

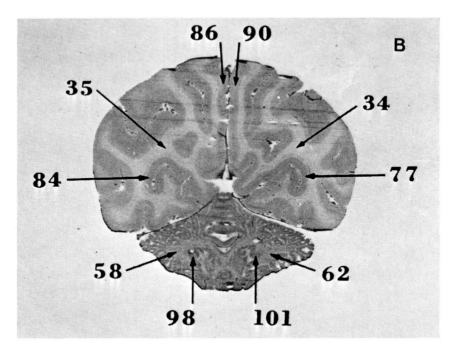

Fig. 11. Autoradiogram of a coronal section (A) at the level of Ammon's horn and (B) through the parieto-occipital area and cerebellum in control fetus no. 1489. Arterial P_{O_2} was 31 mm Hg, P_{CO_2} was 43 mm Hg and pH was 7.31. The regional cerebral blood flow values are in units of ml/100 g/min.

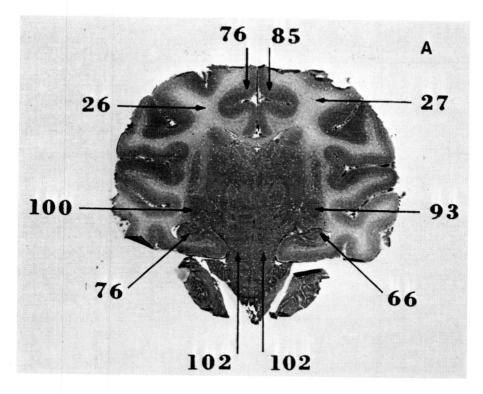

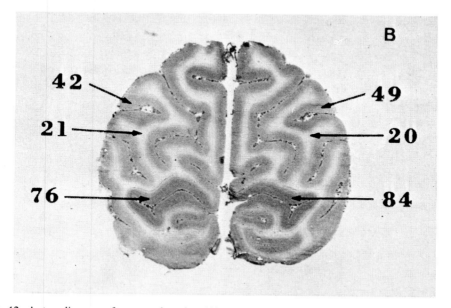

Fig. 12. Autoradiogram of a coronal section (A) at the level of Ammon's horn and (B) through the parieto-occipital area in experimental fetus no. 1497. Arterial P_{O_2} was 16 mm Hg, P_{CO_2} was 100 mm Hg and pH was 6.85.

References pp. 225–228

equal to or below 7.20, 7.00 and 6.90 is shown in the first three columns of this table. The duration of hypercarbia with arterial P_{CO_2} higher than 55 mm Hg and the duration of hypoxia with arterial P_{O_2} lower than 18 mm Hg are shown in the next two columns. In the control animals, fetuses no. 1496, 1498, 1489 and 1491, only fetus no. 1491 experienced a brief period (30 min) of hypercarbia; otherwise no acidosis, hypoxia or hypercarbia in these ranges was produced in these animals. In the experimental series all animals experienced acidosis, hypoxia and hypercarbia for varying periods of time.

In Fig. 11 are shown flow values in ml/100 g/min for various structures in a control animal (fetus no. 1489). The rCBF changes in the experimental animals varied from mild to severe. In fetus no. 1497, which experienced mild acidosis, only mild reductions in rCBF were seen. These changes are shown in Fig. 12. Some evidence of brain swelling was present in this fetus. In addition, hyperemia of the pial vessels is evident, particularly in the parieto-occipital areas. When hematoxyline- and eosin-stained sections adjacent to those used for autoradiography are examined, it is seen that these prominent vessels consist mainly of dilated veins although the arteries are also engorged.

In fetuses nos. 1488 and 1494, which experienced moderate acidosis, a very similar distribution of changes in rCBF was seen (Fig. 13 and Fig. 14). Isolated areas of cortex and underlying white matter had almost no flow. The depths of moderately involved sulci tended to have much greater reductions in flow than the crowns. These areas were mainly situated in the parietal and occipital lobes dorsally with occasional involvement of the inferior temporal and dorsal frontal lobes. In general, the frontal lobes were only mildly affected and the striate cortex tended to be spared. The dorso-medial regions of the thalamus showed isolated regions of severely reduced flow as did the hippocampus and the medial aspect of the globus pallidus. The head of the caudate nucleus also had areas of markedly reduced flow. The cerebellum showed patchy areas of marked reduction in flow involving both the inferior and superior surfaces as well as deep regions. The dorsomedial midbrain had regions of moderate to severe reduction in flow while the lower brain stem was only minimally affected. In addition, these two animals showed moderate brain swelling.

The most severely acidotic fetus was no. 1492. Flow was severely reduced or absent throughout the entire brain. Some regions of the brain stem, hypothalamus and cerebellum had slightly more flow than the rest of the brain but even in these regions flow was markedly reduced (Fig. 15).

The pattern of pathological changes most frequently seen in neonatal hypoxia in man consists of ulegyria, diffuse sclerosis of the white matter and status marmoratus of the basal ganglia (Malamud, 1963 and 1959). The ulegyria is most common in the parietal-occipital region and is predominantly dorsal in location and usually bilaterally symmetrical. In some instances, there are additional independent lesions involving the surface of the cortex which radiate into the underlying white matter. The troughs of sulci rather than the crowns tend to be more severely involved. The diffuse sclerosis of the white matter affects large parts of the central and gyral white matter and predominates in the dorsal regions of the hemispheres usually in a bilaterally sym-

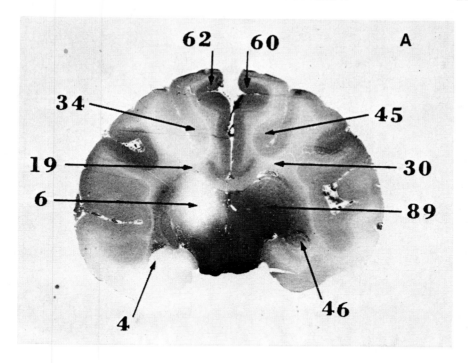

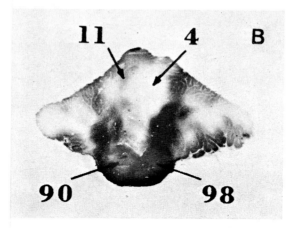

Fig. 13. Autoradiogram of a coronal section (A) at the level of Ammon's horn and (B) through the cerebellum and brain stem in experimental fetus no. 1488. Arterial P_{O_2} was 11 mm Hg, P_{CO_2} was 86 mm Hg and pH was 6.93.

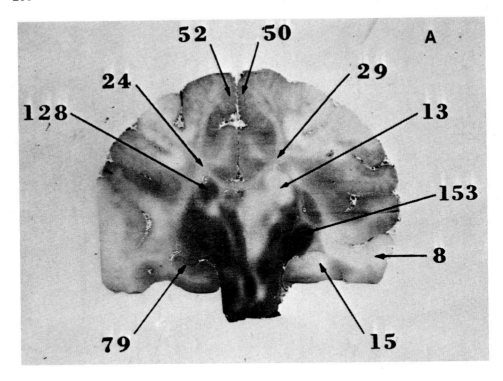

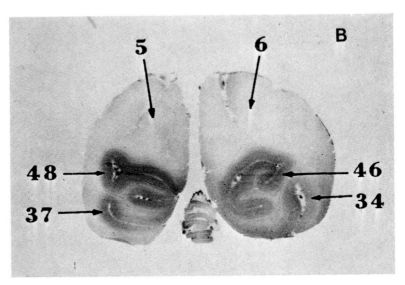

Fig. 14. Autoradiogram of a coronal section (A) at the level of Ammon's horn and (B) through the parieto-occipital area in experimental fetus no. 1494. Arterial P_{O_2} was 16 mm Hg, P_{CO_2} was 80 mm Hg and pH was 6.90.

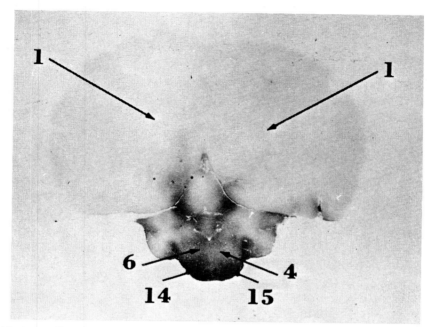

Fig. 15. Autoradiogram of a coronal section through the parietal lobes and brain stem in experimental fetus no. 1492. Arterial P_{O_2} was 24 mm Hg, P_{CO_2} was 68 mm Hg and pH was 6.89.

metrical distribution. Status marmoratus involves primarily the corpus striatum and thalamus. The lesions show a predeliction for the dorsal and lateral parts of the caudate nucleus and putamen. The thalamus is, however, as often involved in its ventrolateral as in its dorsomedial regions. It has been postulated that these lesions are due to a disturbance in venous drainage especially of the great vein of Galen (Marburg and Casamajor, 1944; Norman et al., 1957). This deep system through its anterior and posterior terminal and ventricular tributaries drains the frontal, parietal and occipital white matter, the corpus striatum, the hippocampal region and parts of the thalamus. In addition, interference with the drainage through the superficial dorsal veins, which enter the superior longitudinal sinus and drain the grey matter of the cortex with its immediately underlying white matter, has been postulated (Marburg, 1944).

Malamud (1963) also found atrophy of the cerebellum and sclerosis of Ammon's horn in about 80% of his cases of neonatal hypoxia. He considered these secondary lesions and attributed them to anoxial changes brought about by convulsions that complicated but were not a primary manifestation of the birth trauma. The rCBF changes we have seen in these areas suggest that these changes may in fact be part of the primary injury and not necessarily a secondary phenomenon.

A pathological picture similar to that occurring in the human has been produced in the monkey fetus by partial asphyxia prolonged over several hours (Myers, 1967 a; Myers et al., 1969). If the animal survives, ulegyria is seen primarily in the paracentral region but involving other sulci as well in the parasagittal regions. The involvement is usually bilaterally symmetrical with the severity diminishing further from the central fissures. The depths of sulci appear to be affected first in regions of mild involvement. In addition to cortical lesions, the putamen, head of the caudate nucleus and the lateral and posterior ventral nuclei of the thalamus are involved bilaterally and symmetrically. This is the most typical pattern of involvement seen. In other fetuses, changes in the hemispheral white matter predominating in the prefrontal, posterior parietal and occipital regions are seen.

This pattern of damage produced by prolonged partial asphyxia is quite different from that seen with brief total asphyxia. In the latter situation, it is the brain stem and thalamus which are consistently affected (Windle, 1963).

In the present study, there was a good correlation between the severity of the rCBF changes in a fetus and the hypoxic insult as reflected by the duration of acidosis to which the animal was subjected.

The mildest insult resulted in moderate brain swelling probably with some compromise of venous drainage as indicated by the dilated cortical venous channels seen in this animal. With a more severe insult, more marked brain swelling was present and in addition, a pattern of reduction in rCBF very similar to that of the pathological changes that have been described in neonatal asphyxia both in the monkey and human term fetus.

Is this pattern of impaired flow on the basis of a compromised arterial inflow or disturbed venous drainage from the involved tissue? There are preferential sites of arterial compression associated with brain swelling (Lindenberg, 1955 and 1963). Compression of the sulci interferes with flow through the small terminal branches of the leptomeningeal arteries within the sulci. The tissue in the depths of the sulci is affected before the crown of the convolutions since these deeper portions are further from the parent branch. Initially these lesions are preferentially produced in the parietal lobes. Similarly, terminal branches of the cerebellar arteries may be compressed where they run through the sulci to supply the deeper portions of the cerebellar cortex. Small isolated areas of the cerebral white matter have been found to be affected in the dorsal region of the parietal lobe or in the parietal occipital region. These areas are irrigated by the white matter twigs of the peripheral branches of the main cerebral arteries. It is possible that the lesions are produced by stasis in these "end-arteries" although insufficiency of venous drainage is probably an essential co-factor.

If the brain swelling is severe enough to produce tentorial herniation, other lesions may be added to this. Herniation of the hippocampus can cause compression of cortical branches of the posterior cerebral artery against the sharp tentorial margin producing lesions in Ammon's horn. In addition, the temporal branch of the posterior cerebral artery can become compressed producing ischemia of the lower temporal convolutions. The pallidal branches of the anterior choroidal artery may also be involved by tentorial pressure. These branches supply the medial parts of the pallidum. The lateral portions of the pallidum usually are spared since they are supplied by the striatal branches of the middle cerebral arteries.

With acute generalized brain swelling, it is not uncommon for compression of the interpeduncular fossa to occur with compromise of brain stem branches of the posterior cerebral artery which supply the thalamus and medial tegmentum of the midbrain and upper pons.

Another preferential site of arterial compression involves the distribution of the middle cerebral artery. This vessel may be compressed by brain tissue in the rostral portion of the Sylvian fissure where it passes around the limen of the insula. Its posterior branches may be compressed in the caudal portion of the Sylvian fissure as they emerge to supply the cortex of the convexity of the caudal half of the hemisphere.

The calcarine cortex is supplied by a separate branch of the posterior cerebral artery and may escape damage even though the cortical areas supplied by the other branches of the posterior cerebral artery are involved.

If the cerebellum swells, it may herniate rostrally through the posterior opening of the tentorium compressing the branches of the superior cerebellar arteries against the tentorial margin. The resulting lesions predominantly involve the superior surface of both cerebellar hemispheres. Usually the damage is most severe in the depths of the sulci. Deep branches of the superior cerebellar artery supplying the dentate nuclei may also be involved. If the cerebellum herniates downward through the foramen magnum, the posterior inferior cerebellar arteries may be compressed with lesions over the lower half of the cerebellar hemisphere predominating.

Preferential involvement of these arteries could account for the distribution of flow changes seen in these studies. The changes in rCBF seen in the term fetus subjected to prolonged partial asphyxia could thus be explained on the basis of brain swelling producing increased intracranial pressure and arterial compression. Undoubtedly, impairment of venous drainage also plays some role, however, from the pattern of flow changes seen arterial stasis appears to be the more important factor. The pattern of impaired flow correlates very well with the pattern of pathological changes produced by neonatal asphyxia in the term fetus both in man and the rhesus monkey which strongly suggests that these flow changes are the direct cause of the pathological lesions.

AUTORADIOGRAPHIC METHOD FOR MEASURING REGIONAL CEREBRAL GLUCOSE CONSUMPTION

The development of an autoradiographic technique for the quantitative measurement of regional cerebral glucose consumption would enable the effects of regional metabolic changes on regional blood flow to be directly investigated. An ideal tracer for such a technique would be one which was taken up by the brain at a rate proportional to that of glucose and whose metabolic products remained in the tissue under study. This would allow a relatively simple mathematical model for the uptake of this tracer to be constructed from which the uptake of glucose might be deduced. It was decided to evaluate the use of $[2-^{14}C]$deoxyglucose as such a tracer for the following reasons (Reivich et al., 1970 c). This substance is known to rapidly enter cells (Wick et al., 1955) and to be readily phosphorylated by brain hexokinase (Sols and Crane, 1954). Further metabolism of 2-deoxyglucose-6-phosphate does not appear to occur

(Sols and Crane, 1954; Wick *et al.*, 1957). It is not a substrate for either phospho-hexose isomerase or glucose-6-phosphate dehydrogenase (Crane and Sols, 1953). Thus, if the rate of transfer into cells and subsequent phosphorylation is proportional to that of glucose, the uptake of this tracer would be a measure of glucose uptake in that tissue.

To determine whether this were so, the uptake of 2-deoxyglucose and glucose was studied in cat cerebral cortex slices incubated in modified Ringer's solution containing glucose and [2-^{14}C]deoxyglucose in concentrations varying from 5.6 to 22.2 mM/l and 6.3 to 24.8 μM/l respectively. From the brain slice studies of Tower (1958) it can be estimated that even at the highest concentrations of 2-deoxyglucose used in the present studies that there will be no inhibition of aerobic or anaerobic glycolysis or of oxygen uptake. The slices were cut with a Stadie–Riggs tissue microtome from a freshly removed brain and placed immediately into the incubating flasks which contained 5 ml of medium and were charged with 95 % O_2 and 5 % CO_2. The metabolic rate of the brain slices was varied by incubating them at temperatures ranging from 29.5 to 39.6 °C. Glucose concentration was determined on an aliquot of the medium before and after 2 h of incubation with the tissue. Similar aliquots were also counted in a liquid scintillation counter. As shown in Fig. 16, a significant correlation was found between the uptake of glucose and [2-^{14}C]deoxyglucose under these conditions ($r = 0.70$ and $p < 0.001$).

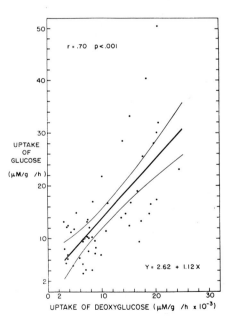

Fig. 16. Uptake of glucose and [2-^{14}C]deoxyglucose by cat cerebral cortex slices *in vitro*. The metabolic rate of the slices was modified by varying the temperature at which they were incubated from 29.5 to 39.6 °C. The regression line as well as its equation and 95 % confidence limits are shown. A significant correlation was present between the uptake of glucose and [2-^{14}C]deoxyglucose under these conditions.

To further compare the uptake of glucose and [2-^{14}C]deoxyglucose *in vivo* studies were performed on a series of 3 cats and 7 dogs which received a constant infusion of [2-^{14}C]deoxyglucose intravenously over a 10–20-min period. The time course of change of glucose and [2-^{14}C]deoxyglucose concentrations in arterial and sagittal sinus venous blood was measured. The highest ratio of [2-^{14}C]deoxyglucose to glucose in the arterial blood in any of these animals was 1 : 1200 or 12 times smaller than that shown to have no effect on glucose consumption *in vitro* by Tower (1958). A typical set of arterial and cerebral venous curves is shown in Fig. 17. From this data, the ratio of the extraction of [2-^{14}C]deoxyglucose to the extraction of glucose by the brain was calculated. As shown in Fig. 18, this ratio approached the value of 1.0

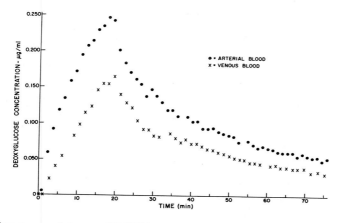

Fig. 17. The time course of change of [2-^{14}C]deoxyglucose in arterial and sagittal sinus venous blood during a 20-min intravenous constant infusion of [2-^{14}C]deoxyglucose and the subsequent 56 min. There is no loss of the tracer from the brain after the infusion is stopped at 20 min, but rather a continuing uptake.

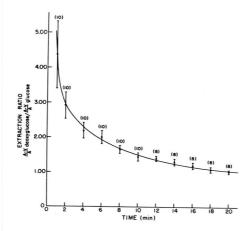

Fig. 18. The ratio of the extractions of [2-^{14}C]deoxyglucose and glucose by the brain in 3 cats and 7 dogs. The number in parenthesis is the number of animals at each point. The symbol $\bar{\mathrm{I}}$ represents the mean and standard error of the values at that point.

References pp. 225–228

by the end of the infusion indicating that the [2-14C]deoxyglucose and glucose were being taken up by the brain at proportional rates.

On the basis of these results, the following model for the uptake of [2-14C]deoxyglucose is suggested (Fig. 19): (1) The rate of delivery of the [2-14C]deoxyglucose

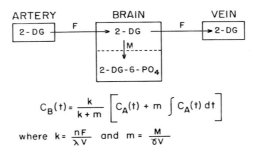

Fig. 19. Mathematical model of uptake of [2-14C]-deoxyglucose for a brain tissue which is homogeneous with regard to flow and glucose uptake. See text for assumptions and definitions of symbols.

to the brain depends on its concentration in the arterial blood and on the cerebral blood flow. (2) The intracellular transfer and phosphorylation of the tracer occurs at a rate proportional to that of glucose. (3) There is little or no back diffusion of [2-14C]deoxyglucose-6-PO_4 out of the tissues. This leads to the following equation for a tissue homogeneous with regard to flow and glucose uptake:

$$C_B(t) = \frac{k}{k + m} \left[C_A(t) + m \int C_A(t)\, dt \right] \tag{7}$$

where $k = nF/\lambda V$ and $m = M/\gamma V$. In these equations $C_B(t)$ equals the concentration of [2-14C]deoxyglucose in the brain in the phosphorylated plus the non-phosphorylated forms, $C_A(t)$ equals the concentration of [2-14C]deoxyglucose in the arterial blood, V is a unit volume of brain, λ equals the tissue–blood partition coefficient for 2-deoxyglucose, n equals the diffusion constant for 2-deoxyglucose, F equals the blood flow of the tissue, M equals the rate of glucose uptake of the tissue and γ equals the ratio of the concentrations of 2-deoxyglucose and glucose in the arterial blood.

Using a version of this model, data were analyzed from a series of 6 dogs in which a [2-14C]deoxyglucose infusion and 85Kr by inhalation were administered simultaneously. The cerebral uptake of glucose was calculated with the model and compared with the measured cerebral uptake of glucose. The results are shown in Table 4. On the basis of these favorable observations, further development of this technique is being pursued. If this method can be validated in animal studies, it may be possible to modify it so that it will be applicable for studies in man. For instance, if [2-14C] deoxyglucose could be prepared the clearance of this substance from the brain in man could be determined by means of collimated scintillation detectors and a measure of regional cerebral glucose consumption obtained.

TABLE 4

CEREBRAL GLUCOSE CONSUMPTION

Animal No.	Measured CMR_{gl} mg/100 g/min	Calculated CMR_{gl} mg/100 g/min	Error %
1	5.51	5.18	−8
2	3.34	3.51	+5
3	4.07	2.74	−33
4	5.05	4.32	−14
5	3.78	4.08	+8
6	4.26	4.32	+1

SUMMARY

The blood flow of the brain is markedly heterogeneous and the changes which occur in cerebral perfusion in various physiologic and pathophysiologic conditions are often focal in nature. This chapter deals with a quantitative method for measuring such regional changes in cerebral blood flow (rCBF) and delineates those changes that occur in cerebral hemodynamics under various conditions. The normal values for rCBF in awake cats are presented. The effect of slow wave sleep and rapid eye movement sleep on these flow values is discussed in relation to the distribution of changes seen and the possible mechanism responsible for these changes.

Studies in cats following cerebral trauma are reported which demonstrate a focal loss of the normal autoregulatory capacity of the cerebral vessels.

Prolonged partial asphyxia in the term monkey fetus and its effect on rCBF was also studied. The mechanism of production of these flow changes and their relation to the pathologic changes seen in these animals is discussed.

Finally, preliminary results from the development of an autoradiographic technique for measuring regional cerebral glucose consumption *in vivo* utilizing [2-14C]deoxy-glucose are presented.

APPENDIX

The relationship between the true arterial time course of isotope concentration, $C_a(t)$, and this function after it has been smeared through the sampling system, $\acute{C}_a(t)$, was determined by introducing a step function change in isotope concentration, $_1(t)$, into the sampling system and determining the output function, $f_0(t)$, as described above. Empirically, it was found that the function $f_0(t)$ could be adequately described by an equation of the form:

$$f_0(t) = 1 - A_1e^{-r1t} + A_2e^{-r2t} \qquad (8)$$

Therefore, the transfer function, T, (*i.e.*, that function which when convoluted on the

References pp. 225–228

input function produces the output function) which in the s domain is defined as:

$$T = \frac{F_0(s)}{F_1(s)} \tag{9}$$

is described by the equation

$$T = 1 - A_1 \frac{s}{(s + r_1)} + A_2 \frac{s}{(s + r_2)} \tag{10}$$

or since $1 - A_1 + A_2 = 0$

$$T = \frac{A_1 r_1}{s + r_1} - \frac{A_2 r_2}{s + r_2} \tag{11}$$

Assuming the first derivative of $f_0(t)$ is zero at time zero, then

$$A_1 r_1 - A_2 r_2 = 0 \tag{12}$$

and

$$T = \frac{r_1 r_2}{s^2 + (r_1 + r_2) s + r_1 r_2} \tag{13}$$

or in the time domain

$$C_a(t) = \left[\frac{1}{r_1 r_2} D^2 + \frac{r_1 + r_2}{r_1 r_2} D + 1 \right] C_a'(t) \tag{14}$$

where $C_a(t)$ is the input function and $C_a'(t)$ the output function.

Substituting equation (14) into equation (1) above

$$C_i(T) = \lambda_i K_i \int_0^T \left[\frac{1}{r_1 r_2} D^2 + \frac{r_1 + r_2}{r_1 r_2} D + 1 \right] C_a'(t) e^{-k_i(T-t)} \, dt \tag{15}$$

which after separation into three integrals and integrating by parts produces the final solution:

$$C_i(T) = \frac{\lambda_i k_i (k_i - r_1)(k_i - r_2)}{r_1 r_2} \int_0^T C_a'(t) e^{-k_i(T-t)} \, dt - \frac{\lambda_i k_i (k_i - r_1 - r_2)}{r_1 r_2} C_a'(T) +$$

$$\frac{\lambda_i k_i}{r_1 r_2} \cdot \frac{dC_a'(T)}{dt} \tag{16}$$

The one assumption made in deriving the operator shown in equation (14) does not limit the solution as can be tested by operating on the generalized function:

$$f(t) = 1 + Ae^{-r_1 t} + Be^{-r_2 t}$$

The operator

$$\left[\frac{1}{r_1 r_2} D^2 + \frac{r_1 + r_2}{r_1 r_2} D + 1 \right]$$

converts this function to a step function.

REFERENCES

BALDY-MOULINIER, M. N. AND FREREBEAU, PH. (1969) Cerebral blood flow in cases of coma following severe head injury. In: BROCK, M., FIESCHI, C., INGVAR, D. H., LASSEN, N. A. AND SCHURMANN, K. (Eds.), *Cerebral Blood Flow*, Springer-Verlag, New York, p. 216–218.

BAUST, W. (1967) Local blood flow in different regions of the brain-stem during natural sleep and arousal. *Electroenceph. Clin. Neurophysiol.*, **22**, 365–372.

BENDA, P. AND BROWNELL, G. L. (1960) The fate of radioactive emboli injected into the cerebral circulation, the brain as a filter. *J. Neuropathol. Exp. Neurol.*, **19**, 383–406.

BIZZI, E., POMPEIANO, O. AND SOMOGZI, I. (1964) Vestibular nuclei; activity of single neurons during natural sleep and wakefulness. *Science*, **145**, 414–415.

BIZZI, E. (1965) Discharge patterns of lateral geniculate neurons during paradoxical sleep. *Assoc. Psychophysiol. Study Sleep, Washington.*

BREBBIA, D. R. AND ALTSHULER, K. Z. (1965) Oxygen consumption rate and electroencephalographic stage of sleep. *Science*, **150**, 1621–1623.

BRODIE, B. B. AND AXELROD, J. (1950) The fate of antipyrine in Man. *J. Pharmacol. Exp. Therap.*, **98**, 97–104.

BROWN, G. W., BROWN, M. L. AND HINES, H. M. (1952) Effect of experimental concussion on blood flow, arterial pressure and cardiac rate. *Amer. J. Physiol.*, **170**, 294–300.

BROWN, G. W. AND BROWN, M. L. (1954) Cardiovascular responses to experimental cerebral concussion in the rhesus monkey. *Arch. Neurol. Psychiat.*, **71**, 707–713.

CAMPBELL, A. C. P. (1938) The vascular architecture of the cat's brain. *Res. Publ. Assoc. Res. Nervous Mental Disease*, **18**, 69–93.

COPPERMAN, R. (1951) Cited by KETY, S. S. (1951).

COURTNEY, J. W. (1899) Traumatic cerebral edema: Its pathology and surgical treatment – a clinical study, *Boston Med. Surg. J.*, **140**, 345–348.

COURVILLE, C. B. (1942) Structural changes in the brain consequent to traumatic disturbances to intracranial fluid balances. *Bull. Los Angeles Neurol. Soc.*, **7**, 55–76.

CRANE, R. K. AND SOLS, A. J. (1953) The association of hexokinase with particulate fractions of brain and other tissue homogenates. *J. Biol. Chem.*, **203**, 273–292.

DENNY-BROWN, D. AND RUSSELL, W. R. (1941) Experimental cerebral concussion. *Brain*, **64**, 93–164.

DURET, H. (1878) Etudes experimentales et cliniques sur les traumatismes cerebraux. *Publ. Progr. Med.*, Paris.

EVANS, J. P. AND SCHEINKER, I. M. (1945) Histologic studies of brain following head trauma. *J. Neurosurg.*, **2**, 306–314.

EVARTS, E. V. (1962) Activity of neurons in visual cortex of the cat during sleep with low voltage fast EEG activity. *J. Neurophysiol.*, **25**, 812–816.

EVARTS, E. V. (1964) Temporal patterns of discharge of pyramidal track neurons during sleep and waking in the monkey. *J. Neurophysiol.*, **27**, 152–171.

FICK, A. (1871) Über die Messung des Blutquantums in den Herzventrikeln. *Sitzungsv. d. phys. med. Gesselsch. zu Würtzb.*, p. 16.

FIESCHI, C. (1964) Blood flow measurements in the brain of cats by analysis of the clearance curves of hydrogen gas with implanted electrodes and of Kr^{85} with external counting of gamma activity. In: *Proc. 2nd Intern. Symp. Question of Cerebral Circulation, Salzburg*, p. 180–186.

FOG, M. (1968) Autoregulation of cerebral blood flow and its abolition by local hypoxia and/or trauma. *Scand. J. Clin. Lab. Invest.*, Suppl. **102**.

FORBES, H. S. (1928) The cerebral circulation. *AMA Arch. Neurol. Psychiat.*, **19**, 751–761.

GERMAN, W. J., PAGE, W. R. AND NIMS, L. F. (1947) Cerebral blood flow and cerebral oxygen consumption in experimental intracranial injury. *Trans. Amer. Neurol. Assoc.*, **72**, 86–88.

HASEGAWA, T., RAVENS, J. R. AND TOOLE, J. F. (1967) Precapillary arterial-venous anastomoses. *Arch. Neurol.*, **16**, 217–224.

HUTTENLOCKER, P. R. (1961) Evoked and spontaneous activity in single units of medial brain stem during natural sleep and waking. *J. Neurophysiol.*, **24**, 451–468.

HYDEN, H. AND LANGE, P. W. (1965) Rhythmic enzyme changes in neurons and glia during sleep and wakefulness. In: AKERT, K., BALLY, C. AND SCHADÉ, J. P. (Eds.), *Sleep Mechanisms, Progress in Brain Research*, Vol. **18**, Elsevier, Amsterdam, p. 92.

INGVAR, D. H. AND LASSEN, N. A. (1962) Regional blood flow of the cerebral cortex determined by $Krypton^{85}$. *Acta Physiol. Scand.*, **54**, 325–388.

INGVAR, D. H., CRONQVIST, S., EKBERG, R., RISBERG, J. AND HOEDT-RASMUSSEN, K. (1965) Normal values of regional cerebral blood flow in man, including flow and weight estimates of grey and white matter. *Acta Neurol. Scand.*, Suppl. **14**, 72–82.

KANZOW, E., KRAUSE, D. AND KUHNEL, H. (1962) Die Vasomotorik der Hirnrinde in den Phasen desynchronisierter EEG-Aktivität im naturlichen Schlaf der Katze, *Pflügers Arch. Ges. Physiol.*, **274**, 593–607.

KAWAMURA, H. AND SAWYER, C. (1965) Elevation in brain temperature during paradoxical sleep. *Science*, **150**, 912–913.

KETY, S. S. (1951) The theory and applications of the exchange of inert gas at the lungs and tissues. *Pharm. Rev.*, **3**, 1–41.

KETY, S. S. (1960) Measurement of local blood flow by the exchange of an inert diffusible substance. In: BRUNER, H. D. (Ed.), *Methods in Medical Research*, Vol. **8**, Year Book, Chicago, p. 228–238.

KETY, S. S. (1965) Measurement of local circulation within the brain by means of inert diffusable tracers; examination of the theory, assumptions and possible sources of error. *Acta Neurol. Scand.*, Suppl. **14**, 20–23.

LANDAU, W., FREYGANG, W. H., JR., ROWLAND, L. P., SOKOLOFF, L. AND KETY, S. S. (1955) The local circulation of the living brain; values in the unanesthetized and anesthetized cat. *Trans. Amer. Neurol. Assoc.*, **80**, 125–129.

LANGFITT, T. W., MARSHALL, W. J. S., KASSELL, N. F. AND SCHUTTA, H. S. (1968 a) The pathophysiology of brain swelling produced by mechanical trauma and hypertension. *Scand. J. Clin. Lab. Invest.*, Suppl. **102**.

LANGFITT, T. W., TANNANBAUM, H. M. AND KASSELL, N. F. (1966) Etiology of acute brain swelling following experimental head injury. *J. Neurosurg.*, **24**, 47–56.

LANGFITT, T. W., WEINSTEIN, J. D., SKLAR, F. H., ZAREN, H. A. AND KASSELL, N. F. (1968 b) Contribution of intracranial blood volume to three forms of experimental brain swelling. *Johns Hopkins Med. J.*, **122**, 261–270.

LASSEN, N. S. AND INGVAR, D. H. (1961) The blood flow of the cerebral cortex determined by radioactive Krypton[85]. *Experientia*, **17**, 42–43.

LEWIS, H. T., RAMIREZ, R. AND MCLAURIN, R. L. (1968) Intracranial blood volume after head injury. *Surg. Forum*, **19**, 433–435.

LINDENBERG, R. (1955) Compression of brain arteries as pathogenetic factor for tissue necroses and their areas of predilection. *J. Neuropathol. Exp. Neurol.*, **14**, 223–243.

LINDENBERG, R. (1963) Patterns of CNS vulnerability in acute hypoxaemia, including anaesthesia accidents. In: SCHADÉ, J. P. AND MCMENEMEY, W. H. (Eds.), *Selective Vulnerability of the Brain in Hypoxaemia*, F.A. Davis Company, Philadelphia, p. 189.

MALAMUD, N. (1959) Sequelae of perinatal trauma, *J. Neuropathol. Exp. Neurol.*, **18**, 141–151.

MALAMUD, N. (1963) Pattern of CNS vulnerability in neonatal hypoxaemia. In: SCHADÉ, J. P. AND MCMENEMEY, W. H. (Eds.), *Selective Vulnerability of the Brain in Hypoxaemia*, F.A. Davis Company, Philadelphia, p. 211.

MANGOLD, R., SOKOLOFF, L., CONNER, E., KLEINERMAN, J., THERMAN, P. G. AND KETY, S. S. (1955) The effects of sleep and lack of sleep on the cerebral circulation and metabolism of normal young men. *J. Clin. Invest.*, **34**, 1092–1100.

MARBURG, O. AND CASAMAJOR, L. (1944) Phlebostasis and phlebothrombosis of the brain in the newborn and in early childhood. *Arch. Neurol. Psychiat.*, **52**, 170–188.

MEYER, J. S. AND DENNY-BROWN, D. (1955) Studies of cerebral circulation in brain injury, II. Cerebral concussion, *Electroenceph. Clin. Neurophysiol.*, **7**, 529–534.

MEYER, J. S., KONDO, A., NOMURA, F., SAKAMOTO, K. AND TERAURA, T. (1969) Cerebral hemodynamics and metabolism following brain trauma. Demonstration of luxury perfusion following brain stem laceration. In: BROCK, M., FIESCHI, C., INGVAR, D. H., LASSEN, N. A. AND SCHURMANN, K. (Eds.), *Cerebral Blood Flow*, Springer-Verlag, New York, p. 199–201.

MYERS, R. E. (1967 a) Patterns of perinatal brain damage in the monkey. In. JAMES, L. S. AND MYERS, R. E. (Eds.), *Fifty-seventh Ross Conference: Brain Damage in the Fetus and Newborn from Hypoxia or Asphyxia*, Ross Laboratories, Columbus, Ohio, p. 17.

MYERS, R. E. (1967 b) Models of asphyxial brain damage in the newborn monkey. Presented at the *Second Pan-American Congress of Neurology*, San Juan, Puerto Rico, Oct. 22–28.

MYERS, R. E. (1968) The clinical and pathological effects of asphyxiation in the fetal rhesus monkey. In: ADAMSONS, K. (Ed.), *Diagnosis and Treatment of Fetal Disorders*, Springer-Verlag, New York, p. 226.

MYERS, R. E., BEARD, R. AND ADAMSON, K. (1969) Brain swelling in the newborn rhesus monkey following prolonged partial asphyxia. *Neurology*, **19**, 1012–1017.

NORMAN, R. M., URICH, H. AND MCMENEMEY, W. H. (1957) Vascular mechanisms of birth injury. *Brain*, **80**, 49–58.

RANCK, J. B. AND WINDLE, W. F. (1959) Brain damage in the monkey, *Macaca mulatta*, by asphyxia neonatorum. *Exp. Neurol.*, **1**, 130–154.

RAND, C. W. AND COURVILLE, C. B. (1931) Histologic studies of the brain in cases of fatal injury to the head. II. Changes in the choroid plexus and ependyma. *Arch. Surg.*, **23**, 357–425.

REIVICH, M., ISAACS, G., EVARTS, E. AND KETY, S. S. (1968) The effect of slow wave sleep and REM sleep on regional cerebral blood flow in cats. *J. Neurochem.*, **15**, 301–306.

REIVICH, M., JEHLE, J., SOKOLOFF, L. AND KETY, S. S. (1969) Measurement of regional cerebral blood flow with antipyrine-^{14}C in awake cats. *J. Appl. Physiol.*, **27**, 296–300.

REIVICH, M., BRANN, A. W., JR., SHAPIRO, H. AND MYERS, R. E. (1970 a) Regional cerebral blood flow during prolonged partial asphyxia in the term monkey fetus. Presented at the *Fifth Salzburg Conf. Cerebral Blood Flow*. Salzburg, Austria, Sept. 23–27.

REIVICH, M. AND MARSHALL, W. J. S. (1970 b) Regional changes in autoregulation following cerebral trauma. In: MEYER, J. S., REIVICH, M., LECHNER, H. AND EICHHORN, O. (Eds.), *Research on the Cerebral Circulation*, Fourth Intern. Salzburg Conference, Charles C. Thomas, Springfield, Ill., p. 130–136.

REIVICH, M., SANO, N. AND SOKOLOFF, L. (1970 c) Development of an autoradiographic method for the determination of regional glucose consumption. Presented at the *Intern. Cerebral Blood Flow Symposium*, London, Sept. 17–19.

ROWBOTHAM, G. F. AND LITTLE, E. (1965) A new concept of the circulation and the circulations of the brain. *Brit. J. Surg.*, **52**, 539–542.

SCHARRER, E. (1940) Arteries and veins in the mammalian brain. *Anat. Rec.*, **78**, 173–196.

SCHEATZ, G. C. (1965) Electrode holders in chronic preparations. A. Multilead techniques for large and small animals. In: SHEER, D. E. (Ed.), *Electrical Stimulation of the Brain*, University of Texas Press, Austin, p. 45–50.

SCHMIDT, C. F. AND HENDRIX, J. P. (1937) The action of chemical substances on cerebral blood vessels. *Res. Publ. Assoc. Res. Nervous Mental Disease*, **18**, 229–276.

SCHUTTA, H. S., KASSELL, N. F. AND LANGFITT, T. W. (1968) Brain swelling produced by injury and aggravated by arterial hypertension – A light electron microscopic study. *Brain*, **91**, 281–294.

SNYDER, F., HOBSON, J. A., MORRISON, D. R. AND GOLDFRANK, F. (1964) Changes in respiration, heart rate, and systolic blood pressure in human sleep. *J. Appl. Physiol.*, **19**, 417–422.

SOKOLOFF, L. (1961) Local cerebral circulation at rest and during altered cerebral activity induced by anesthesia or visual stimulation. In: KETY, S. S. AND ELKES, J. (Eds.), *Regional Chemistry Physiology and Pharmacology of the Nervous System*, Pergamon Press, Oxford, p. 107–117.

SOLS, A. AND CRANE, R. K. (1954) Substrate specificity of brain hexokinase. *J. Biol. Chem.*, **210**, 581–595.

SWANK, R. L. AND HAIN, R. F. (1952) The effect of different sized emboli on the vascular system and parenchyma of the brain. *J. Neuropathol. Exp. Neurol.*, **11**, 280–299.

TAYLOR, R. R. AND BELL, T. K. (1966) Slowing of cerebral circulation after concussional head injury. *Lancet*, **2**, 178–180.

TAYLOR, A. R. (1969) Disturbance of autoregulation following head injury – acute and chronic observations. In: BROCK, M., FIESCHI, C., INGVAR, D. H., LASSEN, N. A. AND SCHURMANN, K. (Eds.), *Cerebral Blood Flow*, Springer-Verlag, New York, p. 202–204.

TOWBIN, A. (1970) Central nervous system damage in the human fetus and newborn infant. *Amer. J. Diseases Childhood*, **119**, 529–542.

TOWER, D. B. (1958) The effects of 2-deoxy-D-glucose on metabolism of slices of cerebral cortex incubated *in vitro*. *J. Neurochem.*, **3**, 185–205.

WHITE, J. C., BROOKS, J. R., GOLDTHWAIT, J. C. AND ADAMS, R. D. (1943) Changes in brain volume and blood content after experimental concussion. *Ann. Surg.*, **118**, 619–633.

WICK, A. N., DRURY, D. R. AND MORITA, T. N. (1955) 2-Deoxy-glucose. A metabolic block for glucose. *Proc. Soc. Exp. Biol. Med.*, **89**, 579–582.

WICK, A. N., DRURY, D. R., NAKADA, H. I. AND WOLFE, J. B. (1957) Localization of the primary metabolic block produced by 2-deoxyglucose. *J. Biol. Chem.*, **224**, 963–969.

WINDLE, W. F., JACOBSON, H. N., ROBERT DE RAMIREZ DE ARELLANO, M. I. AND COMBS, C. M. (1962) Structural and functional sequelae of asphyxia neonatorum in monkeys *(Macaca mulatta)*.

Res. Publ. Assoc. Res. Nervous Mental Disease, **39**, 169–182.

WINDLE, W. F. (1963) Selective vulnerability of the central nervous system of rhesus monkeys to asphyxia during birth. In: SCHADÉ, J. P. AND MCMENEMEY, W. H. (Eds.), *Selective Vulnerability of the Brain in Hypoxaemia*, F.A. Davis Company, Philadelphia, p. 251.

WURTZ, R. H. (1967) Physiological correlates of steady potential shifts during sleep and wakefulness. II. Brain temperature, blood pressure, and potential changes across the ependyma. *Electroenceph. Clin. Neurophysiol.*, **22**, 43–53.

On the Regulation of Cerebral Blood Flow and Metabolic Activity in Coma. Clinical and Experimental Studies

M. N. SHALIT

Department of Neurosurgery, Hadassah University Hospital, Jerusalem (Israel)

Observations on cerebral circulatory and metabolic phenomena in comatose patients have aroused considerable interest because of their importance in understanding the factors participating in the regulation of cerebral blood flow (CBF). The effects of cerebral acidosis, cerebral edema, increased intracranial pressure, and regional brain ischemia on CBF have been investigated, in many cases in comatose patients. Little is known, however, about the behavior of CBF and cerebral metabolic activity in comatose patients in different stages of coma. Most studies have been based on isolated observations of these parameters without a cerebral circulatory and metabolic follow-up.

Such studies may have both theoretical and practical significance especially in regard to comatose patients suffering from different forms of head injury. These patients may remain comatose for prolonged periods with no apparent change in their clinical condition. Depending on the localization and extent of the damage in the brain, some eventually recover, others remain in a chronic vegetative state and others die.

It may therefore be expected that CBF and cerebral metabolic activity would be affected by the site of the damage, and furthermore would differ in different stages of coma. In this respect, the patients with brain stem lesions may be regarded as the most interesting group, perhaps providing the key to the understanding of the role of the brain stem in the regulation of CBF and cerebral metabolism in physiological and pathological conditions.

A. CEREBRAL BLOOD FLOW AND OXYGEN CONSUMPTION AFTER BRAIN STEM LESIONS

It has long been known that comatose patients suffering from increased intracranial pressure have a reduced cerebral blood flow and cerebral metabolic rate for oxygen ($CMRO_2$) (Kety *et al.*, 1948). Marked decrease in CBF and $CMRO_2$ have also been observed in man (Ingvar *et al.*, 1964; Shalit *et al.*, 1969; Shalit *et al.*, 1970 a) and experimental animals (Fujishima *et al.*, 1970; Shalit *et al.*, 1967) with lesions restricted to the upper brain stem but with normal intracranial pressure and no detectable histological damage to total brain tissue.

References pp. 242–243

It is generally agreed that the decrease in CBF which occurs when the intracranial pressure is raised above a critical value is mainly the result of mechanical pressure on the cerebral vessels. Considerable difference of opinion exists, however, as to the explanation of the reduction of CBF found in humans and animals with pure brain stem lesions. This controversy originates in different basic concepts with regard to the intrinsic regulation of CBF in physiological and pathological conditions – namely whether CBF is primarily regulated by the reaction of the vascular smooth muscle to its chemical milieu or whether the diameter of the cerebral vessels is determined also, or mainly by neural regulatory mechanisms which require functional integrity of the brain stem.

The factors which influence the diameter of the cerebral vessels are in many cases also operative in the peripheral circulation. Anoxia, hypercarbia and acidosis have potent vasodilatory effects in both the peripheral and cerebral vessels (Haddy, 1966; Hilton and Eicholtz, 1925; Gremeels and Starling, 1926; Berne et al., 1957; Guz et al., 1960; Fleisch et al., 1932). Autoregulation of blood flow is also a common phenomenon in various organs (Autoregulation of Blood Flow, Symposium, 1963). The rich innervation of the walls of the peripheral vessels is similar in many respects to the innervation found in cerebral vessels (Falck et al., 1968; Nelson and Rennels, 1968; White, 1963). A regulation of vascular tonus by a combination of local metabolic effects and central neurogenic control is known to be effective in the peripheral vascular system. Nevertheless, the possibility of an active neural control of the cerebral vessels analogous to that of the peripheral vessels (Aoki and Brody, 1966; Bard, 1960; Oberholzer, 1960; Unväs, 1960) is denied by many investigators. Lack of an effective response of the cerebral vessels to neural stimulation of various nerves on the one hand (Roy and Sherrington, 1890; Forbes, 1958; Putnam and Ask Upmark, 1934) and their sensitivity to both regional and total cerebral metabolic changes on the other (Schmidt et al., 1945; Ingvar, 1958; Schieve and Wilson, 1953; Himwich et al., 1947; Homburger et al., 1946; Shalit, 1966; White et al., 1961; Jasper and Erickson, 1941; Malmlund, 1968) have led to the view that, unlike peripheral vessels, the diameter of the cerebral vessels is determined solely or mainly by the effects of the electrochemical constituents in the extracellular fluid of the vascular smooth muscle (Lassen, 1968). This muscle would react by relaxation to increased P_{CO_2} and acidosis, and by contraction to decreased P_{CO_2} and alkalosis. Since CO_2 is a principal cerebral metabolic end-product, it has been generally accepted that the local vascular effect of CO_2 or the consequent changes in pH are the means whereby the cerebral circulation is adjusted to the regional and total cerebral metabolic requirements. This theory is supported by numerous studies which showed that CBF is indeed related to regional and total cerebral metabolic activity, and to the CSF pH which is in equilibrium with cerebral extracellular pH (CBF and CSF International Symposium, 1968; Lassen, 1968). Evidence in support of this theory was presented by Ingvar et al. (1964) in their studies of a comatose patient with upper brain stem infarction. At a normal arterial CO_2 tension, the CBF of the patient was reduced to 12 ml/100 g/min while the $CMRO_2$ was only 0.8 ml/100 g/min. Cortical biopsy revealed no pathological findings and the extreme reduction of CBF was considered to be a result of the upper brain stem lesion.

The loss of activation from brain stem reticular formation depressed neuronal activity and a reduction of oxygen uptake followed. The circulatory effects were considered to be secondary to the metabolic changes, since the intrinsic control of the CBF implies that this flow is very accurately regulated by the functional activity

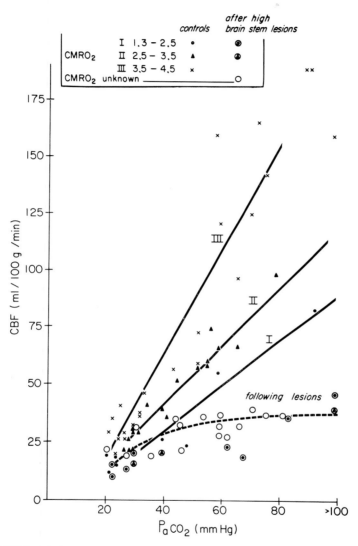

Fig. 1. The CBF in relation to the Pa_{CO_2}, as influenced by different levels of $CMRO_2$ before and after high brain stem lesions. The controls indicate findings in 35 animals. The levels of $CMRO_2$ are probably affected by the depth of anesthesia. An approximate line is drawn to aid in separation of the groups according to $CMRO_2$. Note that after high brain stem lesions the $CMRO_2$ no longer exerts the same influence on the relationship of CBF to Pa_{CO_2} (from Shalit *et al.*, (1967) Carbon dioxide and cerebral circulatory control, III. The effects of brain stem lesions. *Arch. Neurol.*, 7, 342, reproduced by courtesy of the editor).

References pp. 242–243

of the nervous tissue to maintain a constant "milieu interieur" of the brain. The fact that completely normal values of cerebral venous oxygen saturation and CO_2 tension were found, was interpreted as an indication that this very basic control of CBF was functioning in a normal fashion.

On the other hand, this example may be regarded as a potent reason for questioning the validity of the whole theory.

It must be considered that when the measurements were carried out, the patient was in a steady state of prolonged cerebral metabolic depression. Although his cerebral vessels were presumably surrounded by a normal chemical environment, they nevertheless remained markedly constricted, indicating that the mechanism controlling their diameter was functioning abnormally.

It appears, therefore, that another factor, possibly linked to the high brain stem pathology must have modified the normal constant relationship observed between the cerebral vascular diameter and the cerebral extracellular electrochemical environment.

This assumption was investigated in a group of 18 mongrel dogs in which CBF, $CMRO_2$ and the response of CBF to CO_2 were determined before and after lesions induced in various parts of the brain. It was found that extensive lobectomies of the frontal and occipital lobes, as well as destructive lesions (produced either by section,

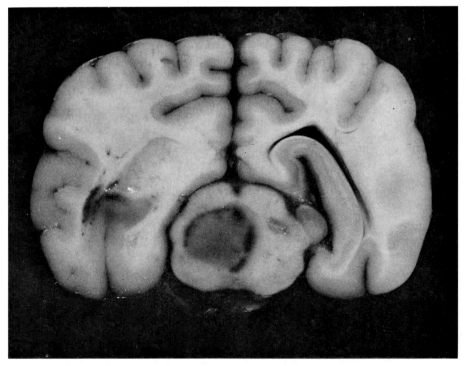

Fig. 2. A typical high brain stem lesion produced by local freezing to $-180\,^{\circ}C$ by the use of Cooper Cryosurgical system (from Shalit et al., see legend to Fig. 1; reproduced by courtesy of the editor).

coagulation or regional freezing) in the medulla, cerebellum and thalamus did not affect CBF and $CMRO_2$ or the response to the stimulus of exogenously administered CO_2. When the lesions were produced in the upper brain stem, a considerable decrease in CBF and $CMRO_2$ followed, with a concurrent decrease in the response of CBF to CO_2 (Shalit *et al.* 1967) (Figs. 1 and 2). Similar findings were observed in patients with high brain stem lesions in the terminal stages of their illness, when $CMRO_2$ was depressed to lower levels (Shalit *et al.*, 1970 a). The following case demonstrates the findings in one of these patients.

A 45-year-old woman was diagnosed as having a glioma of the left posterior thalamic region with infiltration into the upper brain stem. One month after admission her condition deteriorated and she gradually became comatose, but still responded to painful stimuli. At this stage the CBF was 38.8 ml/100 g/min at Pa_{CO_2} of 38 mm Hg. Inhalation of 5% CO_2 in oxygen increased the Pa_{CO_2} to 45 mm Hg, with a concomitant increase in CBF to 48.3 ml/100 g/min.

$CMRO_2$ at that time was 1.74 ml/100 g/min. Two weeks later, when the second study was performed, her clinical condition remained unchanged. The CBF and $CMRO_2$ values were similar to the previous values and the cerebrovascular response to inhaled CO_2 was still evident. About two weeks later her condition worsened. She

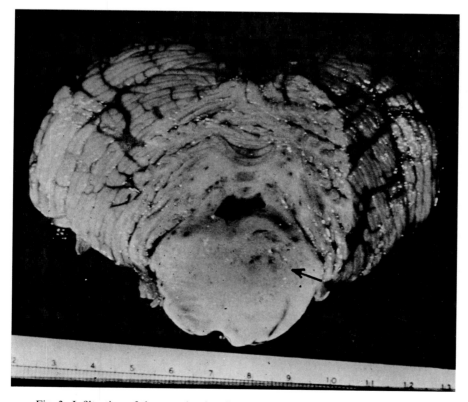

Fig. 3. Infiltration of the pons by the glioma of the left posterior thalamic region.

References pp. 242–243

no longer responded to stimuli, her pupils were widely dilated and artificial respiratory assistance was required. Lumbar puncture disclosed normal pressure. At that time her CBF was somewhat decreased and the $CMRO_2$ was 1.2 ml/100 g/min. Inhalation of a CO_2–oxygen mixture, which increased Pa_{CO_2} from 35 to 59 mm Hg, failed to increase CBF. The patient died five days after the last study (Fig. 3).

Recent observations in dogs after experimental thrombosis of the basilar artery revealed similar findings (Fujishima et al., 1970).

In the clinical and experimental observations cited above, cerebral venous P_{CO2} and pH were normal. Cerebral extracellular pH could nevertheless theoretically be alkaline due to an increase in bicarbonate ion concentration. This possibility was investigated in five chronic vegetative patients with traumatic brain stem damage. In all of them a normal intracranial pressure was found and gross hemispheric pathology was excluded by roentgenological contrast examinations. In the acute phase of their illness CBF was in a few instances normal or above normal, while later, in the chronic phase, it was decreased to very low levels (see Fig. 4). In all instances, cerebral venous P_{CO_2} and pH, and CSF P_{CO_2}, pH and bicarbonate ion concentration were within normal levels in the chronic stage.

The following report illustrates a typical case: a 19-year-old female was admitted a few hours after a car accident. She was deeply comatose with widely dilated non-

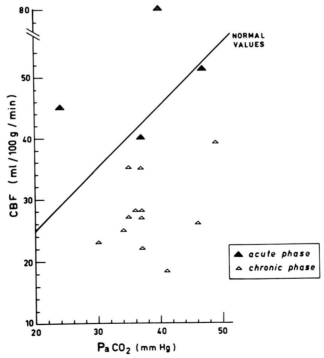

Fig. 4. Correlation between CBF and Pa_{CO_2} in 5 chronic vegetative patients suffering from brain stem injury. (From Shalit et al. (1970) Critical values for cerebral oxygen utilization in man. Proc. Intern. Cerebral Blood Flow Symposium, London, September 17–19, 1970.)

reacting pupils, spasticity and decerebrate rigidity. Bilateral carotid angiography was interpreted as normal. Shortly after the admission she developed diabetes insipidus, which lasted about four days, and her body temperature fell spontaneously to 32°. EEG recordings showed diffuse slowing and depression of the electrical activity. The patient gradually developed the typical manifestations of chronic vegetation. CBF and $CMRO_2$ were studied six times during a two-month period, and CSF pH and bicarbonate ion concentration were determined concurrently (Fig. 5).

The suppression of total cerebral metabolic activity, which in these patients presumably followed inactivation of the reticular formation in the brain stem, was not manifested in the cerebral vascular extracellular space. The cerebral vessels nevertheless remained constricted, despite a completely normal extracellular environment. The constrictive effect of the upper brain stem lesion on the cerebral vessels must therefore be mediated by a mechanism unrelated to local metabolic processes and their products.

The increase of CBF following brain stem stimulation (Geiger and Sigg, 1955; Ingvar and Soderberg, 1958; Meyer et al., 1969) is considered by the generally accepted theory to be secondary to the increase in total cerebral metabolic activity and the consequent liberation of CO_2 and acidification of cerebral tissue. Little is known at present about the time required for the chain of events which follows the stimulation – a sequence which includes the transfer of the stimulus by neural or humoral pathways to the cortex (Ingvar, 1955; Purpura, 1956), the resulting activation of the neurons and neuronal biochemical reaction, the intracellular accumulation of CO_2 and its

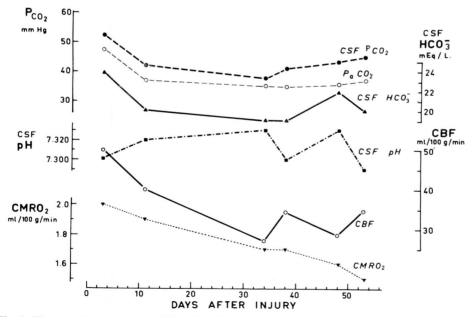

Fig. 5. The correlation between CBF, CMRO₂, Pa_{CO_2} and CSF pH, P_{CO_2} and bicarbonate ion concentration in a chronic vegetative patient after traumatic high brain stem damage. (From Shalit et al., see legend to Fig. 4.)

diffusion to the vascular extracellular space. It was observed that abrupt changes in arterial P_{CO_2} tend to modify jugular venous P_{CO_2} with a certain time lag (Severinghaus and Lassen, 1967). A similar delay might therefore be expected for the diffusion of CO_2 from the metabolically activated neurons to reach an effective concentration in the perivascular compartments. The effect of brain stem stimulation on CBF is, however, instantaneous, suggesting an action of a neural reflex arc mechanism rather than a relatively slow chain reaction of cellular and extracellular metabolic processes (Langfitt and Kassel, 1968).

Metabolic changes occurring in the brain stem may be followed under certain circumstances by an increased CBF with no increase in total brain metabolic activity. This was demonstrated experimentally in cats where the injection of sodium thiopentone into the vertebral artery was followed in many cases by an increase in cortical blood flow in spite of a suppression of cortical electrical activity (Shalit, 1970 b). (Fig. 6). The explanation for these changes remains unknown, but one may speculate that barbiturates under certain circumstances affect cerebro-vasoregulatory centers in the brain stem and thus produce vascular phenomena independent of total brain metabolic levels. Smaller amounts of barbiturates have been shown to produce desynchronization of the EEG, presumably by blocking inhibitory centers (Alema et al., 1966; Magni et al., 1959; Rosina and Mancia, 1966; Rossi, 1965). A similar mechanism may be considered for the explanation of the cerebral vascular effects.

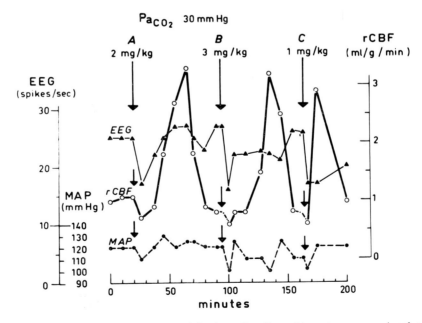

Fig. 6. The effect of intravertebral artery injection of sodium thiopentone on regional cerebral blood flow in a cat. Note the marked increase in flow in spite of depression of EEG activity which follows each injection (From M. N. Shalit (1970) The variable relationship between EEG and cerebral blood flow after selective intra-arterial injections of barbiturates. *Proc. Intern. Cerebral Blood Flow Symp., London, September 17–19, 1970*).

B. CRITICAL VALUES OF CMRO$_2$ IN COMA

Determination of the level of cerebral metabolic activity in comatose patients was found to be of considerable interest, not only for its theoretical implications but also in the assessment of the clinical status and prognosis of comatose patients suffering from cerebral damage. The latter evaluation may be extremely difficult, especially in traumatic cases. It may be impossible to distinguish between a patient who will die within a short time and one who will eventually recover completely. Although two such patients may seem clinically similar and have the same EEG pattern, one of them may have a brain which has been severely and irreversibly injured while the other suffers only a transient functional loss. Because of the inadequacy of the conventional clinical and laboratory methods, an attempt was made to use cerebral oxygen consumption – an expression of the level of cerebral metabolic activity – as an index of brain vitality and of the seriousness of the pathological processes within the brain.

Two critical values of CMRO$_2$ were sought; the lowest value above which coma might be still reversible, and a still lower value which indicates that the brain is dead. CMRO$_2$ values between these two critical values would, therefore, indicate that the coma is, in all cases, irreversible and that the patient would remain comatose for varying periods of time and eventually die.

These critical values were investigated in comatose patients suffering from various cerebral pathological conditions (Shalit *et al.*, 1970 b). CMRO$_2$ and CBF were determined 46 times in 24 patients. As many as six studies were carried out during a period of several months up to one year. At the same time the patients were given a complete neurological examination with EEG recordings and measurements of intracranial pressure by a lumbar puncture.

The lowest values of CMRO$_2$ associated with reversible coma and subsequent return to consciousness were found in two young males who suffered from through-and-through gun-shot wounds of the head.

The first patient B.F. an 18-year-old male, was wounded by a bullet which entered his skull in the left occipital region, with the exit in the right parietal region. On admission he was deeply comatose with wide non-reacting pupils. The systolic blood pressure was 70 mm Hg. Spontaneous respiration was inadequate and artificial respiratory assistance was required. X-ray of the skull revealed several linear fractures extending in different directions in various parts of the skull (Fig. 7). At operation a large intracerebral hematoma was evacuated. The brain tissue was found to be severely edematous with numerous lacerations and petechiae. On the third day after admission, while no change in his clinical condition could be observed, the CMRO$_2$ was found to be 1.4 ml/100 g/min. The patient gradually regained consciousness within a few weeks and recovered. A second study performed one year later, at which time the patient was fully conscious but with residual triplegia, revealed a normal value of CMRO$_2$.

The second patient, N.H. an 18-year-old male was wounded by a bullet which penetrated his skull in the right temporal region and emerged in the left temporal

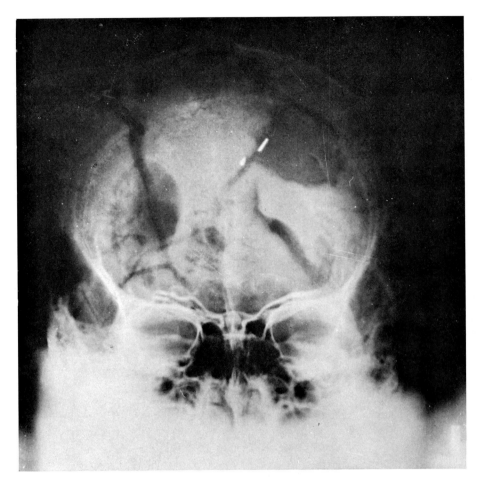

Fig. 7. Skull X-ray of the patient taken after the operation. The multiplicity of the fractures indicates the sudden marked increase in the intracranial pressure consequent to the penetration of the bullet. (From Shalit, see legend to Fig. 4.)

region. On admission he was deeply comatose with wide non-reacting pupils. At operation the brain was found to be markedly edematous with multiple small and large hemorrhages and lacerations. A large intracerebral hematoma was evacuated. Two further operations were performed during the first week for evacuation of recurrent hematoma. Three weeks after his admission, while he was still deeply comatose, the $CMRO_2$ was found to be 1.5 ml/100 g/min. The patient slowly regained consciousness and recovered. Six months later he was fully conscious with a left hemiparesis. A repeated study could not be obtained. The clinical and laboratory findings of the two patients are shown in Table 1.

The findings in the above two patients indicate that coma may still be reversible in spite of severe cerebral metabolic depression due to diffuse parenchymatous damage. $CMRO_2$ values as low as 50% of normal are apparently still compatible with an

TABLE 1

CLINICAL AND LABORATORY FINDINGS IN TWO PATIENTS WITH GUN SHOT
WOUNDS IN THE HEAD

Patient	1. B.F.		2. N.H.	
Time after injury	3 days	1 year	21 days	6 months
State of consciousness	deep coma	conscious	deep coma	conscious
Size of pupils	wide	medium	wide	medium
Type of respiration	artificial	spontaneous	spontaneous	spontaneous
Response to stimuli	absent	normal	absent	normal
Arterial P_{CO_2} (mm Hg)	35.0	38.5	45.0	
(A–V)O_2 (Vol %)	5.3	4.9	4.0	
CBF (ml/100 g/min)	26	67	37	
CMRO$_2$ (ml/100 g/min)	1.4	3.3	1.5	

eventual full recovery of consciousness. The fact that the total CMRO$_2$ finally returns to normal suggests that the viable regions regain normal metabolic activity, while the irreversibly damaged tissue gradually liquefies or undergoes gliosis and no longer participates in cerebral perfusion.

In a few instances relatively high initial values of CMRO$_2$ were found in patients who remained unconscious in a chronic vegetative state or died after varying periods of time. A follow-up of their cerebral metabolic level revealed a persistent gradual decrease of CMRO$_2$. This pattern of deterioration was found especially in patients suffering from traumatic brain stem lesions. It appears, therefore, that coma which follows brain stem lesions might be an active and dynamic process, in which brain damage may be progressive and reach its climax long after the direct traumatic damage is induced. High initial values of CMRO$_2$ do not, therefore, necessarily indicate a favourable prognosis in such cases. Only repeated determinations of cerebral metabolic status may give a true indication of the patients' prognosis.

The correlation between the values of CMRO$_2$ and the accepted clinical phenomena indicating brain functional level were explored in 9 comatose patients (Shalit et al., 1970 a). The lowest values of CMRO$_2$ at which some viability of the brain was still preserved (as indicated by preservation of any EEG activity, spontaneous respiration and naturally maintained blood pressure) were in the region of 1 ml/100 g/min. When the brain oxygen consumption reached levels lower than one third of the normal values (lower than 1 ml/100 g/min), a total breakdown of the vital brain functions occurred. At this critical level, spontaneous respiration ceased, the blood pressure fell, the pupils began to dilate and muscle tone was lost. These severe signs did not all appear simultaneously but developed gradually within the narrow margins of CMRO$_2$ between 1 and 1.3 ml/100 g/min.

One of the last signs of brain function to disappear was its electrical activity. This was still maintained, although very much depressed, when all other signs were abolished. In this respect, the isoelectric EEG can be regarded as one of the best criteria of brain death.

References pp. 242–243

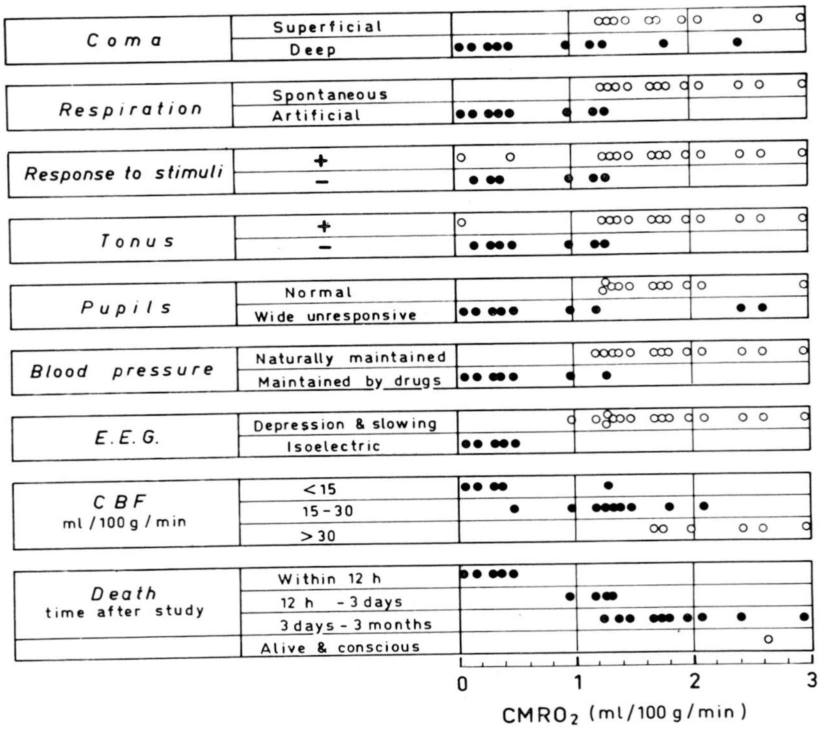

Fig. 8. Correlation between the clinical signs, CBF and CMRO₂ in nine comatose patients. Full circles indicate decompensation. Open circles indicate preservation of brain function. (From M. N. Shalit et al., "The blood flow and oxygen consumption of the dying brain", Neurology, 20: 740, 1970, reproduced by courtesy of the editor).

The clinical criteria of brain death were found in patients having $CMRO_2$ values of 0.6 ml/100 g/min or lower.

It is conceivable that all the criteria of brain death, although they may appear as transitory phenomena in different pathological situations, are not reversible when accompanied by a value of $CMRO_2$ below 0.6 ml/100 g/min.

Other clinical signs such as the depth of coma evaluated by clinical examination, the response to painful stimuli, muscle tonus and the width of the pupils were found to have no constant correlation with the status of brain activity (Fig. 8).

The patients studied included a group of chronic vegetative patients in whom the $CMRO_2$ levels were in the range of 1.3–2 ml/100 g/min. No full recovery was seen when the $CMRO_2$ remained at this level for a few months. The relationship between the clinical status of the 24 comatose patients and the $CMRO_2$ values is summarized in Fig. 9.

Considering these observations, it appears that the use of a direct and objective estimation of cerebral metabolic status when combined with the conventional clinical and laboratory methods may be used as an index for the evaluation of brain damage and the prognosis of the patient.

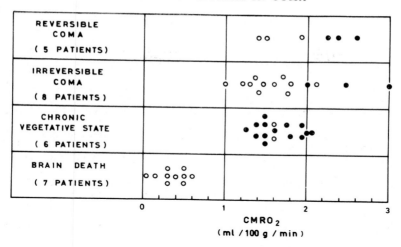

Fig. 9. Correlation between the clinical status of all 24 patients studied and the values of CMRO₂. Some patients appear in more than one category if their condition changed during the studies.

SUMMARY

The correlation between cerebral blood flow (CBF), cerebral oxygen consumption (CMRO₂) and the clinical status was explored in 24 comatose patients suffering from various pathological conditions of the brain. The lowest values of CMRO₂ at which signs of any brain viability could still be detected were in the region of 1 ml/100 g/min. When CMRO₂ was suppressed to lower values than 0.6 ml/100 g/min, the accepted criteria of brain death were manifested. When the damage was induced mainly in the cerebral hemispheres, coma was at times reversible in spite of an initial severe metabolic depression expressed by CMRO₂ values of 1.5 ml/100 g/min. On the other hand, patients with brain stem damage with relatively higher initial values of CMRO₂ usually deteriorated gradually and either remained in a chronic vegetative state with corresponding CMRO₂ values in the range of 1.3–2 ml/100 g/min or eventually died.

In five chronic vegetative patients suffering from trauma restricted mainly to the brain stem, successive determinations of CBF, CMRO₂ and CSF pH, P_{CO_2} and bicarbonate ion concentration over a period of several months were performed. It was found that CBF and CMRO₂ were markedly decreased while the CSF parameters remained within normal values. When CMRO₂ was further decreased in progressive brain stem damage, the response of CBF to the stimulus of CO₂ was decreased or abolished. This phenomenon was also observed in animals in which high brain stem lesions were induced experimentally.

It is suggested, therefore, that cerebral blood flow and the response of cerebral vessels to changes in arterial P_{CO_2} and cerebral extracellular pH require brain stem functional integrity.

References pp. 242–243

REFERENCES

ALEMA, G., PERRIA, L., ROSADINI, G., ROSSI, G. F. AND ZATTONI, J. (1966) Functional inactivation of human brain stem related to the level of consciousness. *J. Neurosurg.*, **24**, 629–639.

AOKI, V. S. AND BRODY, M. J. (1966) Medullary control of vascular resistance. *Circulation Res.*, **18** and **19**, *Suppl.* 1, June.

BARD, P. (1960) Anatomical organization of the central nervous system in relation to control of the heart and blood vessels. In: *Proc. Symp. Central Nervous System Control of Circulation*, Washington, D.C., 1959, *Physiol. Rev.*, **40**, *suppl.* 4, 3.

BERNE, R. M., BLACKMAN, J. R. AND GARDNER, T. H. (1957) Hypoxemia and coronary blood flow. *J. Clin. Invest.*, **36**, 1101–1106.

FALCK, B., NIELSON, K. C. AND OWMAN, CH. (1968) Adrenergic innervation of the pial circulation. *Scand. J. Lab. Clin. Invest.*, *Suppl.* **102**, VI B.

FLEISCH, A., SIBUL, I. AND PONOMEREV, V. (1932) Kohlensäure und Sauerstoffmangel als auslösende Reize. *Pfluegers Arch. Ges. Physiol.*, **230**, 814.

FORBES, H. S. (1958) Regulation of the cerebral vessels; new aspects. *Arch. Neurol. Psychiat.*, **80**, 689–695.

FUJISHIMA, M., SCHEINBERG, P. AND REINMUTH, O. M. (1970) Effects of experimental occlusion of the basilar artery by magnetic localization of iron filings on cerebral blood flow and metabolism and cerebrovascular responses to CO_2 in the dog. *Neurology*, **20**, 925–932.

GEIGER, A. AND SIGG, E. B. (1955) The significance of the hypothalamus in the regulation of the metabolism of the brain. 80th Ann. Meeting, *Trans. Amer. Neurol. Assoc.*, **1955**, 117–120.

GREMEELS, H. AND STARLING, E. H. (1926) On the influence of hydrogen ion concentration and of anoxemia upon heart volume. *J. Physiol.*, **60**, 61–297.

GUZ, A., KURLAND, G. S. AND FREEDBERG, A. S. (1960) Relation of coronary flow to oxygen supply. *Amer. J. Physiol.*, **199**, 179.

HADDY, F. J. (1966) Role of chemicals in local regulation of vascular resistance. *Circulation Res.*, **18** and **19**, *Suppl.* 1, June, 14–22.

HIMWICH, W. A., HOMBURGER, E., MARESCA, R. AND HIMWICH, H. E., (1947) Brain metabolism in man: Unanesthetized and in pentothal narcosis. *Amer. J. Psychiat.*, **103**, 689–696.

HILTON, R. AND EICHHOLTZ, F. (1925) Influence of chemical factors on the coronary circulation. *J. Physiol.*, **59**, 413.

HOMBURGER, E., HIMWICH, W. A., ETSTEN, B., YORK, R., MARESCA, R. AND HIMWICH, H. E., (1946) Effect of pentothal anesthesia on canine cerebral cortex. *Amer. J. Physiol.*, **147**, 343–345.

INGVAR, D. H. (1955) Extra neuronal influence upon the electrical activity of isolated cortex following stimulation of the reticular activating system. *Acta Physiol. Scand.*, **33**, 169–193.

INGVAR, D. H. (1958) Cortical state of excitability and cortical circulation. In: JASPER, H. H. (Ed.), *Reticular Formation of the Brain*, Little Brown and Co., Boston, Mass., pp. 381–408.

INGVAR, D. H., HAGGENDAL, E., NILSSON, N. J., SOURANDER, P., WICKBORN, I. AND LASSEN, N. A., (1964) Cerebral circulation and metabolism in a comatose patient. *Arch. Neurol.*, **11**, 13–21.

INGVAR, D. H. AND SODERBERG, U. (1958) Cortical blood flow related to EEG patterns evoked by stimulation of the brain stem. *Acta Physiol. Scand.*, **42**, 130–143.

INGVAR, D. H., LASSEN, N. A., SIESJÖ, B. K. AND SKINHOJ, E. (Eds.) (1968) Cerebral blood flow and cerebro spinal fluid. Third Intern. Symp. Lund–Copenhagen, May 9–11, 1968, *Scand. J. Clin. Lab. Invest.*, *Suppl.* **102**.

JASPER, H. H. AND ERICKSON, T. C. (1941) Cerebral blood flow and pH in excessive cortical discharge induced by Metrazol and electrical stimulation. *J. Neurophysiol.*, **4**, 333–347.

JOHNSON, P. C. (Ed.) (1963) Autoregulation of blood flow. In: *Proc. Intern. Symp., Indianapolis, June 10–12, 1963.* American Heart Association, Monograph No. **8**.

KETY, S. S., SHENKIN, H. A. AND SCHMIDT, C. F. (1948) Effects of increased intracranial pressure on cerebral circulatory functions in man. *J. Clin. Invest.*, **27**, 493–499.

LANGFITT, T. W. AND KASSEL, N. T. (1968) Cerebral vasodilatation produced by brain stem stimulation: Neurogenic control *vs.* autoregulation. *Amer. J. Physiol.*, **215**, 90–97.

LASSEN, N. A. (1968) Brain extracellular pH: The main factor controlling cerebral blood flow. *Scand. J. Clin. Lab. Invest.*, **22**, 247–251.

MAGNI, F., MORRUZZI, G., ROSSI, C. F. AND ZANCHETTI, Z. (1959) EEG arousal following inactivation of the lower brain stem by selective injections of barbiturate into the vertebral circulation. *Arch. Ital. Biol.*, **97**, 33–46.

MALMLUND, H. O. (1968) Cerebral blood flow and oxygen consumption in barbiturate poisoning. *Acta Med. Scand.*, **184**, 373–377.

MEYER, J. S., NOMURA, F., SAKAMOTO, K. AND KONDO, A. (1969) Effect of stimulation of the brain stem reticular formation on cerebral blood flow and oxygen consumption. *Electroencephalog. Clin. Neurophysiol.*, **26**, 125–132.

NELSON, E. AND RENNELS, M. (1968) Electron microscopic studies on intracranial vascular nerves in the cat. *Scand. J. Clin. Lab. Invest.*, *Suppl.* **102**, VI A.

OBERHOLZER, R. J. H. (1960) Circulatory centers in medulla and midbrain. Proc. Symp. central nervous system control of circulation, Washington, D.C., 1959. *Physiol. Rev.*, **40**, *Suppl.* 4, 179.

PURPURA, D. P. (1956) A neurohumoral mechanism of reticulo-cortical activation. *Amer. J. Physiol.*, **186**, 250–254.

PUTNAM, T. J. AND ASK UPMARK, E. (1934) Cerebral circulation XXIX. Microscopic observations of the living choroid plexus and ependyma of the cat. *Arch. Neurol. Psychiat.*, **32**, 72–80.

ROSINA, A. AND MANCIA, M. (1966) Electrophysiological and behavioural changes following selective and reversible inactivation of lower brain stem structures in chronic cats. *Electroencephalog. Clin. Neurophysiol.*, **21**, 157–167.

ROSSI, C. F. (1965) Some aspects of the functional organization of the brain stem: Neurophysiological and neurosurgical observations. *Excerpta Medica*, No. 93, 117–122.

ROY, C. S. AND SHERRINGTON, C. S. (1890) On the regulation of the blood supply of the brain. *J. Physiol.*, **11**, 85–108.

SCHIEVE, J. F. AND WILSON, W. P. (1953) The influence of age, anesthesia and cerebral arteriosclerosis on cerebral vascular activity to CO_2. *Amer. J. Med.*, **15**, 171–174.

SCHMIDT, C. F., KETY, S. S. AND PENNES, H. H. (1945) The gaseous metabolism of the brain of the monkey. *Amer. J. Physiol.*, **143**, 33–52.

SEVERINGHAUS, J. W. AND LASSEN, N. (1967) Step hypocapnia to separate arterial from tissue pCO_2 in the regulation of cerebral blood flow. *Circulation Res.*, **20**, 272–278.

SHALIT, M. N., BELLER, A. J., FEINSOD, M., DRAPKIN, A. J. AND COTEV, S. (1970 a) The blood flow and oxygen consumption of the dying brain. *Neurology*, **20**, 740–748.

SHALIT, M. N., BELLER, A. J., FEINSOD, M. AND COTEV, S. (1969) Cerebral oxygen consumption: another indicator of brain death. In: PENIN, H. AND KÄUFER, C. (Eds.), *Der Hirntod*, Georg Thieme Verlag, Stuttgart, p. 56–61.

SHALIT, M. N., REINMUTH, O. M., SHIMOJYO, S. AND SCHEINBERG, P. (1967) Carbon dioxide and cerebral circulatory control: III. The effects of brain stem lesions. *Arch. Neurol.*, **17**, 342–353.

SHALIT, M. N. (1966) The effect of metrazol on the hemodynamics and impedance of the cats brain cortex. *J. Neuropathol. Exp. Neurol.*, **24**, 75–84.

SHALIT, M. N. (1970) The variable relationship between EEG and cerebral blood flow after selective intra arterial injections of barbiturate. *Proc. Intern. Cerebral Blood Flow Symp.*, London, September 17–19, 1970.

SHALIT, M. N., BELLER, A. J., FEINSOD, M., ZEIGLER, M. AND COTEV, S. (1970 b) Critical values for cerebral oxygen consumption in man. *Proc. Intern. Cerebral Blood Flow Symp.*, London, September 17–19, 1970.

UNVÄS, B. (1960) Central cardiovascular control. In: FIELD, J., MAGOUN, H. W. AND HALL, V. E. (Eds.), *Neurophysiology, Handbook of Physiology*, Vol. II, section I, chap. 44. American Physiological Society, Washington, D.C.

WECHSLER, R. L., DRIPPS, R. D. AND KETY, S. S. (1951) Blood flow and oxygen consumption of the human brain during anesthesia produced by thiopental. *Anesthesiology*, **12**, 308–314.

WHITE, J. C. (1963) Nervous control of the cerebral vascular system. *Clin. Neurosurg.*, **9**, 67–87.

WHITE, P. T., GRANT, P., MOSIER, J. AND GRAIG, A., (1961) Changes in cerebral dynamics associated with seizures. *Neurology*, **11**, 354–361.

Spinal Cord Blood Flow*

H. FLOHR, M. BROCK AND W. PÖLL

Department of Physiology, 53 Bonn and Department of Neurosurgery, University of Hannover, 3 Hannover-Buchholz (W. Germany)

The high vulnerability of the spinal cord to blood flow disturbances has been well known since the investigations by Stenon (1667) and Swammerdam (1667), and has been the subject of numerous investigations from that time until today (Haller, 1756; Legallois, 1830; Schiffer, 1869; Luchsinger, 1878; Fredericq, 1889; Colson, 1890; Tureen, 1936, 1938; Rexed, 1940; van Harreveld, 1941, 1944; Krogh, 1950; Blasius, 1950; Blasius and Zimmermann, 1957; Kirstein, 1951; Gelfan and Tarlov, 1955; Murayama and Smith, 1965).

The significance of disturbances of the spinal cord flow for the formation and development of neurological diseases was recognized early (Vulpian, 1875; Marie, 1892; Lewandowsky, 1911). Since about 1950 a great number of clinical and pathological investigations on disturbances of the spinal cord circulation have been published (Bodechtel and Schrader, 1957; Sarteschi and Giannini, 1960; Corbin, 1961; Nunes-Vicente, 1964; Jellinger, 1966; Neumayer, 1967). Our present knowledge of the physiology of spinal blood flow however is based on a small number of experimental investigations. Only recently quantitative values have been obtained, and some insight in the circulatory control mechanisms has been achieved.

Field *et al.* (1951) investigated the influence of arterial blood pressure, asphyxia and hypercapnia on the blood flow of the thoracic and lumbosacral cord of anaesthetized rabbits using heat clearance probes. They found that the blood flow is substantially independent of arterial pressure. Asphyxia led to a measurable increase of the blood flow, but there was no evidence to indicate a specific vasodilator role for CO_2 in the cord. In contrast Otomo *et al.* (1960) through direct observation of pial vessels in dogs came to the conclusion that the chief factor controlling spinal cord flow is the systemic blood pressure.

Similarly Capon (1961) concluded that CO_2 has a less obvious vasodilator action in the cord and plays a less important role compared with the brain.

Palleske and Herrmann (1968) investigated the blood flow of the lumbosacral cord of dwarf pigs using heat clearance probes. They found no evidence of any fundamental difference between brain and spinal cord so far as their circulatory control mechanisms and the effects of systemic pressure, Pa_{O_2} and Pa_{CO_2} are concerned.

---

* The work was supported by the Deutsche Forschungsgemeinschaft.

References pp. 260–262

Wüllenweber (1969, 1968), measuring spinal cord flow of humans during neuro-surgical operations, Flohr *et al.* (1970 c) in experiments on cats, Kindt *et al.* in experiments on rhesus monkeys and Tschetter *et al.* (1970) in experiments on dogs arrived at similar conclusions.

Quantitative data about the amount of the blood flow of the spinal cord were first made known by Sokoloff (1961) using an autoradiographic technique to determine the rate of uptake of a radioactive indicator following its injection into the blood stream. In the cervical cord of rats the blood flow of the grey matter in the case of non-narcotized animals was measured as 63 ml/100 g · min, the flow through the white matter as 14 ml/100 g · min. In the case of narcotized animals values of 53 or 15 ml/100 g · min respectively were measured.

Mandel *et al.* (1963) calculated flow values from the uptake of Iodoanti-pyrine of 0.28 ml/g · min for the cord compared with 0.41 ml/g · min for the brain.

Smith *et al.* (1969) determined local blood flow in different segments of the spinal cord of goats by means of a ^{133}Xe clearance technique. The mean value of all measurements was 16.2 ± 1.2 S.E. ml/100 g · min.

Flohr *et al.* (1969) in experiments with cats obtained values of 20.3 ml/100 g · min for the cervical cord, 16.5 ml/100 g · min for the thoracic cord, and of 23.7 ml/100 g · min for the lumbosacral cord.

Tschetter *et al.* (1970) presented similar values for the dog. For the cervical, thoracic and lumbosacral cord they obtained values of 15.1, 13.5 and 19.2 ml/100 g · min respectively.

The latter values were obtained by the particle distribution technique (Flohr, 1968; Neutze *et al.*, 1968; Tschetter *et al.*, 1968). The introduction of this method has extended the possibilities of measuring regional blood flow in various organs and offers certain practical advantages. In principle it is possible to measure quantitatively the blood flow of all parallel circuits of the systemic circulation simultaneously. It is therefore possible to determine the perfusion of organs which had not hitherto been accessible and to perform comparative measurements of regional flow to different structures of complex organs.

The present report summarizes results obtained by this technique. Blood flow to different segments of the spinal cord and different parts of the brain (prosencephalon, cerebellum and brain-stem) were measured simultaneously under varying conditions. The effects of Pa_{O_2}, Pa_{CO_2} and the mean arterial blood pressure on blood flow to the different regions were assessed and comparatively analysed.

METHODS

The particle distribution method represents an application of the principle of measuring the fractional distribution of cardiac output by measuring the distribution of an indicator during the first transit (Sapirstein, 1956). According to the Fick principle the blood flow of an organ is:

$$F_n = \frac{Q_n}{\int\limits_0^\infty (C_{an} - C_{vn})\,dt} \tag{1}$$

where

F_n = blood flow in ml/min

Q_n = added quantity of indicator

C_{an} = concentration of the indicator in the arterial blood of the organ n

C_{vn} = concentration of the indicator in venous blood of the organ n

For the cardiac output the following is valid:

$$CO = \frac{Q}{\int\limits_0^\infty (C_a - C_v)\,dt} \tag{2}$$

CO = cardiac output in ml/min

Q = the quantity of indicator added to the total organism

C_a = concentration of the indicator in the blood of the left ventricle

C_v = concentration of the indicator in the blood of the right ventricle

If an indicator is so added that it is fully mixed with the blood leaving the left ventricle and remaining mixed with the flowing blood, then the following equation is valid:

$$C_a = C_{an} \tag{3}$$

The indicator spreads itself during the first passage of the blood through the periphery to the particular regions according to the different blood flow values. With an indicator which does not recirculate, but which during the first passage through the capillaries is quantitatively eliminated from the flowing blood, the following equation is valid:

$$C_{vn} = 0, \tag{4}$$

and the distribution pattern of the first passage remains. From this follows:

$$\frac{F_i}{CO} = \frac{Q_n}{Q} \tag{5}$$

or

$$F_i = \frac{Q_n}{C_q} \cdot CO \tag{6}$$

F_i = blood flow in ml pro g tissue and min

C_q = regional indicator-concentration

CO = cardiac output

If cardiac output at the time of the injection is measured independently the following parameters can be calculated:

1. the percentage of the cardiac output flowing through an organ or section of an organ;

2. the total blood flow of an organ in ml/min;

3. the flow in ml/100 g · min.

In a series of methodical investigations (Flohr 1968; Neutze *et al.*, 1968; Phibbs *et al.*, 1967) it was shown that certain small radioactively labelled particles provide such an indicator substance and fulfill the above described conditions adequately. For the present investigations, ^{131}I-labelled macro-aggregated albumin was used. These particles were produced according to a modification of a technique described by Taplin (1964). The particle diameter lay between 10 and 50 μ. The investigations were carried out on cats. The animals were given 40 mg of nembutal/kg. They were tracheotomized and after relaxation ventilated by means of a Starling pump. The animals were so thoracotomized that the left ventricle lay exposed.

Arterial blood pressure was continuously registered with Statham pressure gauge-transducers by means of a polyvinyl catheter inserted in the A. femoralis. For the determination of the end-expiratory carbon dioxide content an infrared analyser (Hartmann & Braun) was used. The arterial P_{CO_2} and the arterial pH were measured according to the micro-method of Astrup. The arterial oxygen pressure was determined by Clark Electrodes (P_{O_2} Electrode E 5046, Radiometer). Cardiac output was measured by means of the thermo-dilution technique. A computer designed by Slama and Piiper (1964) was used for rapid automatic evaluation of the curves and this enabled many quick consecutive determinations to be performed.

Five groups of experiments were carried out. In group 1 ($n = 13$) the animals were ventilated normally. Arterial blood pressure, cardiac output, Pa_{O_2}, Pa_{CO_2} and pH of arterial blood were kept in the normal range.

In group 2 ($n = 15$) the animals were ventilated at a normal rate and normal tidal volume with N_2/O_2 mixtures of different oxygen content to obtain different degrees of reduced Pa_{O_2}.

In group 3 ($n = 6$) the animals were hyperventilated so that different degrees of reduced Pa_{CO_2} were maintained.

In group 4 ($n = 15$) 3–5% CO_2 were added to the inspired air so that different degrees of Pa_{CO_2} were maintained.

In group 5 ($n = 17$) the mean arterial blood pressure was varied by withdrawal and reinjection of systemic blood at various rates. Pa_{O_2} and Pa_{CO_2} were kept in the normal range.

The indicator suspended in isotonic NaCl was injected by means of direct punction of the left ventricle. 50–100 μC MAA were given. Double determinations of cardiac output and blood gas values were performed immediately before and after the injection.

Four to six minutes after finishing the indicator injection in the left ventricle the animal was sacrificed by means of an intravenous KCl injection. The whole CNS was removed and dissected into the following parts: 1. prosencephalon, 2. cerebellum, 3. brain-stem, 4. cervical cord, 5. thoracic cord, 6. lumbosacral cord. These segments so taken were at once weighed after preparation. The activity of the particular preparations was measured in an Armac scintillation counter (Picker).

The following values were calculated:

1. *The relative blood flow* of the particular segments in % of *CO*

$$Qr = \frac{Io}{I}$$

Qr = relative blood flow in % of the *CO*
Io = regional activity
I = total applied activity

   2. *the blood flow of the particular segments* in ml/min

$$Qn = Qr \cdot CO$$

Qn = blood flow in ml/min
CO = cardiac output in ml/min

   3. *the regional blood flow values*

$$Qi = \frac{Q_n}{W_n} \cdot 100$$

Qi = regional blood flow values in ml/100 g · min
Wn = weight of the region n

From the mean arterial blood pressure and the regional blood flow values the regional resistance was calculated:

$$PR = \frac{MABP}{Qi}$$

Analogously the total body resistance was calculated:

$$TPR = \frac{MABP}{CO}$$

RESULTS

The results are summarized in Table 1 and Figs. 1–12.

1. Spinal cord flow on maintaining normal values for Pa_{O_2}, Pa_{CO_2} and MABP

The results of group 1 are summarized in Table 1. The blood flow of the whole spinal cord was in the normally ventilated group 19.28 ($\pm$ 1.67 S.E.) ml/100 g · min. This correspondents to relative blood flow of 0.68 ($\pm$ 0.057 S.E.) % of the cardiac output and a flow of 1.33 ($\pm$ 0.087) ml/min for the whole spinal cord. The mean resistance for the total spinal cord was a 6.95 ($\pm$ 0.745 S.E.), PRU.

Blood flow and resistance of the particular segments of the spinal cord are different. For the cervical cord a blood flow value of 19.92 ($\pm$ 1.66 S.E.) ml/100 g · min was determined. The values for the thoracic cord and lumbosacral cord were 16.79 ($\pm$ 1.45 S.E.) ml/100 g · min and 22.05 ($\pm$ 2.37 S.E.) ml/100 g · min.

References pp. 260–262

TABLE 1

REGIONAL SPINAL CORD AND BRAIN FLOW UNDER NORMAL CONDITIONS

	Weight g	CO ml/100 g·min	MABP mmHg	Pa_{CO_2} torr	Pa_{O_2} torr	pH	Blood flow ml/100 g·min						
							SC	CC	TC	LC	P	C	BS
1	1900	13.16	145	27.0	110	7.38	15.1	17.4	12.3	16.0	45.0	46.0	28.0
2	3200	9.28	160	25.7	118	7.35	13.4	14.0	11.1	16.0	45.0	46.0	
3	2380	6.80	100	27.2	110	7.17	10.4	9.0	10.0	13.0	33.0	40.0	38.4
4	2200	7.95	95	26.5	90	7.32	19.0	21.0	17.0	19.1	48.2	47.0	27.4
5	2000	9.50	115	30.0	115	7.24	28.3	28.2	27.0	30.0	53.0	74.0	55.3
6	2200	8.73	145	30.0	130	7.30	24.4	26.0	19.1	32.3	53.1	59.1	42.0
7	3320	6.17	95	32.5	110	7.27	21.2	22.0	20.0	22.0	64.0	84.0	66.3
8	2300	7.39	65	27.8	92	7.22	19.0	20.5	16.8	19.3		42.0	
9	2400	7.79	155	28.0	88	7.30	21.4	24.2	20.0	19.9	43.3	65.0	42.0
10	3000	6.67	145	28.5	110	7.25	20.5	22.5	18.1	21.1	50.9	41.0	24.1
11	2880	4.79	95	27.0	146	7.34	12.6	13.0	11.0	14.0	42.6	62.9	43.3
12	3000	9.47	135	29.3	93	7.30	30.4	27.1	23.5	43.7	48.1	69.0	16.5
13	3285	8.34	150	27.3	100	7.40	14.9	14.0	12.4	19.5	52.3		
$\bar{x}$	2620	8.118	123.1	28.22	108.6	7.295	19.28	19.92	16.79	22.05	47.15	55.92	37.33
S.D.	507	2.078	30.3	1.83	16.7	0.054	6.03	5.00	5.23	8.54	8.83	16.18	15.33

SC total spinal cord flow　　P prosencephalon
CC cervical cord　　　　　　C cerebellum
TC thoracic cord　　　　　　BS brain-stem
LC lumbosacral cord

Statistically the differences in the blood flow of cervical cord and thoracic cord as well as between the lumbosacral cord and the thoracic cord are significant ($P < 0.001$).

The blood flow of the forebrain was in this group 47.44 ($\pm$ 2.55 S.E.), that of the cerebellum 55.92 ($\pm$ 4.67 S.E.), that of the brain stem 37.33 ($\pm$ 4.85 S.E.) ml/100 g · min. The differences are statistically significant ($P < 0.001$).

2. The effect of the arterial P_{CO_2}

The arterial P_{CO_2} is with the cat lower than with other species (Koeppen *et al.*, 1967). In our investigations it was with cats chosen at random in slight nembutal narcosis and with spontaneous breathing 28–29 torr. In the normoventilated group of these investigations, it was a mean 28.29 ($\pm$ 0.48 S.E.) torr. In the hyperventilated group it was a mean 21.05 ($\pm$ 1.23 S.E.), in the hypercapnic group the mean Pa_{CO_2} was 47.33 ($\pm$ 3.26 S.E.) torr.

The relation of Pa_{CO_2} to the flow in the different regions is shown in Figs. 1–4. On observing the whole material we see a statistically significant ($P < 0.001$) positive correlation between Pa_{CO_2} and spinal blood flow values. The blood flow of the total spinal cord fell in the hyperventilation to a value of 11.20 ($\pm$ 2.396 S.E.) and increased in hypercarbia to 63.66 ($\pm$ 9.81 S.E.) ml/100 g · min. The relative blood flow, *i.e.* the percentage of the cardiac output which flows through the spinal cord, increases also with increased Pa_{CO_2} and falls with the reduced Pa_{CO_2}. With normo-ventilation the mean relative blood flow was 0.679 % of the cardiac output, with hyperventilation

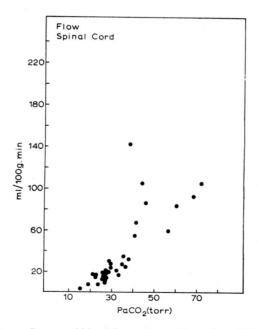

Fig. 1. Relationship between Pa_{CO_2} and blood flow to the total spinal cord. In this as in the following diagrams each point represents one measurement in one animal.

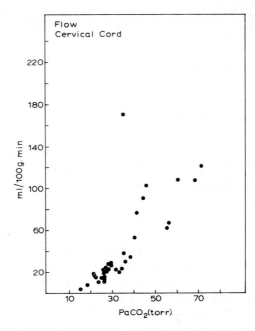

Fig. 2. Relationship between Pa_{CO_2} and blood flow to the cervical cord.

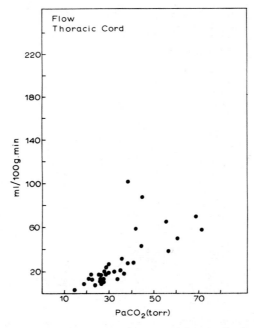

Fig. 3. Relationship between Pa_{CO_2} and blood flow to the thoracic cord.

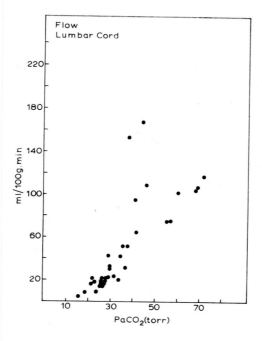

Fig. 4. Relationship between Pa_{CO_2} and blood flow to the lumbar cord.

it fell to a value of 0.421 % and increased in hypercarbia to a value of 1.243 % of the cardiac output (Fig. 5).

The same data is valid for all segments of the spinal cord as well as for all other investigated sections of the CNS (Fig. 6–7). The relationship between Pa_{CO_2} and blood flow values can, as shown by computer analysis, be described approximately by means of a linear regression for the range studied (Fig. 9).

The vascular resistance of the spinal cord and brain sections falls absolutely and in relation to the total body resistance with increased Pa_{CO_2}, and it increases absolutely and relatively with falling Pa_{CO_2}. The relationship between resistance and Pa_{CO_2} in the first approximation is described by means of a right-angled hyperbola the assymptotes of which lie parallel to the co-ordinates (Fig. 10).

3. The effect of the arterial oxygen partial pressure

The arterial oxygen partial pressures were, in group 2, between 60 and 146 torr. Its relationship to the blood flow values of cervical, thoracic and lumbosacral cord is illustrated in Fig. 12. Statistically no significant correlation was found for this range of Pa_{O_2}.

4. The effect of the mean arterial blood pressure

The mean arterial blood pressure in group 5 lay within a range of 65–160 mm Hg.

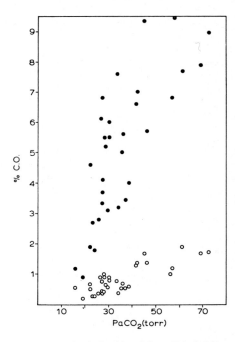

Fig. 5. Relationship between Pa_{CO_2} and relative blood flow ($\%$ of *CO*) to the prosencephalon (dots) and to the spinal cord (open circles).

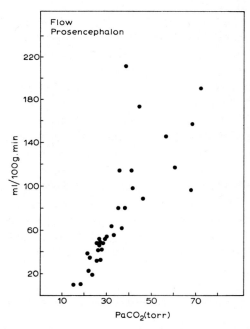

Fig. 6. Relationship between Pa_{CO_2} and blood flow to the prosencephalon.

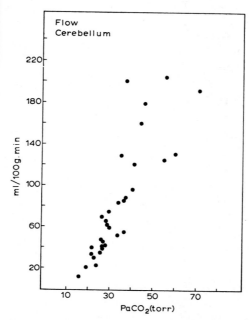

Fig. 7. Relationship between Pa_{CO_2} and blood flow to the cerebellum.

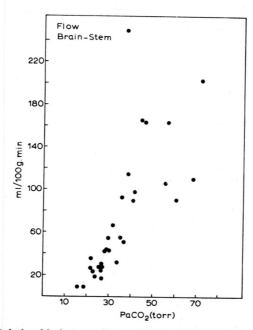

Fig. 8. Relationship between Pa_{CO_2} and blood flow to the brain-stem.

References pp. 260–262

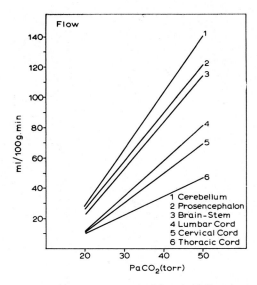

Fig. 9. Regressions of the Pa_{CO_2} response of flow in different parts of the CNS. The regressions for the particular segments are:

forebrain	: $Y = 3.09\,x - 34.13$;
cerebellum	: $Y = 3.83\,x - 48.89$;
brain-stem	: $Y = 3.19\,x - 42.41$;
cervical cord	: $Y = 2.25\,x - 37.62$;
thoracic cord	: $Y = 1.25\,x - 14.90$;
lumbosacral cord:	$Y = 2.39\,x - 37.02$.

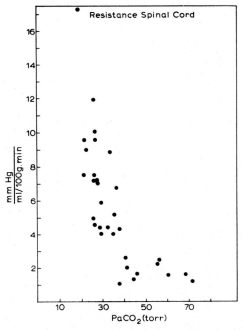

Fig. 10. Total spinal cord vascular resistance at different Pa_{CO_2} values.

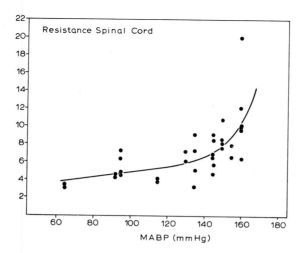

Fig. 11. Resistance of the cervical and lumbar cord at different mean arterial blood pressures.

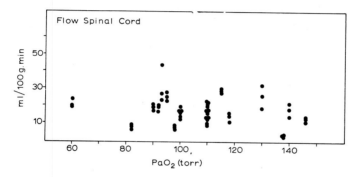

Fig. 12. Relationship between Pa_{O_2} and blood flow in the cervical, thoracic and lumbar cord.

Pa_{O_2} and Pa_{CO_2} were kept in the normal range. No significant relationship between MABP and blood flow values of the different CNS segments was observed. The resistance increases with increased pressure (Fig. 11).

DISCUSSION

The flow values for the spinal cord and the different brain regions are in the same range as those previously reported (Mandel *et al.*, 1963; Flohr *et al.*, 1969; Smith *et al.*, 1969; Tschetter *et al.*, 1970; Roth *et al.*, 1970). The values obtained for the cervical cord are in accordance with values that can be calculated from the data of Sokoloff (1961) if the relation of grey and white matter in the cervical cord is taken into account (Stilling, 1859). The data also agree with the value range which should be expected from measurements of spinal cord oxygen uptake *in vitro* (Himwich *et al.*, 1941; McIlwain, 1959). Table 2 summarizes the values for the spinal cord flow in different species known up till now.

References pp. 260–262

TABLE 2

QUANTITATIVE DATA ON SPINAL CORD FLOW

Ref.	Method	Species	Flow (ml/100 g · min)	
1 Sokoloff, 1961	CF_3-^{131}I uptake	cat	c	21.8*
			th	—
			l	—
2 Mandel et al., 1963	Antipyrine uptake	rat	c	
			th }	28.0
			l	
3 Flohr et al., 1969	Particle distribution	cat	c	19.9
			th	16.8
			l	22.1
4 Smith et al., 1969	^{133}Xe Clearance	goat	c	
			th }	16.2**
			l	
5 Tschetter et al., 1970	Particle distribution	dog	c	15.1
			th	13.5
			l	19.2

* Calculated values
** Mean value of all determinations in different segments.

According to Kety (1960) all factors which affect the blood flow of the CNS can be divided according to their mechanism, into such which influence the perfusion pressure and such which change the vascular resistance.

The perfusion pressure of the CNS is essentially determined by the arterial pressure (Kety, 1960). While it was once supposed that the blood flow passively depended on this, since the investigations by Rapela and Green (1964), Lassen (1964), Häggendahl and Johansson (1966), it is reckoned as certain that cerebral blood flow is subjected to autoregulation. The present observations agree with this view. The existence of an autoregulation could be shown for each of the brain regions.

For the spinal cord as a whole as for each of the single sections the same statement is valid. No correlation exists between flow and mean arterial pressure if the latter is varied in a range of 60–160 torr. These findings agree with the observations by Wüllenweber (1968, 1969) and Palleske and Herrmann (1968).

No attempt was made in this investigation to study the effects of hypercapnia and hypoxia on spinal cord autoregulation. From previous experiments, however, it can be concluded that autoregulation of the cord flow is effected by the Pa_{CO_2} in the same manner as in the brain and disappears with high Pa_{CO_2} (Flohr et al., 1970 c).

Among the factors which direct the vascular resistance of the brain, the arterial CO_2 partial pressure is the decisive one (Lennox and Gibbs, 1932; Schmidt, 1934; Kety and Schmidt, 1946; Noell and Schneider, 1944; Noell, 1944; Reivich, 1964). All other chemical factors are, under physiological conditions, of minor importance for the regulation of the CNS resistance (Sokoloff and Kety, 1960).

The present observations on the fore-brain, cerebellum and brain-stem agree fully with this view. The response of the blood flow in the different brain regions to changes in Pa_{CO_2}, however, was much steeper than that observed with other techniques (Harper et al., 1968; Reivich, 1964).

Spinal cord vascular resistance is effected in essentially the same way by the Pa_{CO_2}. The resistance decreases with increased Pa_{CO_2} absolutely and relatively to the total body resistance; it increases absolutely and relatively with decreasing Pa_{CO_2}.

There are, however, quantitative differences in the CO_2 response of the particular segments of the CNS. The absolute sensitivity of the various parts in ml/100 g · min/mm Hg CO_2 was 3.09 for the prosencephalon, 3.83 for the cerebellum, 3.19 for the brain stem, 2.25 for the cervical cord, 1.25 for the thoracic cord and 2.39 for the lumbosacral cord (Fig. 9). Apparently $dF/d\,Pa_{CO_2}$ of the different regions is related to its flow and $CMRO_2$ under normal conditions.

According to our present knowledge the arterial O_2 pressure affects the vascular resistance of the brain if there are values of less than 50 torr. Within normal partial pressure ranges there is no dependence of the blood flow on Pa_{O_2} (Lambertsen et al., 1959; Lambertsen, 1961; Shimojyo et al., 1968).

In the present investigation the measured arterial O_2 partial pressures were between 60 and 140 torr. With normal Pa_{CO_2} no influence of Pa_{O_2} on brain flow was found for this range. Again the same statement is valid for the cord.

A comparison of the effects of Pa_{O_2}, Pa_{CO_2} and mean arterial blood pressure on spinal cord and brain flow indicates that there is apparently no fundamental difference: the main factor controlling spinal cord vascular resistance is the CO_2 partial pressure, arterial oxygen tension is without significant influence if varied between 60–146 torr, and the existence of autoregulation of spinal cord blood flow can be demonstrated.

From this follows that the mechanisms involved in the regulation of local flow are virtually the same at all levels in the CNS.

SUMMARY

The blood flow of the spinal cord, fore-brain, cerebellum and brain-stem were measured on anaesthetized cats using the particle distribution technique.

With normal arterial blood pressure, normal CO_2 partial pressure and O_2 partial pressure, and with normal pH, the mean blood flow value of the total spinal cord is 19.28 ml/100 g · min. This correspondents to 0.68% of the cardiac output under resting conditions. The blood flow value of the particular segments of the spinal cord differs; for the cervical cord there was a value of 19.92, for the thoracic cord 16.79 and for the lumbosacral cord 22.05 ml/100 g · min. The blood flow values determined in the same experiment for the fore-brain, cerebellum and brain-stem were 47.15, 55.92 and 37.33 ml/100 g · min respectively.

The effects of Pa_{O_2}, Pa_{CO_2} and arterial blood pressure on blood flow through the different segments of the spinal cord and the different parts of the brain were studied comparatively. Spinal cord vascular resistance is closely correlated to arterial carbon dioxide tension but there are quantitative differences in the CO_2 response at different levels on the CNS. No significant correlation between arterial oxygen tension and spinal cord blood flow was observed when Pa_{O_2} varied between 60–146 torr and Pa_{CO_2} was kept in the normal range.

The existence of autoregulation of spinal cord blood flow was demonstrated.

It is concluded from these observations that the mechanisms involved in the regulation of local blood flow are virtually the same at all levels in the CNS.

REFERENCES

BLASIUS, W. (1950) Das gesetzmässige Verhalten der Funktions- und Erholungsfähigkeit der Vorderhornganglienzelle bei zeitlich abgestufter Aortenabklemmung. *Z. Biol.*, **103**, 209–252.

BLASIUS, W. AND ZIMMERMANN, H. (1957) Vergleichende Untersuchungen über die funktionellen, strukturellen und histochemischen Veränderungen an den Vorderhornganglienzellen des Kaninchenrückenmarkes bei zeitlich abgestufter Ischämie. *Pflügers Arch. Ges. Physiol.*, **264**, 618–650.

BODECHTEL, G. AND SCHRADER, A. (1957) Die Zirkulationsstörungen am Rückenmark einschliesslich des Rückenmarkstraumas und der Caisson-Krankheit. In: *Handbuch der Inneren Medizin* Vol. V, Springer-Verlag Berlin, Göttingen, Heidelberg, p. 545.

CAPON, A. (1961) Les régulations vasculaires dans la moelle épinière. *Acta Neurol. Psychiat. Belg.*, **61**, 227–232.

CARLYLE, A. AND GRAYSON, J. (1955) Blood pressure and the regulation of the brain blood flow. *J. Physiol.*, **127**, 15 p.

COLSON, C. (1890) Recherches physiologiques sur l'occlusion de l'aorte thoracique. *Arch. Biol. Paris*, **10**, 431–439.

CORBIN, J. C. (1961) *Anatomie et Pathologie Artérielles de la Moelle*, G. Masson, Paris.

FIELD, E. J., GRAYSON, J. AND ROGERS, A. F. (1951) Observations on the blood flow in the spinal cord of the rabbit. *J. Physiol.*, **114**, 56–70.

FLOHR, H. (1968) Methode zur Messung regionaler Durchblutungsgrössen mit radioaktiv markierten Partikeln. *Pflügers Arch. Ges. Physiol.*, **302**, 268–274.

FLOHR, H., BROCK, M. AND PÖLL, W. (1969) Quantitative Messung der Durchblutung des Rückenmarkes an der anaesthesierten Katze. *Pflügers Arch. Ges. Physiol.*, **312**, R 38.

FLOHR, H., BROCK, M. AND PÖLL, W. (1970 a) Untersuchungen zur Regulation der Durchblutung des Rückenmarkes. *Pflügers Arch. Ges. Physiol.*, **316**, R 56.

FLOHR, H., PÖLL, W. AND BROCK, M. (1970 b) Regulation of spinal cord blood flow. *Intern. Symp. Cerebral Blood Flow*, London, in press.

FLOHR, H., BROCK, M., CHRIST, R., HEIPERTZ, R. AND PÖLL, W. (1970) Arterial P_{CO_2} and blood flow in different segments of the central nervous system of the anaesthetized cat. In: LASSEN, N. A., INGVAR, D. H., FIESCHI, C., BROCK, M. AND SCHÜRMANN, K. (Eds.), *Cerebral Blood Flow*, Springer-Verlag, Berlin–New York, p. 86–88.

FRÉDERICQ, L. (1889) L'anémie expérimentale comme procédé de dissociation des propriétés motrices et sensitives de la moelle épinière. *Arch. Biol. Paris*, **10**, 131–139.

GELFAN, S. AND TARLOV, J. M. (1955) Differential vulnerability of spinal cord structures to anoxia. *J. Neurophysiol.*, **18**, 170–188.

HÄGGENDAHL, E. AND JOHANSSON, B. (1966) Effects of arterial carbon dioxide tension and oxygen saturation on cerebral blood flow autoregulation. *Acta Physiol. Scand.*, **66**, Suppl. **258**, 27–53.

HALLER, H. V. (1756) *Deux Mémoires sur le Mouvement du Sang*, Lausanne.

HARPER, A. M., JENNET, W. B. AND LITTLEJOHN, J. G. (1968) Simultaneous measurement of beta and gamma clearance curves of radioactive inert gases from the monkey brain. In: BAIN, W. H. AND HARPER, H. M. (Eds.), *Blood Flow through Organs and Tissues*, Livingstone, Edinburgh and London, p. 214–220.

HIMWICH, H. E., SYKOWSKI, P. AND FAZEKAS, J. F. (1941) A comparative study of excised cerebral tissues of adult and infant rats. *Amer. J. Physiol.*, **132**, 293–299.

JELLINGER, K. (1966) *Zur Orthologie und Pathologie der Rückenmarksdurchblutung*, Springer-Verlag, Wien-New York.

KETY, S. S. (1960) The cerebral circulation. In: *Handbuch der Physiologie*, **III**, p. 1751.

KETY, S. S. AND SCHMIDT, C. F. (1946) The effects of active and passive hyperventilation on cerebral blood flow, cerebral oxygen consumption, cardiac output and blood pressure of normal young men. *J. Clin. Invest.*, **25**, 107–116.

KIRSTEIN, L. (1951) Early effects of oxygen lack and carbon dioxide excess on spinal reflexes. *Acta Physiol. Scand.*, **23**, Suppl. **80**, 1–54.

KOEPPEN, F., DIECKHOFF, D., KANZOW, E. AND KOTSERONIS, I. (1967) Über die CO_2-Spannung im arteriellen Blut nicht narkotisierter Katzen. *Verh. Deut. Physiol. Ges.*, *Würzburg*, R. 49.

KROGH, E. (1950) The effect of acute hypoxia on the motor cells of the spinal cord. *Acta Physiol. Scand.*, **20**, 263–292.

LAMBERTSEN, C. J. (1961) Chemical factors in respiratory control. In: *Medical Physiology*, St. Louis, p. 633.

LAMBERTSEN, C. J., OWEN, S. G., WENDEL, H., STRAUD, M. W., LURIE, A. H., LOCHNER, W. AND CLARK, G. F. (1959) Respiratory and cerebral circulatory control during exercises at 0.21 and 2.0 atmospheres inspired P_{O_2}. *J. Appl. Physiol.*, **14**, 966–982.

LASSEN, N. H. (1964) Autoregulation of cerebral blood flow. *Circulation Res.*, **15**, Suppl. **1**, 201–204.

LEGALLOIS, A. (1830) *Expériences sur le Principe de la Vie*, Paris.

LENNOX, W. G. AND GIBBS, E. L. (1932) The blood flow in the brain and the leg of man and the changes induced by alteration of blood gases. *J. Clin. Invest.*, **11**, 1155–1159.

LEWANDOWSKY, M. (1911) Rückenmarkserkrankungen durch Störungen der Zirkulation. In: *Handbuch der Neurologie*, Vol. 2/I, Springer-Verlag, Berlin, p. 550.

LUCHSINGER, B. (1878) Zur Kenntnis der Funktionen des Rückenmarkes. *Arch. Ges. Physiol.*, **16**, 510–516.

MANDEL, M. J., ARCIDIACON, O. F. AND SAPIRSTEIN, L. H. (1963) Jodoantipyrine and 86-Rb Cl uptake by brain, cord and sciatic nerve in the rat. *Amer. J. Physiol.*, **204**, 327–329.

MARIE, P. (1892) *Leçons sur les Maladies de la Moelle*, G. Masson, Paris.

McBROOKS, C. AND ECCLES, J. C. (1947) A study of the effects of anaesthesia and asphyxia on the monosynaptic pathway through the spinal cord. *J. Neurophysiol.*, **10**, 349–354.

McILWAIN, H. (1959) *Biochemistry and the Central Nervous System*, Churchill, London.

MURAYAMA, S. AND SMITH, C. M. (1965) Rigidity of the hind limbs of cats produced by occlusion of spinal cord blood supply. *Neurology (Minn.)*, **15**, 565–569.

NEUMAYER, E. (1967) Die vasculäre Myelopathie. Springer-Verlag, Wien-New York.

NEUTZE, J. M., WYLER, F. AND RUDOLPH, A. M. (1968) Use of radioactive microspheres to assess distribution of cardiac output in rabbits. *Amer. J. Physiol.*, **215**, 486–495.

NOELL, W. (1944) Über die Durchblutung und Sauerstoffversorgung des Gehirns. V. Einfluss der Blutdrucksenkung. *Pflügers Arch. Ges. Physiol*, **247**, 528–575.

NOELL, W. AND SCHNEIDER, M. (1944) Über die Durchblutung und die Sauerstoffversorgung des Gehirns. IV. Die Rolle der Kohlensäure. *Pflügers Arch. Ges. Physiol.*, **247**, 514–527.

NUNES-VICENTE, A. (1964) *Enfarte medular. Contribuiçao Experimental e Anatomo-Patologia*, Coimbra.

OPITZ, E. (1960) Energieumsatz des Gehirns in situ unter aeroben und anaeroben Bedingungen. In: *Die Chemie und der Stoffwechsel des Nervensystems*, Springer-Verlag, Berlin-Heidelberg, p. 66.

OTOMO, E., WOLBARSHT, M. L., VAN BURSKIRK, C. AND DAVIDSON, M. (1960) A comparison of spinal cord, cortical and superficial circulation. *J. Nervous Mental Disease*, **131**, 418.

PALLESKE, H. AND HERRMANN, D. H. (1968) Experimental investigations on the regulation of blood flow in the spinal cord. *Acta Neurochir.*, **19**, 73.

PHIBBS, R. H., WYLER, F. AND NEUTZE, J. (1967) Rheology of microspheres injected into circulation of rabbits. *Nature*, **216**, 1339–1340.

RAPELA, C. E. AND GREEN, H. D. (1964) Autoregulation of canine cerebral blood flow. *Circulation Res.*, **15**, Suppl. I, 205–215.

REIVICH, M. (1964) Arterial P_{CO_2} and cerebral hemodynamics. *Amer. J. Physiol.*, **206**, 25–35.

REXED, B. (1940) Some observations on the effect of compression of short duration of the abdominal aorta in the rabbit. *Acta Psychiat.*, **15**, 365–371.

ROTH, J. A., GREENFIELD, A. J., KAIHARA, S. AND WAGNER, H. N. JR. (1970) Total and regional cerebral flow in unanaesthetized dogs. *Amer. J. Physiol.*, **219**, 96–101.

SAPIRSTEIN, L. H. (1956) Fractionation of the cardiac output of rats with isotopic potassium. *Circulation Res.*, **4**, 689–692.

SARTESCHI, P. AND GIANNINI, H. (1960) *La Patologia Vasculare del Midollo Spinale*, Giardini, Pisa.

SCHIFFER, J. (1869) Über die Bedeutung des Steno'schen Versuches. *Zbl. Med. Wiss.*, **7**, 579–587.

SCHMIDT, C. F. (1934) The intrinsic regulation of the circulation in the hypothalamus of the cat. *Amer. J. Physiol.*, **110**, 137–1502.

Shimojyo, S., Scheinberg, P., Kogure, K. and Reinmuth, D. M. (1968) The effects of graded hypoxia upon transient cerebral blood flow and oxygen consumption. *Neurology (Minn.)*, **18**, 127–133.

Slama, H. and Piiper, J. (1964) Direktanzeigendes Rechengerät zur Bestimmung des Herzzeitvolumens mit der Thermoinjektionsmethode. *Z. Kreislaufforsch.*, **53**, 322.

Smith, H. C., Pender, J. W. and Alexander, S. C. (1969) Effects of P_{CO_2} on spinal cord blood flow. *Amer. J. Physiol.*, **216**, 1158–1163.

Sokoloff, L. and Kety, S. S. (1960) Regulation of cerebral circulation. *Physiol. Rev.*, **40**, *Suppl.* **4**, 38–44.

Sokoloff, L. (1961) Local cerebral circulation at rest and during altered cerebral activity induced by anaesthesia or visual stimulation. In: Kety, S. S. and Elkes, J. (Eds.), *Regional Neurochemistry, Proc. 4th Intern. Neurochem. Symp.* Pergamon Press, London, p. 107–117.

Stenon, W. (1667) *Elementorum Myologiae Specimen*, Amsterdam.

Stilling, B. (1859) *Neue Untersuchungen über den Bau des Rückenmarkes*, H. Hotop-Verlag, Kassel.

Swammerdam, J. (1667) *Tractatus de Respiratione*, Ludg. Batav.

Taplin, G. V., Johnson, D. E., Dore, K. E. and Kaplan, H. S. (1964) Suspension of radioalbumin aggregates for photoscanning liver, spleen, lung, and other organs. *J. Nucl. Med.*, **5**, 259–264.

Tureen, L. L. (1936) Effect of experimental temporary vascular occlusion on the spinal cord. I. Correlation between structural and functional changes. *Arch. Neurol. Psychiat.*, **35**, 789–795.

Tureen, L. L. (1938) Circulation of spinal cord and the effect of vascular occlusion. *Res. Publ. Assoc. Nervous Mental Disease*, **18**, 384–389.

Tschetter, T. H., Klassen, A. C., Resch, J. N. and Meyer, M. W. (1970) Blood flow in the central peripheral nervous system of dogs using a particle distribution method. *Stroke*, **1**, 370–374.

Van Harreveld, (1944) Survival of reflex contraction and inhibition during cord asphyxiation. *Amer. J. Physiol.*, **141**, 97–101.

Vulpian, A. (1875) *Leçons sur l'Appareil Vasomoteur. XVII. Les Nerfs Vasomoteurs de la Moelle Épinière*, Paris.

Wüllenweber, R. (1969) Untersuchungen der spinalen Durchblutung mit Thermosonden beim Menschen. *Deutsch. Z. Nervenheilk.*, **195**, 33–42.

Wüllenweber, R. (1968) First results of measurements of local spinal blood flow in man by means of heat clearance. In: *Blood Flow Through Organs and Tissues*, Livingstone, Edinburgh, pp. 176–180.

Radiocirculography – A Profile of Cerebral Circulation Clinical Uses and Limitations

A. R. TAYLOR, H. A. CROCKARD AND T. K. BELL

Royal Victoria Hospital, Belfast (Northern Ireland)

The term "radiocirculography" was first used by Eichhorn (1959) and describes the graphic representation of the cerebral blood flow profile following intravenous injection of a gamma-emitting isotope, in his case ^{51}Cr. Oldendorf (1961) independently developed a similar method but focussed attention on the first derivative or rate of change curve, from which was derived the mode circulation time (MCT). A similar method has been employed in this clinic since 1962, making use of data from both primary and differentiated curves and combining them, at different times, with flow curves taken from over the heart or ear lobe (dye with a photoelectric sensor) to give information about cardiac output, systemic circulation time and extracranial circulation. $[^{131}I]$Hippuran was injected in the earlier years and has lately been replaced by ^{99m}Tc as pertechnetate which has a shorter half-life and gives a better signal for a given dose.

Over 3000 observations have been made and analyzed and it has become clear from the data what are the functions and limitations of the studies in a clinical setting. No endeavour has been made to assess a patient's blood flow in digital terms, the radiocirculogram is assessed as a flow profile, much as the radiologist assesses a profile of stomach-emptying, the conclusions being a matter of judgement as well as measurement. The questions asked of the records are of the type – "Is this patient's blood flow faster or slower than that anticipated from a normal patient?" or "Is the blood flow better or worse than it was (a) yesterday, (b) before treatment, (c) before inhalation of CO_2 or change in blood pressure?" It has not been thought necessary or worth while to make observations on regional blood flow because such flow cannot be influenced therapeutically in a predictable manner by any chemical or biological agent in a clinical, as distinct from an experimental, setting. Nor is it possible to repeat regional observations with the necessary frequency because they require carotid artery puncture, a procedure not without risk.

This chapter is devoted to a consideration of the usefulness of radiocirculography (RCG) in general diagnosis, patient management and prognosis.

METHOD

Intracranial gamma-ray activity is observed by two detecting systems, each containing a collimated Sodium Iodide crystal, 1.5″ diameter. The axes of the crystals are inclined to each other at an angle of 20° and the collimators are on a fixed mounting with the mid-line between them directed through the occiput on a level with the inion towards a point 7 cm above the glabella, Fig. 1. There is very little "cross-talk" between the detectors and the fields of view are shown in Fig. 2.

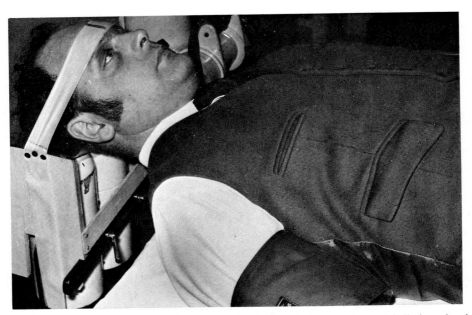

Fig. 1. Position of patient and skull in relation to twin scintillation counters. Glabella is under the central mark on the headband ensuring symmetry of brain fields viewed by the counters.

Gamma-rays detected by the crystals produce electrical pulses in the coupled photo-multiplier tubes and these are fed into ratemeters operating with a time constant of 0.5 seconds. A chart recorder is linked to each ratemeter and the resultant primary activity curves are displayed on paper charts, moving at 15 cm/min. In addition signals from each ratemeter are fed into separate differentiation units, the outputs of which provide the rate of change curves and these are also displayed on the appropriate chart recorders. Before beginning the investigations both detecting systems are adjusted to be equally sensitive to the radioisotope being used.

The radioisotope, 50 microcuries (μC)[^{131}I]hippuran, or 500 μC ^{99m}Tc in 1 to 2 ml saline is loaded into a shielded syringe for injection into an antecubital vein in the arm. The technique is important. With the patient lying supine and his head resting on the detector, the vein is distended for 30 sec by holding a sphygmomanometer cuff at 100 mm Hg. This raises the intravenous pressure to about that level. The needle is then inserted and the cuff pressure raised above the patient's systolic pressure. The injectate now introduced remains in the antecubital vein until the cuff is suddenly released (Figs. 3, 4). It is then abruptly deposited in the right heart by the accumulated pressure wave and remains together as a much more compact bolus

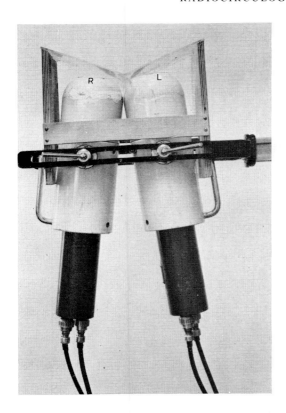

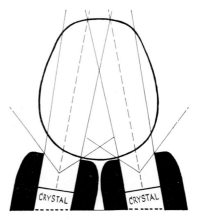

Fig. 2. (a) The scintillation counters.
(b) Outline of right and left fields viewed, showing the very small overlap.

than if it were injected in the conventional way. After passage through lungs and left heart, the radioactive stream can then approach the head through the four main arteries. By now it is 12–15 sec long. The densest concentration of radioactivity is in the centre and it tails off to either end. As the first half of the bolus enters the field viewed, the curve climbs to a peak. Shortly after the dense central part has entered, the curve begins to decline. The rate of change curve has two peaks, positive and negative, corresponding to the entry and exit times of the dense part of the bolus. The period of time between the peaks is the Mode Circulation Time, which has been shown to vary little from the Mean Circulation Time (Fig. 5). This is the time taken to turn

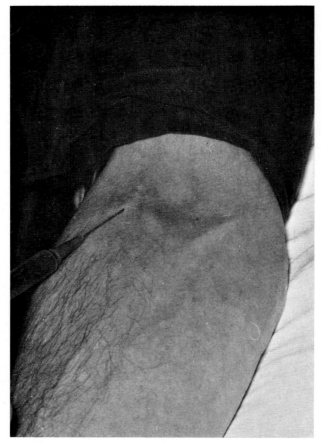

Fig. 3. Position of arm and sphygmomanometer cuff inflated above the patient's systolic pressure.

over or exchange the Cerebral Blood Volume (CBV). The MCT is therefore reciprocally related to the Cerebral Blood Flow (CBF) but, as the CBV varies within narrow limits but unpredictably, the CBF cannot be reliably calculated from the MCT.

The rising arm of the circulation curve is altered in length and slope by increased intracranial pressure or multiple arteriosclerotic lesions in the major cranial vessels. The descending arm, or clearance side, is lengthened by the two factors above as a direct consequence of slow entry, or by anything which increases the size of the capillary bed or causes venous distension. The total transit time (TT) and the mean circulation time (MCT) are therefore increased by the presence of a vascular tumour, arteriosclerotic small vessel disease, cerebral oedema or the cerebral vasoconstriction which accompanies hypocapnia. The maximum height (h.max) of the curve decreases with the increase in circulation time. The only disorder which decreases the circulation time and increases the h.max is an arteriovenous communication (Fig. 6). Hypercapnia from a lung condition causing CO_2 retention increases the h.max, but does not decrease the circulation time (Fig. 7).

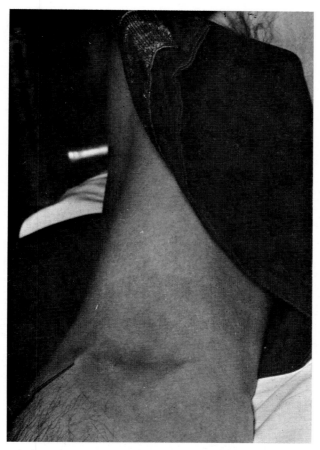

Fig. 4. Cuff released abruptly, allowing propulsion of bolus rapidly to the right heart from the previously distended antecubital vein.

RCG as part of an atraumatic screening test battery

The RCG being safe, atraumatic, repeatable and easy to interpret at the time of examination, makes it an ideal test for use in out-patient screening. Following history taking and clinical examination, if the diagnosis is in doubt, EEG, EchoEG, and brain scans can be done. Circulation times are observed during intravenous injection of technetium for brain scanning. If all these tests give normal results it is very unlikely that the patient requires further investigation at that time to exclude a structural or vascular cerebral lesion. 107 consecutive patients were studied in this way and in 88% the correct diagnosis was made without resort to further investigation (Swallow et al., 1968). RCG's were considered positive if either of the circulation times were increased or the h.max decreased, and negative if the dimensions of the curves lay in the normal range. In 85% of cases they were correct, there were 8% false positives and 7% false negatives; only one cerebral tumour gave a false negative result, the

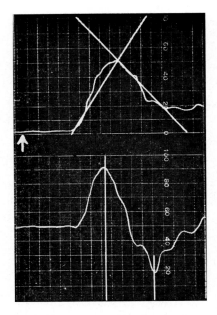

Fig. 5. Normal primary and rate of change curves, showing the shape and amplitude of the primary curve and the method of estimating the mode circulation time (MCT).

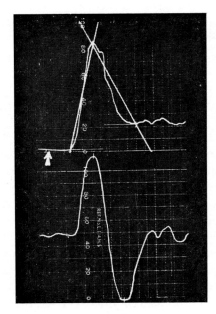

Fig. 6. The steep curve and rapid circulation in an arteriovenous malformation.

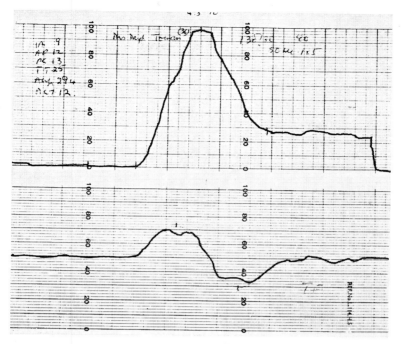

Fig. 7. Curve of high amplitude but increased transit time (TT) in a patient with chronic bronchitis and CO_2 retention.

remainder being patients with cerebral vascular accidents. Only one patient in this series had an A–V malformation and the RCG was diagnostic. The general usefulness of the test at this early stage is that it may obviate the necessity to carry out further "traumatic" investigations, in particular angiography.

Diagnosis

As an isolated piece of evidence the RCG is never aetiologically diagnostic except in patients with A–V malformations. It does, however, increase the degree of likelihood

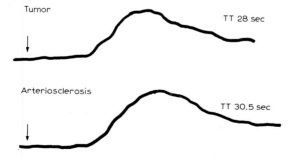

Fig. 8. A comparison of curves from patients with cerebral arteriosclerosis and a cerebral tumour, showing their similarity.

References p. 283

that a patient does or does not harbour a structural intracranial lesion. For example, a patient with headaches or migraine, who has a normal RCG, is unlikely to have a cerebral tumour. In the acute situation a patient in unexplained coma, with gross slowing of the circulation, is more likely to have an intracranial haemorrhage than barbiturate or some other intoxication. It is, however, not possible to distinguish between the flow profiles of a cerebral tumour or a cerebral vascular accident in an arteriosclerotic subject – both have increased TT's and diminished h.max (Fig. 8).

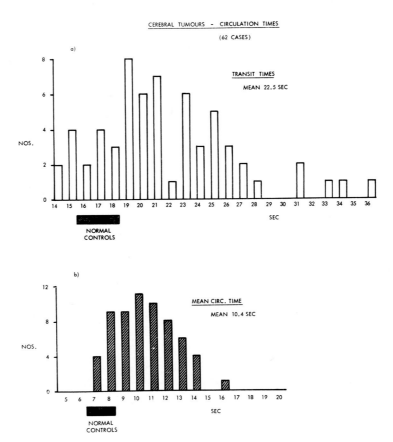

Fig. 9. The scatter of circulation times in a series of 62 consecutive cerebral tumours, compared with the distribution in normal controls.

If a tumour is present the TT will be increased in 85% of cases (Fig. 9). The greatest increase occurs in the presence of increased intracranial tension and there is a roughly linear relationship between the size of the tumour and the length of the TT. Among the tumour patients with normal TT's and MCT's more than half presented with a history of epilepsy and no neurological deficit. Under these circumstances, the tumour causing the epilepsy is often so small that it cannot be detected by brain scanning and has not a sufficient vascular bed to alter the cerebral circulation profile.

RCG as a guide to patient management

It is in the field of patient management that the RCG plays its most useful role because it is both reproducible and almost indefinitely repeatable.

Investigation of subarachnoid haemorrhage has shown a very close correlation between circulation times and the degree of intracranial vascular spasm (Table 1). Vascular spasm, with its attendant infarction, is the main immediate cause of death

TABLE 1

ANGIOGRAPHIC SPASM AND CIRCULATION TIMES

	No.	TT	MCT
Without spasm	49	18.53	8.95
With spasm	31	23.16	11.58
No angiogram	10	25.10	11.80

The patients without arterial spasm seen on angiograms had circulation times within the normal range. Patients with angiographic spasm showed a 30–40% mean increase in circulation time.

and disablement following subarachnoid haemorrhage. Direct surgical intervention or artery ligation is much more dangerous while vascular spasm persists, so it is very important that the surgeon be aware of the state of the cerebral circulation when he is deciding on the best time to intervene. Circulation may be slowed by intracranial haematoma or a co-existing cerebral arteriosclerosis as well as by arterial spasm following subarachnoid haemorrhage but, after the initial RCG and arteriogram have established the existence of vascular spasm, serial RCG's will accurately reflect the state of the cerebral circulation and enable the surgeon to intervene at the optimum time when the circulation times are approaching normal. Fig. 10 shows the effect on the angiogram and RCG of an episode of arterial spasm three days after haemorrhage from a posterior communicating aneurysm. Fig. 11 shows the progressive improvement in circulation in the weeks after haemorrhage.

Aneurysms on the internal carotid artery can, in most cases, be prevented from bleeding again by ligation of the common carotid artery on the same side. Ligation in an unselected series of patients carries a complication rate of 30%, and only if the collateral circulation through the circle of Willis is adequate can ligation be performed safely. Adequacy has been assessed from the patient's clinical state and EEG with the artery manually compressed in the neck. Cross circulation can also be seen angiographically. An RCG recorded from the right and left hemispheres under normal conditions and with the artery to be ligated compressed in the neck gives an accurate picture of the immediate results which will follow ligation. If the circle of Willis is functioning normally, carotid compression will not alter the RCG. If it is not, compression will result in a sharp reduction on the side of the compression, indicating that it is not safe to tie the artery. As it is not possible to compress the carotid artery

References p. 283

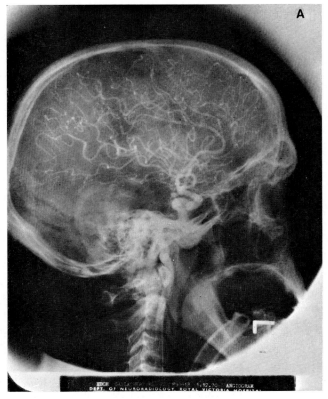

Fig. 10. RCG's in a patient with a posterior communicating aneurysm before (A & B) and after (C & D) an episode of intracranial vascular spasm following a subarachnoid haemorrhage. The spasm causes a very great increase in TT and reduction in h. max.

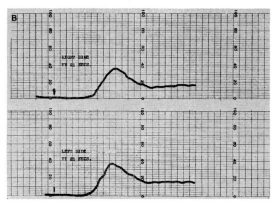

Fig. 10B.

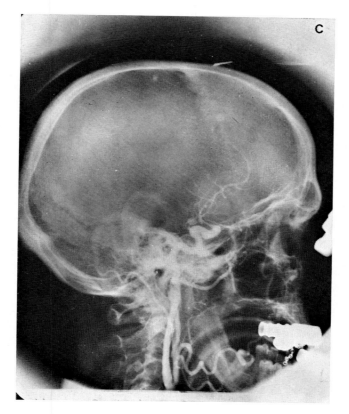

Fig. 10C.

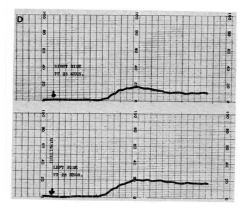

Fig. 10D.

without simultaneously occluding the internal jugular vein, time must be given after compression is begun (20 sec) to allow venous drainage to be directed to the opposite jugular vein and intracranial pressure to return to normal before the RCG is recorded. Fig. 12 shows the effect of carotid compression on a patient with a normal circle of Willis whose carotid artery was ligated with safety and Fig. 13 a patient with an

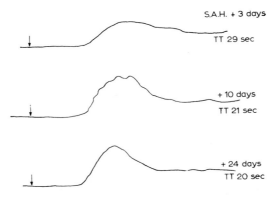

S.A.H. + 3 days

TT 29 sec

+ 10 days

TT 21 sec

+ 24 days

TT 20 sec

Fig. 11. A series of RCG's in a patient following subarachnoid haemorrhage, showing the gradual improvement in blood flow as the vascular spasm subsides. Top – 3 days after ictus, second – after 10 days, third – after 24 days.

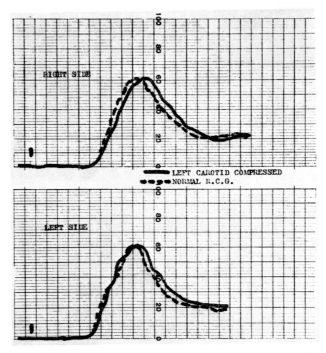

Fig. 12. Unchanged blood flow curves following carotid compression in a patient with a normally functioning circle of Willis.

inefficient circle of Willis. The latter showed a pronounced fall in circulation of the ipsilateral cerebral hemisphere. It was unsafe to treat this patient by carotid artery ligation and the aneurysm was approached directly and occluded by clipping.

Increased intracranial pressure

Increased intracranial pressure is a problem requiring direct treatment in patients with cerebral tumours pre- and post-operatively and following head injury. It is increasingly possible to monitor the intracranial pressure directly without catheterizing the ventricles; but where this is not possible, serial recording of RCG's will give the same information. Intravenous injection of hyperbaric solution is often used to reduce intracranial pressure where a dangerous state of pressure exists threatening consciousness and vital functions. It is important for the clinician to know how effective the administration of such a solution is. Fig. 14 shows angiograms and RCG's done on a patient with a cerebral tumour before and after the intravenous injection of 30% urea.

The pre-injection X-ray shows that blood is entering and remaining in the tumour bed and that the normal veins are not filled, presumably because they are compressed

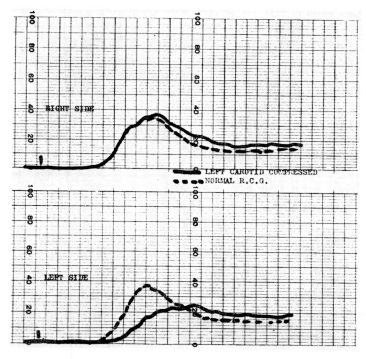

Fig. 13. The effect of carotid compression on hemisphere blood flow in a patient with an inefficient collateral circulation. Unsafe to tie the common carotid artery.

References p. 283

by the swollen normal brain. After reduction in brain volume the intracranial pressure is reduced and the draining veins fill and function normally. Repeated RCG's indicate any necessity for further intravenous therapy. Similarly, the state of intracranial pressure in response to dexamethonium can be assessed from the behaviour of the blood flow. It is important to keep intracranial pressure down while investigations into a case of cerebral tumour are proceeding before a definite decision about treatment has been made. Although the clinical response of a patient frequently supplies all the necessary information about the effectiveness of steroid treatment, the state of the cerebral circulation is useful corroborative evidence. A similar situation exists after intracranial operation because the occurrence of post-operative oedema is somewhat unpredictable and may reach a peak on the second or third day. Even simple removal of a subdural haematoma is not followed immediately by the restoration of a normal blood flow pattern (Fig. 15). Recovery of flow is not, therefore, a simple function of changing intracranial pressure, and monitoring blood circulation can give more useful clinical information in the post-operative period than direct monitoring of intracranial pressure.

Care of the acutely head-injured patient is a more complicated matter because a sudden deceleration force acts differently on brain function than do the slowly changing foci of an expanding intracranial tumour abscess or haemorrhage. It is known that, following cerebral infarction, the area round the infarcted brain may show an increased circulation which can be detected angiographically or by multiple

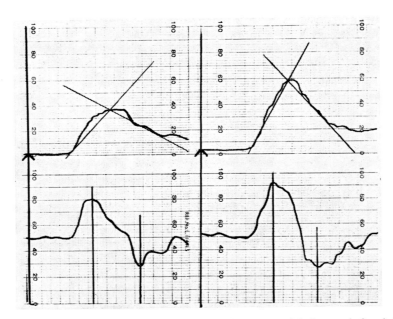

Fig. 14. Angiogram and RCG in a patient with a cerebral tumour: a–b before; c–d after, intravenous injection of mannitol solution. Note the release of pressure on the venous system with decrease in circulation time.

small scintillation detectors recording regional [133]Xenon or [85]Krypton wash-out curves (Lassen, 1966). Further, these hyperaemic areas do not respond normally to changing systemic blood pressure or arterial CO_2. Increasing P_{CO_2}, which normally results in an increased cerebral blood flow, causes a reduction of flow in the peri-infarcted area. The same response is found generally for some time after injury in the brains of severely head-injured patients. It seems likely that these patients have diffuse hypoxic areas resulting from widespread spasm or actual vessel damage from shearing stresses and the combined effect is to cause a total reduction of cerebral blood flow. Recording of cerebral circulation times and their response to inhaled CO_2 should be part of the routine investigation of severely head-injured patients, particularly as it has been suggested that hyperventilation – or positive pressure respiration with detectable reduction of P_{CO_2} – is a useful measure in the treatment of coma (Gordon and Rossanda, 1968). Sufficient information has not been accumulated in this clinic about the effectiveness of hyperventilation in improving the quality of survival in severe head trauma, but investigations into vascular responses are continuing. Patients who are unconscious following trauma, whose cerebral circulations respond paradoxically to inhaled CO_2 (Fig. 16), are treated by positive pressure ventilation reducing the P_{CO_2} to 25–30 mg/100 ml. If this results in an improved circulation curve after 10–12 h (Fig. 17), than hyperventilation is continued until signs of clinical improvement appear. The state of the cerebral circulation, the blood gasses and CSF chemistry are also monitored daily as the hyperventilation continues.

Other head-injured patients whose blood responses must be known if they are to be intelligently treated, are those who hyperventilate to a state of hypocapnia; but who, in spite of a high minute volume, remain hypoxic, presumably because of a pulmonary condition of widespread microatalectasis, which prevents efficient oxidation in the alveolar bed (Froman, 1968). Theoretically such patients may have cerebral vasoconstriction from hypocapnia, cerebral vasodilation because of a low

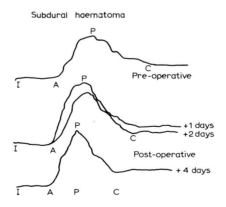

Fig. 15. RCG's before and up to four days after operative removal of a subdural haematoma. The blood flow does not return to normal until the fourth day.

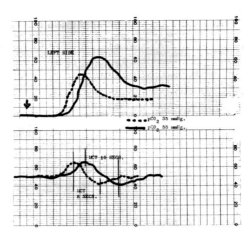

Fig. 16. RCG's, (a) resting and (b) after inhalation of 8% CO_2, in a patient in coma following head injury. A rise in P_{CO_2} causes an abnormal response, decrease in blood flow with increase in circulation time.

arterial P_{O_2}, or may be reacting paradoxically to blood gas changes as a result of head injury as described above. It is essential that the physician know what the cerebral circulation times of these patients are and how they respond to inhaled CO_2 and hyperventilation. The correct treatment (again theoretically) is to supply an oxygen-rich mixture and adjust the physiological dead space in the circuit so that the blown off CO_2 is restored and the end tidal CO_2 returns to normal. The response of the cerebral circulation to these measures must be ascertained by serial RCG's.

RCG in prognosis

Head injury

Investigation of RCG following head injury (Taylor and Bell, 1966) showed that patients with the common post-traumatic complaints of headaches, dizziness, anxiety, irritability, poor effort tolerance, etc., had greater increase in cerebral circulation time and reduced h.max compared with a matched series of controls (Fig. 18). It was further shown that the reduction or disappearance of these symptoms was preceded by a return of the cerebral circulation time to normal. Recording of RCG is therefore a useful part of the investigation of a patient with post-traumatic symptoms. It can be said with some confidence that a patient who, one to two weeks after head injury, (in the absence of neurological deficit), has a normal RCG is unlikely to have post-traumatic symptoms. If the RCG is found to be abnormal the prognosis for the early disappearance of symptoms should be guarded and the investigation should be repeated at monthly intervals until it returns to normal. It should be noted that this investigation is not of much value in the first two days after injury because it is often found that the increase in circulation time does not appear until after the third day. The reason for this latent interval of normality is not known.

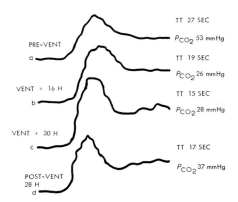

Fig. 17. Effect of hyperventilation: (a) before hyperventilation; (b) 16-h hyperventilation; (c) 30-h hyperventilation; (d) 28 hours after ventilation ceased. Increase in cerebral blood flow after hyperventilation in a patient in coma after head injury, who reacted paradoxically to CO_2 inhalation. The improvement in blood flow was maintained after ventilation had ceased.

Prognosis in cerebral vascular disease

The patient with an acute stroke usually has an abnormal RCG with reduced h.max and increased circulation time. The significance of this cannot be immediately known as the slowing may be caused either by local or diffuse arteriosclerotic plaques in the great or small vessels, by complete obstruction of a major vessel, or by oedema and decreased perfusion in the infarcted area if it is large enough. The response of the cerebral circulation, either to treatment or the "vis medicatrix naturae" is, however, all important prognostically, and daily RCG's will, after 2 to 3 days, allow a fairly accurate forecast to be made. If the first observation shows a near normal circulation profile, the outlook is good. If it is abnormal and improves rapidly it is similarly good. If it starts slow and of poor amplitude and remains so or worsens, then the outlook is bad because, either there is no evident response from the collateral circulation, or continuing hypoxia is resulting in increasing swelling with the establishment of a vicious circle of hypoxia–swelling–more hypoxia–more swelling, which cannot readily be broken. It is in the presence of the last progression that hyperventilation could play a decisive role in the management of increased intracranial pressure and progressive oedema, but, as in the head injury situation, the response of the circulation to changes in P_{CO_2} must be known and observed by serial RCG's before a decision to hyperventilate the patient can be arrived at.

More confidence can be placed in prognosis concerning patients with transient ischaemic attacks. After such an attack the circulation time, if increased at all, rapidly returns to its pre-attack level. The important factor is the basic level of the circulation profile. If it is normal it is probable that the ischaemic attacks can be stopped or reduced by attention to the causative factors – coagulability, triglyceride levels, diet, exercise, respiratory function or neck movement. If the basic RCG shows an increase in TT or decreased h.max, the probability is that the attacks cannot be reduced and that a major cerebral vascular accident will follow within a short period of time.

The end result of spontaneous internal carotid artery thrombosis is readily assessable on the basis of a single RCG done shortly after the event and even more accurately by a series of RCG's done at intervals during the first weeks (Garg *et al.*, 1968). In favourable cases, where the collateral circulation is good and dilates rapidly,

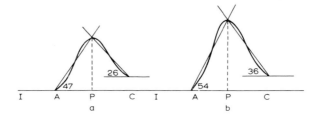

Fig. 18. The mean blood flow profile in 70 patients (a) after head injury compared with those of 70 controls (b). The patients' circulation time is increased and h.max reduced.

INTERNAL CAROTID ARTERY THROMBOSIS

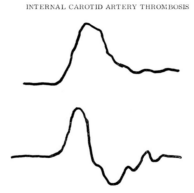

Fig. 19. RCG approaching normal in a patient following spontaneous internal carotid artery thrombosis. Good recovery.

INTERNAL CAROTID ARTERY THROMBOSIS

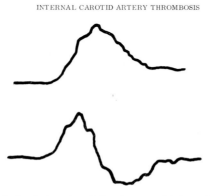

Fig. 20. RCG with increased circulation time following carotid thrombosis. Recovery very limited.

there will be little if any slowing in circulation from the beginning (Fig. 19). Such patients will almost certainly recover without paralysis or dysphasia. If the circulation is slow at the outset and does not recover rapidly, the patient will have a residual neurological deficit (Fig. 20).

Disobliteration of major extracranial vessels

Surgery for major stenoses of extracranial arteries is sometimes carried out with the aim of increasing total cerebral blood flow and preventing further episodes of regional ischaemia. RCG's can help in the selection of patients for operation. A patient with a significant slowing of cerebral circulation, particularly if the slowing is great on the "input" side, almost certainly has small vessel disease and a poor run off area in addition to the stenosis seen on the angiogram, and will not benefit from surgery unless it be from the removal of an ulcerated area in the stenotic plaque from which emboli are originating. On the other hand, a patient whose circulation time is only slightly increased pre-operatively is not likely to have significant vascular disease beyond that seen on an angiogram and will benefit from surgery at least prognostically by an increase in his total circulatory reserve. Improvement in circulation time or h.max is, however, not always found after disobliterative operations.

MISCELLANEOUS

RCG's in therapeutic trials

Double blind trials of drugs said to improve cerebral function by increasing cerebral blood flow can be assisted by serial RCG's done before, during and after therapy in treated and control patients (Ball and Taylor, 1967). By correlating blood flow changes with changes in intellectual function test scores, such drugs can be classified into:

    i. Drugs which increase cerebral blood flow and improve intellectual and/or physical function.

    ii. Drugs which do not significantly alter blood flow, but improve function.

    iii. Drugs which increase flow but do not improve function.

    iv. Drugs which do not alter blood flow or function.

    This information is of practical use both to the geriatric physician and the pharmaceutical chemist.

RCG's in neuroradiology

Injection of hyperbaric solutions – usually radio-opaque iodine compounds – for cerebral angiography may have important effects on cerebral vasomotor tone and capillary permeability resulting in changes in circulation time and blood flow which the physician or surgeon in clinical charge of the patient should know about. Patients with cerebral tumours frequently show an increase in cerebral blood flow after angiography (Donaldson and Brown, 1970), which may cause increased supratentorial pressure and precipitate tentorial herniation. Such an increase, if observed in the post-angiogram RCG, indicates the necessity for measures to reduce intracranial pressure – hyperbaric solutions or dexamethasone. Following angiography in patients with subarachnoid haemorrhage, cerebral blood flow has been found to decrease significantly in the first hour. Presumably this reduction is caused by reactive spasm of the vessels already hypertonic in the area of the ruptured aneurysm. The possibility of avoiding this reduction of blood flow by employing hyperventilation before or during injection, or by intravenous or intra-arterial injection of a drug known to cause cerebral vasodilation, is at present under investigation. An RCG done immediately before angiography will inform the radiologist of the time elapsing between appearance and maximum concentration of isotope in the head. This will enable him to time the serial X-ray exposure to give the best concentration of contrast medium.

DISCUSSION AND SUMMARY

Observation of the cerebral blood flow profile following intravenous injection of a gamma-emitting isotope is a safe, atraumatic and almost indefinitely repeatable method of obtaining clinically useful information about the cerebral circulation which is immediately available and readily interpreted by the responsible physician. Tests can be done on out-patients and in any clinical condition up to the very sick patients, without moving them from their beds.

The method is not useful except in general terms for diagnosis. However, screening patients to determine whether the circulation pattern is normal or not can assist materially the decision whether to subject them to the more traumatic radiological investigations of angiography or air encephalography. The RCG in patients with A–V malformation is absolutely diagnostic and can only be partly simulated by severe thyrotoxicosis.

The usefulness of the method is due mainly to its being reproducible and repeatable. Twenty examinations can be done before the radioactive dose level of a single brain scan is reached and it is therefore possible to make daily estimations over three weeks if necessary, in the interests of efficient management. The state of spasm of the intra-cerebral vessels can be followed after subarachnoid haemorrhage without recourse to further angiography. This helps the surgeon to choose the optimum time for operative intervention. Observations made during carotid compression indicate whether or not it is safe to ligate the artery proximal to an aneurysm. The management of intracranial hypertension is facilitated by a knowledge of the behaviour of the cerebral circulation in response to treatment by operation, intravenous hypertonic solutions and steroids. In the acute head injury maintenance or loss of autoregulation in response to changing blood pressure or arterial P_{CO_2} is an important guide to the use of positive pressure ventilation in the treatment of hypoxia. This function can be serially investigated by RCG.

At a late stage after head injury the behaviour of the circulation is a prognostic guide to the likely persistence and severity of post-traumatic symptoms.

Cerebral vascular disorders can be investigated both in the acute and chronic stages of cerebral deprivation, and the RCG profile, basic and in response to treatment, is a valuable guide both to immediate therapy and prognosis.

During radiological contrast studies RCG can assist the radiologist in timing the X-ray exposures following injection and can inform him whether injection has temporarily increased or decreased blood flow.

Serial examinations can be used during trials of new drugs which allegedly improve mental function by increasing cerebral blood flow or release spasm following subarachnoid haemorrhage.

The method may also find a place in the investigation of patients dying from cerebral or other causes in whom it is suspected that the cerebral circulation has been so reduced as to be incompatible with survival of cerebral function.

REFERENCES

BALL, J. A. C. AND TAYLOR, A. R. (1967) Effect of Cyclandelate on mental function and cerebral blood flow in elderly patients. *Brit. Med. J.*, **3**, 525.

DONALDSON, A. A. AND BROWN, A. S. (1970) The effect of X-ray contrast medium (angiografin) on regional cerebral blood flow. *Intern. Cerebral Blood Flow Symposium, London.*

EICHHORN, O. (1959) Die Radiocirculographie, ein klinische Methode zur Messung der Hirndurchblutung. *Wien. Klin. Wochschr.*, **71**, 499.

FROMAN, C. (1968) Alterations of respiratory function in patients with severe head injury. *Brit. J. Anaesthesia*, **40**, 354.

GARG, A. G., GORDON, D. S., TAYLOR, A. R. AND GREBBELL, F. S. (1968) Internal carotid artery thrombosis secondary to closed craniocerebral trauma. *Brit. J. Surg.*, **55**, 4.

GORDON, E. AND ROSSANDA, M. (1968) The importance of CSF acid base status in the treatment of unconscious patients with brain lesions. *Acta Anaesthesiol. Scand.*, **12**, 51.

LASSEN, N. A. (1966) The luxury perfusion syndrome and its possible relation to acute metabolic acidosis localised within the brain. *Lancet*, **i**, 1113.

OLDENDORF, W. H. AND CRANDALL, P. H. (1961) Bilateral circulation curves obtained by intravenous injection of radioisotopes. *J. Neurosurg.*, **18**, 195.

SWALLOW, M. W., TAYLOR, A. R. AND GARG, A. G. (1968) Unpublished observations.

TAYLOR, A. R. AND BELL, T. K. (1966) Slowing of cerebral circulation after concussional head injury. *Lancet*, **ii**, 178.

Relationship of Cerebral Blood Flow and Metabolism to Neurological Symptoms

JOHN STIRLING MEYER AND K. M. A. WELCH

Department of Neurology, Baylor College of Medicine, Houston, Texas 77025 (U.S.A.)

INTRODUCTION

The last two decades have seen the gradual decline of the attitude of pessimism with which the physician approached the problem of treating patients with clinically proven cerebrovascular disease, for it has been during this period that striking advances in the knowledge of the physiology and pathology of the cerebrovascular system have been made by research workers and clinicians in medical centers all over the world.

This is not to say that contributions to this field of study before this time were insignificant. On the contrary, the writings of Galen show us that interest in the cerebral vasculature dates from a much earlier period. More important, enthusiasm of workers in the first half of this century, with knowledge gained using only the simple and limited technical facilities then available, laid the foundation on which the recent inroads in research into cerebrovascular disease have been made. A review of the history of research concerned with the physiological mechanisms regulating cerebral blood flow will be found in the monograph of Meyer and Gilroy in 1968.

For almost two decades the work of our laboratories has been concerned with classification of the pathogenetic mechanisms related to neurological disorders, particularly those responsible for the signs and symptoms of cerebrovascular disease. The remarkable reversibility of many symptoms of cerebral ischemia, *e.g.*, transient ischemic attacks, is well known, and has encouraged research into methods of measuring CBF and metabolism in patients with cerebrovascular disease in the hope that recovery from cerebral ischemia may be hastened or symptoms prevented.

The first section of this communication consists of a review of work done by early investigators to develop methods for measuring CBF and metabolism and the efforts of the numerous workers in our laboratory to refine and improve upon these methods. Experimental animals were first used, and if the techniques proved reliable and appropriate they were applied to the study of patients with cerebrovascular disease. Methods will be reviewed in general terms. Further details may be found in the original papers which are extensively referenced for this purpose.

The second section summarizes the results of such studies in experimental animals and human subjects. The techniques and certain of the special devices were also

References pp. 339–347

found to be applicable to the study of other neurological disorders such as epilepsy, and the results of these applications will also be discussed. However, this section deals mainly with the physiology and pathophysiology of cerebrovascular function in health and disease in light of results from experiments in animals and studies in the patient with stroke.

The third and final section is concerned with present concepts of medical and surgical treatment of patients with cerebrovascular disease, or stroke.

Section I: METHODOLOGY

MEASUREMENT OF CEREBRAL BLOOD FLOW

Skull window observations

Among the earliest techniques for the study of cerebral blood flow was direct exposure of the pial vessels or observations of the pial vessels through windows inserted into the skull. Donders (1850, 1859), a midnineteenth century investigator, was one of the prominent pioneers who employed this approach. Forbes, in 1928, developed a reliable airtight skull window which permitted observation and photography of the pial vessels. Wolff and Lennox (1930) applied this method in their studies of pial blood flow and established the all-important vasodilator effect of carbon dioxide (CO_2). Fog (1934, 1939 a, 1939 b) carried these investigations further and established the vital concept of autoregulation of the cerebral circulation. Autoregulation may be defined as the ability of the brain to maintain its blood flow constant despite changes in perfusion pressure.

A modification of the skull window method was used in our laboratories to observe blood flow in the leptomeningeal vessels following occlusion of the middle cerebral artery (Meyer, 1958 c). A trephine hole was made over the frontal or parietal operculum of the sylvian fissure and a tight-fitting window, after Forbes (1928) and modified later by Sohler et al. (1941), was screwed into place. By recessing the window in a brass frame the glass could be irrigated with saline or cerebrospinal fluid for the purpose of observation and photography. Watertight screws, which could be temporarily removed from holes drilled through the frame of the window, permitted irrigation of the surface of the underlying brain and insertion of polarographic electrodes for measuring the oxygen tension (P_{O_2}) of the area under observation. Phenomena observed in this manner included the establishment of collateral circulation, reversal of flow in bordering vessels near an ischemic area, infarction despite continuing but sluggish circulation, red veins, hyperemia, slow flow, loss of axial flow, platelet aggregation, and formation of thrombi and emboli. The implication of these responses to the genesis and recovery from neurological deficits will be discussed in Sections II and III.

Polarographic methods

Davies and Brink (1942) were the first to employ electropolarography to provide physiological measurements of brain P_{O_2}, although the method had been used in physical chemistry long before this time. The principle of electropolarography is that the unknown P_{O_2} of any solution may be measured with a platinum electrode acting as a cathode and recording the flow of current between it and a nonpolarizable reference electrode (calomel half-cell or silver–silver chloride wire). When the current is plotted as a fraction of the voltage, a plateau is reached at around 0.6 to 0.8 V which is dependent upon the reaction:

$$2H^+ + O_2 + 2\,\text{electrons} \rightarrow H_2O_2$$

Provided the voltage is maintained constant at about 0.6 to 0.8 V, the flow of current is proportional to the P_{O_2} of the solution. Local changes in tissue oxygen were shown to be rapid.

Several modifications of the original platinum electrode were made by Meyer *et al.* (1954) in their study of cerebral collateral circulation. Open-tip electrodes were constructed from a 1-cm length of platinum wire 25 to 50 μ in diameter, soldered to an 8-cm length of silver wire and insulated with Teflon so that only the tip was exposed (Meyer and Hunter, 1957 b). When chronically implanted in the brain, any trauma caused by insertion of the electrodes healed. This usually took three to four days. The electrodes were then shown to give a constant response to inhaled oxygen. The reference electrode consisted of a silver–silver chloride anode, which was also insulated with Teflon except for the 1-cm terminal freshly coated with chloride before use. The development of this anode was a significant improvement over the calomel half-cell which is clumsy to use in chronic preparations.

The simultaneous use of multiple electrodes deployed over the brain was first employed at this time (Meyer *et al.*, 1954), and continuous recording of the P_{O_2} of multiple areas of brain simultaneously on a polygraph allowed spatial and temporal recording of changes of regional brain tissue oxygen availability. The cathodes were

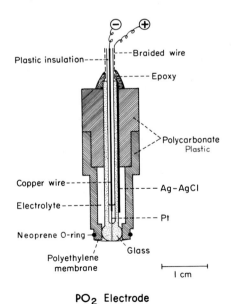

PO₂ Electrode

Fig. 1. Diagrammatic sketch of construction of P_{O_2} electrode. Scale in centimeters is indicated below the electrode.

placed in the desired area of the cortex or white matter to be measured with the anode placed on any convenient cranial tissue adjacent to the operative site.

Later, cathodes were placed in a small quantity of electrolyte solution covered with a thin polyethylene or Teflon membrane so that absolute P_{O_2} measurements of various regions of the brain could be made (Fig. 1). Local cerebral P_{O_2} levels were found to vary according to three variables: local blood flow, local metabolism of oxygen, and arterial oxygen concentration. If metabolic consumption of oxygen (CMRO$_2$) in the area measured was constant, then changes in local P_{O_2} reflected changes in blood flow. CMRO$_2$ may also be measured in semiquantitative terms when the oxygen electrode is combined with regional measurements of CBF.

Such membrane-covered electrodes may also be used for measuring hydrogen gas tensions. Oxygen and hydrogen electrodes may be applied to the arterial and cerebral venous blood to measure average CBF and CMRO$_2$. These methods will be described fully later in this communication.

Thermometric methods

The heat clearance principle may be used for regional cerebral blood flow (rCBF) measurements by the application of a thermistor; *i.e.*, the rate of heat removed or delivered to an area of brain is dependent upon rCBF. Thermistor probes can be applied directly to vessels or placed on adjacent brain to measure changes in rCBF. The most simple thermistor probe consists of a minute glass bead, 0.045 inches in diameter, mounted on a glass stem with connecting wires (Meyer and Denny-Brown, 1955). Thermistors such as these have a resistance range of 100 thousand ohms at 25°C to 34 thousand ohms at 50°C. Current is applied to the electrodes by means of a 6-V battery and potentiometer. The drop of voltage in the circuit is recorded on the graph and the temperature change can be accurately quantitated. Such local temperature changes may be used for measuring relative changes in CBF. The disadvantage of the method is that any alteration of body temperature during the experiment will be a source of artifact.

The heat clearance principle may also be used to measure velocity of flow in a vessel after injection of a bolus of hot or cold saline or intermittent heating of the blood (Meyer *et al.*, 1964 a). This has been applied to man. Two small thermistors mounted on the ends of polyethylene catheters were inserted percutaneously through a 16-gauge needle into the internal jugular vein above the jugular foramen. One thermistor was intermittently heated every 15 seconds for 5 seconds. The second thermistor, connected to a Wheatstone bridge, served as a temperature sensor, and the output from the bridge was measured and recorded on a polygraph. The temperature of the second thermistor depends on the rate of cooling, which varies directly with the velocity of the blood flowing past it. Repeated curves similar to dye dilution curves are produced. The area under this curve is inversely proportional to the velocity of flow regardless of the temperature of the blood; thus, the higher the curve recorded the lower the flow and *vice versa*. Limitations of the method are that calibration curves are difficult to obtain since a model must be set up using the same blood as that from the subject to be measured. For this reason, it is more practical to obtain calibration curves using another method of measuring blood flow such as local dye dilution or the Kety–Schmidt method (1945); otherwise, the measurements derived with the thermistors are only semiquantitative. Movement of the thermistor produces artifacts, and blood clot formation on the thermistor will distort the curves. Continuous monitoring of changes in cerebral venous flow without surgical exposure of the vessels is possible with this method. Changes in temperature of the blood do not influence the results, and since the thermistors placed in the blood stream are small there is negligible disturbance of flow.

Regional dilution methods

A thermistor may be used for the measurement of cerebral venous outflow if a bolus of hot or cold saline solution is injected into the internal jugular blood as an indicator and the resulting dilution curve recorded downstream. When the indicator is thoroughly mixed with the blood, the dilution curve and rate of disappearance will vary directly according to the velocity of blood flow.

Contact of the thermistor on the vessel wall may cause errors, however, and, in practice, the exact temperature of the indicator at the moment of injection is difficult to obtain.

Dye dilution curves may be obtained using a similar principle by drawing the blood continuously from a catheter through a densitometer (Meyer et al., 1964 a). Cardiogreen was found to be a more suitable dye than others, such as Evans blue, since it is not influenced by the oxygen saturation of the blood. Careful calibration of the dye concentrations immediately before or after the study is essential.

With both methods the problem of adequate mixing within the bloodstream can be overcome by using a mechanical injector designed to inject the indicator in a constant and reproducible manner. Dilution methods are simple, may be repeated many times, and permit detection of rapid changes in cerebral venous outflow.

Rheoencephalography

While in the process of evaluating techniques for measuring CBF, workers in our laboratory have at the same time subjected methods developed in other laboratories to critical analysis. One of these methods was rheoencephalography (Perez-Borja and Meyer, 1964). When an alternating current passes through a part of the body, modulated changes of impedance occur due to the pulsatile flow of blood. The principle of rheoencephalography is to attempt to correlate these changes with modifications of the cerebral circulation (Jenkner, 1966). A 2 mA current with an average input of 3 V is passed at a frequency of 30 kc across the head of the patient. Impedance waves are monitored from multiple electrode placements, somewhat like those of an electroencephalogram (EEG). The curves may be analyzed with respect to amplitude, angle of inclination, the time at which the first peak is reached, the wave form, the number of peaks present in a single pulse, the regularity of the wave, and the inclination of the descending part of the curve. Unfortunately, after analysis of the data on 19 control subjects and 28 patients with proven cerebrovascular disease, it was evident that rheoencephalography is unsatisfactory for determining the rate of CBF. It became apparent that a significant proportion of the pulse wave was derived from extracranial blood flow as well as changes in cerebrospinal fluid and blood volume. Rheoencephalography has been more favorably reviewed (Jenkner, 1968), but in our opinion difficulties such as contamination by extracerebral flow render the method an unreliable indication of rCBF.

Electromagnetic flowmeters

The development of electromagnetic flowmeters was a significant contribution to the progress that has been made in the study of CBF since it made possible quantitative and continuous measurements through exposed but unopened vessels. Electromagnetic probes are placed around the blood vessel. An electromagnet within this probe is intermittently excited by a gated sine or square wave current and produces a magnetic field at a right angle to the direction of blood flow. As the flowing blood cuts the magnetic lines of force, a pulsatile voltage develops which is sensed by electrodes located at diametrically opposed points in the lumen of the vessel. The signal is amplified and demodulated and presented as a mean or pulsatile flow indicator which is recorded on the polygraph. Calibration is performed before or after the experiment by recording the rate of flow of blood or isotonic saline pumped through the vessel *in vitro*. Total CBF has been monitored by applying electromagnetic flowmeters about both exposed internal jugular veins and expressing venous outflow as the sum of the two flow values (Table 1) (Meyer *et al.*, 1964 a, 1964 b; Symon *et al.*, 1963 b). Measurement of flow within the internal carotid and vertebral arteries has also been made. When used in combination with the Guyton arteriovenous oxygen analyzer, average CBF and oxygen consumption can be monitored from second to second.

The main disadvantage of using electromagnetic flowmeters is that exposure of

TABLE 1

MEASUREMENT OF CEREBRAL BLOOD FLOW IN THE MONKEY

Method	Cerebral blood flow (ml/min)
Electromagnetic flowmeter	
Arterial outflow (ml/100 g brain/min)	70.0 ± 7.1
Jugular inflow (ml/100 g brain/min)	56.1 ± 1.5
Hydrogen inhalation	
Average (ml/100 g brain/min)	43.5 ± 5.1
Intracarotid hydrogen bolus	
HBF (ml/100 g brain/min)	43.3 ± 4.3
Chronically implanted hydrogen electrodes	
rCBF (ml/g brain/min) white matter	0.230 ± 0.57

the vessels may cause vasospasm. The probes are too large for effective use in animals smaller than monkeys.

Extracorporeal systems analysis for metabolic changes

An effective procedure for continuous monitoring of cerebral metabolism which has been widely used in our laboratory (Gotoh et al., 1966 a) has been the use of flow-through cuvettes and an extracorporeal circulation (Fig. 2). Blood is continuously

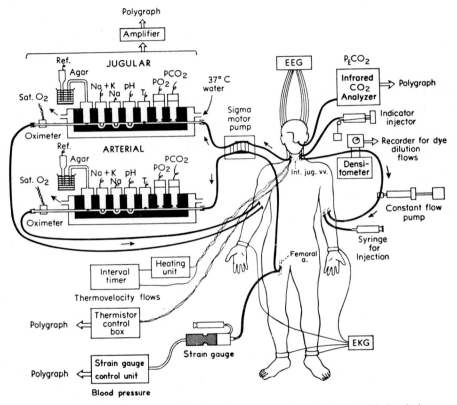

Fig. 2. Diagram illustrating the use of the flow-through cuvette and extracranial circulation as part of an early method employed in this laboratory for measuring CBF by the thermovelocity technique.

sampled from the venous and arterial systems by means of indwelling catheters and a peristaltic pump. The blood is propelled through the cuvettes containing appropriate measuring sensors and is then returned to the systemic circulation via a major vein. The majority of investigators in the past have employed percutaneous needle puncture of the internal jugular bulb to obtain samples of cerebral venous blood, a technique introduced by Myerson et al. (1927). Kety and Schmidt (1945) used a modification of this procedure for their nitrous oxide method. Gotoh and associates (1966 a) further modified the technique, using a catheter instead of a needle, after the method

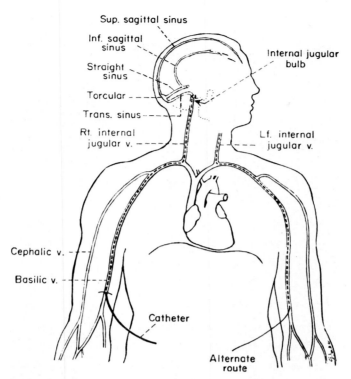

Fig. 3. Schematic drawing illustrating anatomic course followed during insertion of catheters from the left and right basilic veins into the left and right transverse venous sinuses of the brain. (From Meyer *et al.* (1969) *Neurology*, **19**, 353–358).

of Seldinger (1953), since catheters can be inserted above the jugular bulb. A new method of indirect catheterization of the cerebral transverse sinus recently was developed in our laboratory employing principles originally described by Forssman, in 1929, for cardiac catheterization (Meyer *et al.*, 1969 d). The catheters are inserted through a small incision in the skin overlying the right and left antecubital veins and, then, into the right and left transverse sinuses of the brain, using fluoroscopy and image amplifiers for control of placement (Figs. 3 and 4). This approach permits blood sampling from the cerebral venous circulation, mainly from the ipsilateral hemisphere, without the possibility of extracerebral contamination. The brachial artery may be exposed in the same incision and catheters directed into the carotid and vertebral arteries for injecting indicators and contrast media.

The cuvette used for this purpose is shown in Fig. 5. Each cuvette contains seven portholes arranged in a series from inlet to outlet into which appropriate sensors are fitted, depending upon the measurements desired (*e.g.*, pH). When measuring sodium, potassium, and pH, an agar bridge must be incorporated into one of the portholes so that a calomel half-cell used as a reference electrode makes contact with blood flowing through the cuvette. The temperature of the blood as it flows through the cuvettes is maintained at 37 °C by means of a water jacket, and the temperature is monitored

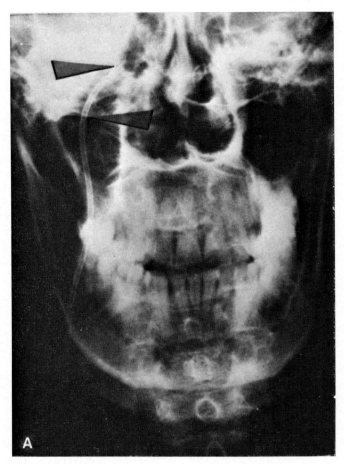

Fig. 4. A. Anteroposterior roentgenogram showing catheter placed in right transverse sinus. Upper arrow indicates tip of catheter in transverse sinus. Lower arrow indicates lower border of jugular fossa where the catheter passes upward beyond the jugular bulb.

by a thermistor mounted in the cuvette. To prevent clot formation, the internal surfaces of the cuvette are coated with silicone and the patient is given 75 to 100 mg of heparin intravenously.

Nitrous oxide method

Kety and Schmidt (1945) made a fundamental contribution when they introduced the nitrous oxide method for measuring average CBF and metabolism using the Fick principle. The Fick principle states that the amount of indicator taken up by tissue per unit of time is equal to the quantity brought to that tissue by the arterial blood less the quantity removed from that tissue by the venous blood. The subject inhales nitrous oxide gas until the arterial and cerebral venous blood is in equilibrium and the brain tissue is saturated. Intermittent sampling of arterial and venous blood during

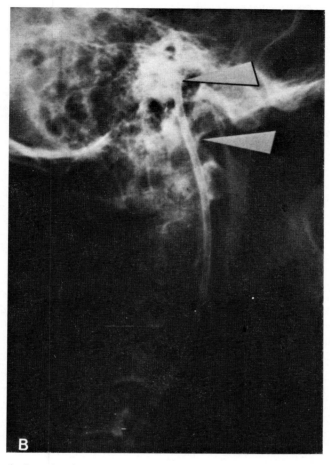

Fig. 4. B. Lateral view showing position of catheter. (From Meyer *et al.* (1969) *Neurology*, **19**, 353–358).

nitrous oxide inhalation makes it possible to produce a saturation curve from which CBF may be calculated using the equation

$$\frac{\mathrm{d}Qi}{\mathrm{d}T} = F_l(Ca - CVi)$$

where Qi is the quantity of indicator in the tissue, F_l is the total blood flow through the tissue, Ca is the arterial concentration of the indicator, and CVi is the venous concentration of the indicator. Kety and Schmidt in their original method used the Van Slyke and Neill apparatus for measuring nitrous oxide levels. This was time consuming, subject to human error, and required frequent sampling of as much as 60 ml of blood for each estimation. To overcome these limitations, workers in our laboratories replaced this apparatus with the extracorporeal circulatory system (Meyer *et al.*, 1967 c). Blood was pumped through a diffusion coil, permitting the

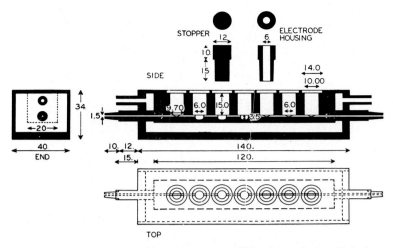

Fig. 5. Transparent acrylic cuvette used in measurement of blood P_{O_2}, P_{CO_2}, pH, hydrogen tension, sodium, and potassium. Dimensions expressed in millimeters.

nitrous oxide gas to diffuse through the inner silastic coil which was continuously measured with an infrared gas analyzer and the blood returned to the patient.

The colorimetric method of Spencer and associates (1961) or gasometry by infrared absorption may also be employed for gas analysis.

Our modification of the Kety–Schmidt method prevents blood loss and enables large volumes of blood to be pumped rapidly through diffusion coils, thus improving the response time and reliability of the nitrous oxide sensor system as more gas is made available for estimation (Meyer *et al.*, 1966 c). In addition, continuous analysis of nitrous oxide gas permits early identification of arterial and venous equilibrium, thereby improving the accuracy of the technique. Saturation and desaturation curves are always obtained and differences between the areas under the arterial and cerebral venous curves can be measured with great accuracy. CBF during saturation is calculated from the formula

$$\text{CBF} = \frac{100\ Vu}{\int_{o}^{v} (A - V)\,\mathrm{d}t}$$

where CBF is cerebral blood flow in ml per 100 grams of brain per minute, A is arterial nitrous oxide content in volume %, V is jugular nitrous oxide content in volume %, and Vu is jugular nitrous oxide content at time u in volume %. During desaturation the following formula is used:

$$\text{CBF} = \frac{100\ (V_o)}{\int_{o}^{v} (V - A)\,\mathrm{d}t}$$

Thus, two CBF values are obtained with every inhalation. The measurements can be repeated many times in the same individual. The absence of blood loss makes this method applicable to small animals as well as humans. The results obtained agree well with values obtained by other investigators who have also used the nitrous oxide technique.

From both theoretical and practical points of view, there are several disadvantages to the nitrous oxide method. Equilibrium of the nitrous oxide gas between cerebral blood and brain tissue might not be complete within 10 minutes, particularly in abnormal brain. Incomplete saturation of brain tissue is a source of error. Furthermore, the method cannot be modified to measure rCBF.

Measurement of cerebral blood flow using hydrogen gas

Measurement of total blood flow by hydrogen inhalation

The hydrogen method for measuring average CBF was developed in our laboratory, utilizing the Fick principle (Gotoh et al., 1966 c, 1966 d). Molecular hydrogen, 2.5%, mixed in air is inhaled as the inert gas indicator. Hydrogen saturates blood rapidly, permitting accurate and almost immediate analysis of partial pressure in blood by the use of hydrogen electrodes. Hydrogen is physiologically inert and causes no significant alterations in arterial and internal jugular venous P_{O_2}, carbon dioxide tension (P_{CO_2}), pH, and oxygen saturation, indicating that the inhaled mixture does not change pulmonary ventilation or cerebral circulation. Furthermore, hydrogen gas in blood does not interfere with hydrogen dissociation, nor was any evidence noted for its combination with the blood constituents. Since hydrogen enters the blood almost entirely in physical solution, its molecular concentration in blood can be determined by monitoring hydrogen gas tension with hydrogen electrodes.

The polarographic principle employed in measuring cerebral P_{O_2} is used in constructing the hydrogen electrode. The electrodes are made in the same manner as the oxygen electrodes developed earlier in our laboratory except that the platinum electrode acts as the anode. Platinum wire is sealed in a glass tube with a surface area of 25 to 100 μ diameter exposed. The surface of the wire is platinized by means of electrolysis shortly before use. The hydrogen electrode is then combined with a silver chloride reference electrode in such a way that both make contact with the film of electrolyte solution. The components are placed in an electrode housing and covered with a 50-μ Teflon membrane held in place with a neoprene ring. A potential of 0.68 V is applied to the platinum anode, a voltage at which the electrode is no longer sensitive to changes in P_{O_2} and becomes a pure hydrogen sensor. The electrode is sensitive and permits the use of the low concentrations of hydrogen. The use of cuvettes in the extracorporeal blood flow system permits continuous monitoring of the arteriovenous hydrogen differences. Arterial and cerebral venous blood samples are propelled through two cuvettes at a rate of 15 ml/minute from catheters placed within the brachial artery and internal jugular veins. Hydrogen electrodes are mounted in these cuvettes to monitor the partial pressure of hydrogen within the arterial and venous blood.

In our studies, a hydrogen gas mixture consisting of 2.5% hydrogen, 21% oxygen, and the balance nitrogen is inhaled from a face mask until jugular venous equilibrium is achieved. The response time of the electrode to this gas mixture is 95% in 20 to 30 seconds, and two electrodes having compatible response times are used. Equilibrium of hydrogen between brain and blood is confirmed when a plateau is observed in the saturation curves (Fig. 6). To check the equality of hydrogen tension, the blood

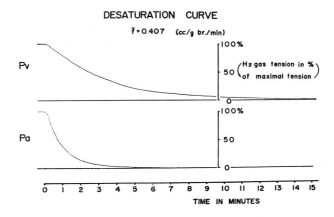

Fig. 6. Photograph of actual recorded curves of hydrogen gas tension in arterial and internal jugular venous blood during desaturation after inhalation of 2.5% hydrogen in air until arteriovenous equilibrium was reached. f̄ is average CBF. (From Tomita, *et al.*, *Research on the Cerebral Circulation*; *3rd Salzburg Conference*. Courtesy of Charles C. Thomas, Publisher, Springfield, Ill.).

samples are switched between the two cuvettes. CBF is calculated from the desaturation curves using the same formula as that for desaturation of nitrous oxide. Simultaneous CBF measurements using both the hydrogen and nitrous oxide gas methods in human subjects during the desaturation phase showed statistically significant correlation. In general, the CBF values obtained with the hydrogen method were about 10% higher than those obtained with the nitrous oxide method.

Advantages of the hydrogen method include: (1) no blood loss; (2) display of arterial and venous hydrogen curves in less than 30 seconds of arteriovenous equilibrium; and (3) rapid tissue and venous hydrogen equilibrium because of the relative insolubility of hydrogen in blood. Furthermore, since equilibrium of hydrogen between blood and brain is directly confirmed, the modified method is more accurate than the original nitrous oxide procedure employed by Kety and Schmidt.

Intracarotid injection of hydrogen gas for hemispheric blood flow measurement

The methods described thus far measure average CBF but do not measure rCBF. The techniques of Lassen and associates (1961, 1963), derived from the clearance curves of radioactive inert gases following intracarotid injection and recorded by means of counters applied over the head, were important landmarks in determining regional cerebral hemodynamics. However, contamination of flow values by extracranial sources such as reflux of the indicator gas into the external carotid artery system, self absorption of the radioisotope, and uncertainty of the exact area measured due to the inverse square law and Compton scattering, are critical drawbacks to an accurate interpretation of the results. As a result, a method first investigated in the monkey and later applied to human subjects was developed whereby a bolus of hydrogen dissolved in saline was injected into the internal carotid artery and clearance curves were recorded from the lateral sinus of the ipsilateral side (Meyer and Shinohara, 1970). In this way, the possibility of contamination of blood from extracerebral sources was overcome. A catheter is inserted into each cerebral transverse or sigmoid sinus via the basilic veins of the forearms (Meyer *et al.*, 1969 d) and blood from each lateral sinus is pumped through two cuvettes via the extracorporeal system. The partial pressure of hydrogen in each lateral sinus is simultaneously recorded by means of two hydrogen electrodes. Hemispheric blood flow (HBF) is calculated from the clearance curve of hydrogen using a formula based on the Stewart–Hamilton principle:

$$F = \frac{\int_o^v P(t)\,\mathrm{d}t}{\int_o^v t\,P(t)\,\mathrm{d}t}$$

where F is the blood flow per gram of tissue and $P(t)$ is the recorded partial pressure of the hydrogen at time (t) of exit.

It has also been possible from these cerebral venous clearance curves to calculate rCBF by height over area analysis and by compartmental analysis. All methods of calculation give comparable results. Extensive theoretical and experimental proofs of the validity of these methods of calculation were reported by Tomita and associates in 1969.

From the hydrogen bolus method of estimating cerebral HBF an index of hemispheric metabolism measured by the arteriovenous differences has been devised. Prior to the development of this method, total cerebral metabolism was calculated from the product of CBF using, for example, the nitrous oxide method and arteriovenous metabolic difference. It became apparent with the hydrogen bolus method that cerebral venous blood sampled from the same side as the injected carotid artery also contained a small portion of blood from the contralateral hemisphere. The amount of mixing differs from one individual to another. A formula was therefore devised to correct for such mixing and to provide a more accurate estimate of hemispheric metabolism:

$$V_1(t) = \frac{bC_1(t) - C_2(t)}{b - 1}$$

where $V_1(t)$ is hemispheric venous content of metabolite at time t and b is the ratio of partial pressure of oxygen appearing in the contralateral sinus after carotid injection of hydrogen gas. $C_1(t)$ and $C_2(t)$ are the concentrations of metabolite in the ipsilateral and contralateral transverse sinuses respectively at time t (Meyer and Shinohara, 1970).

Some comments will be made concerning the validity and advantages of the hydrogen method of measuring HBF and metabolism. The blood flow supplied by one internal carotid artery to cerebral tissue is measured; *i.e.*, the flow measured is almost exclusively that in the ipsilateral hemisphere. In this way, possible errors can be prevented when sampling the blood from an unknown area of drainage from one internal jugular vein, an unavoidable error that occurs when using the Kety–Schmidt method. The hydrogen clearance curves recorded from each lateral cerebral sinus are similar, although the curve is usually larger from the ipsilateral sinus. This fact, plus the high degree of reproducibility in a single individual, provides strong evidence that in the steady state blood flow and blood distribution from each hemisphere into each transverse sinus are constant. Another advantage is that measurements of hemispheric collateral flow in patients with occlusion of the internal carotid artery remain accurate and valid, which is not the case with the Lassen method. When the Stewart–Hamilton principle was applied, the average HBF value in the lightly anesthetized monkey was 41.2 ± 5.2 ml per 200 g of brain per minute (Meyer *et al.*, 1968 c). This was independent of the side injected and was in close agreement with the average CBF measured with the hydrogen inhalation method (see Table 1).

Comparison of the carotid bolus method with inhalation of hydrogen in the human patient revealed important limitations of all inhalation methods. During inhalation, although the shape of the hydrogen curves was identical in the two lateral sinuses, the height of the two were at different partial pressures of hydrogen, indicating incomplete mixing of blood from the two hemispheres. In some instances at least, when samples are drawn from one or the other transverse sinus the average CBF measurement may be influenced by HBF derived from the ipsilateral side. It is common knowledge that regional HBF differs, especially in persons with cerebrovascular disease. In the monkey, the close agreement between the values obtained for average CBF and HBF is due to the normal, healthy state of both cerebral hemispheres, which is not the case in human patients with cerebrovascular disease.

Chronically implanted hydrogen electrodes for regional cerebral blood flow measurement

A newly developed method for measuring rCBF in experimental animals is chronic implantation of open-tip hydrogen electrodes within the cerebral cortex and white matter. Aukland *et al.* (1964) first reported the use of this type of electrode implanted in the kidney. The first attempt to measure rCBF in the brain was made by Fieschi *et al.* (1965). Technical difficulties were encountered due to trauma of the brain tissue surrounding the acutely implanted electrode and recirculation of the hydrogen during desaturation following inhalation. These difficulties were overcome in our laboratories by chronically implanting the electrodes and measuring rCBF following intracarotid injection of a hydrogen-saturated saline solution (Meyer *et al.*, 1971, b). This procedure was carried out after uniform response of the electrodes was demonstrated by brief inhalation of hydrogen gas several days after implantation.

These electrodes are constructed of platinum wire, 250 μ in diameter, coated, and baked with silicone–phenolic resin for insulation except for the tip which is platinized. The reference electrode, which is mounted on the frontal bone, consists of a nickel-plated brass plate. After insertion into the brain, the hydrogen electrodes are held in place with a plastic holder mounted in a hole drilled through the skull. A potential of 0.65 to 0.7 V is applied to the electrode system and the current generated is amplified. The output of each electrode measuring several regional areas of blood flow is then recorded on the polygraph. The response of each electrode during inhalation of a mixture of 2.5 % hydrogen with 21 % oxygen and the balance of nitrogen was found to be constant about three or four days after implantation and remained constant for at least 20 days (the longest interval the tests were carried out). Following intra-carotid injection, the hydrogen clearance curves are recorded simultaneously from each region of the brain in which the electrodes have been implanted. The curve is then replotted against time on semilogarithmic paper and rCBF is calculated using the following formula:

$$f = \frac{0.693}{t\ 1/2}\ \text{ml/g brain/min}$$

where $t\ 1/2$ is one half time in minutes for desaturation of hydrogen, assuming the blood–brain partition coefficient is unity (Meyer et al., 1971, b).

Intracarotid injection of hydrogen is superior to the gas inhalation method since recirculation of hydrogen is overcome. This was confirmed by placing electrodes in the arterial blood and showing that removal of hydrogen from the cerebral venous blood during its first passage through the lungs was complete. Chronically implanted electrodes give consistent responses in situ, unlike acutely implanted electrodes which give inconsistent responses due to trauma of the tissues (Table 2).

Autoradiographic method for measuring regional cerebral blood flow

In our laboratories, investigations have been carried out repeatedly to assess and compare all available methods for measuring CBF. At present studies are underway to compare the values obtained with implanted electrodes with those obtained by autoradiography (Landau et al., 1955). Reivich and co-workers (1969) modified the original autoradiographic method of Landau using ^{131}I-labeled antipyrine intra-venously and were able to measure rCBF with extreme accuracy. Following injection, the animal is sacrificed, the brain frozen and sectioned, and the radioactivity of various sections determined by means of autoradiography. Radio emission in each area is proportional to the blood flow. The major disadvantage is that only one flow measurement can be made per animal and it must be sacrificed, whereas the implanted hydrogen electrodes permit multiple measurements from hour to hour and day to day.

Isotope methods for measuring regional cerebral blood flow

The value of rCBF measurements using intracarotid injection of gamma-emitting radioactive inert gases has been well established (Lassen and Ingvar, 1961; Lassen

TABLE 2

REPRODUCIBILITY OF REGIONAL CEREBRAL BLOOD FLOW MEASUREMENT
BY THE CHRONICALLY IMPLANTED HYDROGEN ELECTRODE

Monkey No.	Electrode	1st Measurement (x)	2nd Measurement (y)
4	C	0.203	0.237
	D	0.233	0.185
	F	0.312	0.297
7	B	0.237	0.231
	D	0.213	0.225
8	F	0.291	0.248
	H	0.325	0.305
	B	0.205	0.216
9	B	0.203	0.213
	A	0.252	0.261
	D	0.181	0.163
12	G	0.225	0.245
14	F	0.177	0.189
	G	0.219	0.238
	H	0.297	0.287
	B	0.213	0.219

Average		0.237	0.235
Mean of two averages $(\bar{x})$		0.236	
S.D.		0.016	
Variation coefficient		6.8%	

$$\text{S.D.} = \sqrt{\Sigma(x - y)^2/2n}$$

$$\text{Variation coefficient } (\%) = \text{SD}/\bar{x} \times 100$$

Blood flow in ml/g brain/min.

et al., 1963; Høedt-Rasmussen et al., 1967; McHenry et al., 1969). Investigators used collimated probes and scintillation detectors placed over the patient's head to monitor the uptake and clearance of isotope. The exact area of study is uncertain, however, due to the overlapping of zones of measurement. To decrease this overlapping, recording devices with better resolution have been developed. The Anger camera (Pho-gamma III, Nuclear, Chicago) has a resolution of 10 to 15 mm (Anger, 1958; Heiss et al., 1968 b; Heiss and Tschabitscher, 1969; Lorenz and Adam, 1967; Westerman and Glass, 1968). Because of the parallel hole collimator, the depth resolution is also superior to that of the cone-shaped single probes.

Heiss and co-workers (1968 a) were the first to describe measurement of rCBF with the Anger camera and multiple channel analyzers following intracarotid injection of ^{133}Xe. This radioisotope technique is currently being used in our laboratories in conjunction with the hydrogen bolus method. Since the flow pattern over the entire hemisphere can be observed and repeatedly "played back" from a tape recorder, up to 160 special areas of interest can be measured after observing total and average

HBF. The measurements obtained with this method are in good agreement with those obtained with the hydrogen method in the same patient. This verifies the previous but unproven assumption that the partition coefficient for ^{133}Xe is unity. The radiation emitted from the ipsilateral hemisphere after intracarotid injection of Technetium can also be visualized and recorded continuously between ^{133}Xe injections. In this way, regional cerebral blood volume can be measured, permitting comparison between regional circulation times and rCBF (*Mathew* et al. 1971).

Cerebral circulation time measured by serial angiography

Methods described up to this point for measuring CBF require special apparatus and training. However, regional circulation time can be calculated following routine arteriography if seriograms are used. This has been done in this laboratory in patients with cerebrovascular disease with valid results (Gilroy *et al.*, 1963). Briefly, standard techniques were developed for timing the arrival and passage of dye through multiple areas of brain after injection of the dye. Cerebral circulation times were calculated from 12 serial exposures at 0.7-second intervals following the injection of a constant volume of contrast material at constant pressure. Circulation times were measured within the areas supplied by both the carotid and vertebrobasilar systems. In patients without stroke, carotid to jugular circulation time was less than 5.6 seconds. Prolonged regional cerebral circulation times were demonstrated in appropriate territories in patients with cerebrovascular disease, although in those with recent thrombosis the circulation time was diffusely slowed. Inhalation of 5% CO_2 was found to decrease the regional circulation times in both normal and abnormal areas.

MEASUREMENT OF CEREBRAL METABOLISM

Electrode methods

Oxygen electrode

The oxygen electrode is constructed on the polarographic principle and has been described earlier in this chapter in connection with indirect measurement or rCBF (Gotoh *et al.*, 1966 a; Meyer *et al.*, 1962 b). Electrodes of this type can be adapted for measurement of hydrogen gas and, when membrane covered, give absolute values for gas tensions.

Carbon dioxide electrode

The CO_2 electrode is constructed on the potentiometric principle with an outer plastic housing and an inner glass pH electrode which makes contact with a weak bicarbonate solution and a calomel half-cell for reference (Fig. 7) (Gotoh *et al.*, 1966 a). The outer housing is made of polycarbonate or acrylic plastic, closed at one end by a Teflon membrane secured with a neoprene-O ring, and fits tightly into the porthole of the cuvette system. The pH electrode is fabricated from a glass membrane mounted on a flint glass tube which is nonreactive to pH change. The glass tube is then filled with 0.1 *N* HCl solution into which a silver–silver chloride wire is immersed. The pH electrode is then mounted into a polycarbonate stopper which fits tightly into the outer plastic housing. The housing is filled with a weak bicarbonate solution containing 0.001 M $NaHCO_2$ and 0.1 M KCl. The pH electrode and stopper are then inserted into this housing with the glass membrane at the tip flush against the Teflon membrane. A thin layer of bicarbonate solution is kept between the Teflon and the glass membrane of the pH electrode. Since the dead space is minimal, response time is rapid (15 seconds). The housing containing the calomel half-cell reference electrode is kept at the same height as the P_{CO_2} sensor so that the surfaces of the solution in one housing are level with those in the other to avoid artifacts from hydrostatic pressure. The output of the P_{CO_2} electrode is amplified with a radiometer and recorded on one

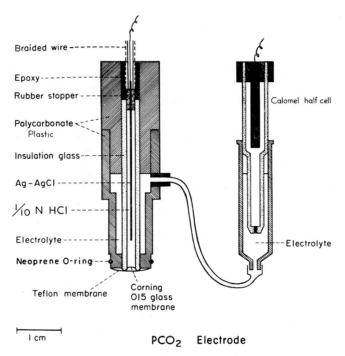

Fig. 7. Diagram illustrating construction of the P_{CO_2} electrode. Scale, in centimeters, is indicated below the electrode. Calomel half-cell and its housing are reduced in size.

channel of the polygraph. Absolute P_{CO_2} values are obtained from the pH scale and converted into millimeters of mercury (mm Hg) from a calibration scale drawn on semilogarithmic paper. Calibration is made at 37 °C by exposing the sensor to water-saturated gas mixtures of known P_{CO_2}. pH readings plotted against known P_{CO_2} calibrations form a straight line on the semilogarithmic paper.

pH electrode

An electrode similar to the CO_2 electrode is used for recording the pH of blood.

The electrode is mounted in a plastic plug and fitted directly into one of the portholes of the cuvette with a calomel half-cell serving as the reference electrode (Gotoh et al., 1966 a). The output of the pH electrode is registered on the scale of a radiometer and recorded on the polygraph. The pH electrode is calibrated at 37 °C with phosphate buffers pumped through the cuvette.

Sodium electrode

The glass pH electrode used for detecting sodium and potassium ions is based on the same principle as that for measuring the concentration of hydrogen ions. According to the Nernst equation (Meyer et al., 1962 b), the electrical potential between two electrolyte solutions separated by a thin membrane is proportional to the logarithm of the ratio of the ionic concentration on either side of the membrane. If the known ionic concentration inside the membrane is kept constant, the ionic activity of an unknown solution can be measured by recording changes in the electrical input of the electrode. A membrane of sodium aluminum silicate (NAS) glass is highly selective for sodium ions. The electrode for measuring the sodium ionic activity of blood is constructed by fusing a 3 mm inert glass stem to a thin membrane of NAS glass. The inside of the electrode is filled with 0.1 N HCl or 0.1 M NaCl and contact is made with a silver–silver chloride wire sealed into the rubber stopper closing the stem. This assembly is then sealed into a plastic plug which fits tightly into the porthole of the cuvette so that the exposed sodium-sensitive glass membrane comes into contact with the flowing blood. The sodium electrode is calibrated at 37 °C by exposing it to flowing saline solutions of known sodium concentration in the same manner used in calibrating the pH electrode. The electrical outputs are plotted in a straight line by means of semilogarithmic paper against sodium ionic concentration, expressed as milliequivalents (mEq). Absolute values of sodium ionic activity thus can be estimated from the recorded potentials in terms of mEq/liter.

A sodium electrode has also been designed in this laboratory for measuring extra-cellular sodium activity at the brain surface (Gotoh et al., 1962; Meyer et al., 1961 b). It is similar in structure to the electrode just described, except that a bulb of thin-walled (3 mm in diameter) sodium-sensitive glass is blown and the entire electrode except for this convex surface is insulated. The convex surface is placed in contact with the brain, and the output from the electrode amplified by the radiometer and recorded on the polygraph (Fig. 8).

Potassium electrode

An ideal potassium electrode is not yet available; however, electrodes which respond to sodium and potassium can also be used to estimate changes in potassium levels provide separate simultaneous recordings are made of sodium levels. Correction for the sodium portion of the output can be made. To measure the potassium activity of the blood, a thin membrane of potassium-sensitive glass is fused to an inert 3-mm glass stem with a plastic jacket so that the electrode can be fitted into the cuvette. The interior of the electrode is filled with a 0.1 M KCl solution and sealed.

The brain surface electrode is constructed from Corning 015 glass covered with a

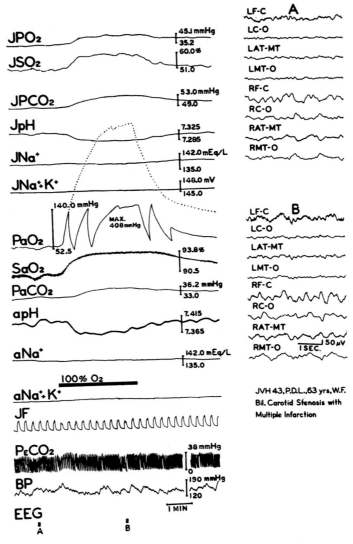

Fig. 8. Simultaneous continuous recording of arterial and internal jugular oxygen tension (P_{O_2}), oxygen saturation (S_{O_2}), carbon dioxide tension (P_{CO_2}), pH, sodium (Na^+) activity, sodium and potassium ionic activity ($Na^+ + K^+$), jugular flow (JF), end tidal CO_2 ($PeCO_2$), blood pressure (BP), and EEG in a patient with bilateral carotid stenosis. The changes from the steady state are produced by inhalation of 100% O_2.

thin collodion membrane (Gotoh *et al.*, 1962; Meyer *et al.*, 1961 b) and responds equally to both potassium and sodium ions. All but the sensitive surface is insulated and the interior of the electrode again filled with 0.1 M KCl solution. The sodium fraction of the output can be similarly corrected. The output is measured with a pH meter connected to a polygraph and calibrated by exposure to electrolyte solutions of known sodium and potassium ionic activity (see Fig. 8).

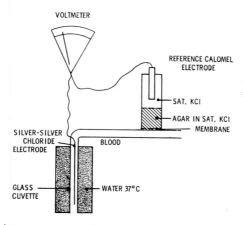

Fig. 9. Diagram illustrating arrangement for measuring plasma chloride using the silver–silver chloride electrode.

Chloride electrode

Chloride electrodes used in earlier studies admittedly were subject to artifacts such as those resulting from changes in blood flow and possibly DC potentials (Gotoh *et al.*, 1962). Recently, an improved electrode has been developed to measure chloride in which a silver wire electrically coated with silver chloride is used (Fig. 9). This electrode is based on the potentiometric principle; *i.e.*, release of silver ions by the electrode is proportional to the chloride ions available in blood (Marx *et al.*, in press). Frequent blood samples should be obtained during measurement so that plasma chloride values estimated by conventional chemical means using the Technicon Auto-Analyzer (Technicon Instrument Co., 1968) may be used to correct for oxidation–reduction potentials generated by free hemoglobin.

A special cuvette consisting of a small vertical glass tube, 2 mm in internal diameter, is used and a silver–silver chloride wire is inserted into it in such a way that the blood is pumped past at a constant rate and surface exposure. The temperature of the electrode system is maintained at 37 °C by a warming bath. The calomel half-cell used for a reference electrode makes contact with the flowing blood by means of an agar bridge inserted into the tubing at a right angle so that bubbles and clots do not lodge beneath. The electrode is calibrated against standard solutions of sodium chloride and the output recorded with a pH meter connected to the polygraph.

Changes in cerebral blood gases, pH, and metabolism

Arteriovenous oxygen differences

Cerebral arteriovenous oxygen (A–V O_2) differences have been continuously recorded in animals by means of catheters inserted into the sagittal sinus and femoral artery (Meyer *et al.*, 1967 e). Blood is pumped through a Guyton* arteriovenous

---

* Oxford Instrument Co., Jackson, Mississippi.

References pp. 339–347

oxygen analyzer and returned to the subject. The apparatus is calibrated using the manometric method of Van Slyke and Neill. The Guyton analyzer permits continuous and rapid measurement of A–V O_2 differences. Since CBF is measured during the same study, $CMRO_2$ can be calculated from the product of CBF and cerebral A–V O_2 differences.

Oxygen saturation

The oxygen saturation of arterial (SaO_2) and cerebral venous ($CVSO_2$) blood can be monitored with two catheter cuvette oximeters (Kipp**, Model 3). These oximeters are calibrated with blood samples using the manometric method of Van Slyke and Neill and their output adapted for continuous recording on the polygraph. These instruments have been widely applied to human subjects in our laboratory (see Fig. 8).

Carbon dioxide

The total CO_2 content of whole blood can be continuously recorded with an infra-red absorption CO_2 gas analyzer (Godart capnograph*, type KK) (Meyer *et al.*, 1971, a). Blood is pumped from cerebral arteries and veins at the rate of 0.1 ml/minute and mixed with 1 N lactic acid pumped at 2 ml/minute to the mixing coil. This mixture is then pumped into the inner silastic lumen of a diffusion coil which is highly permeable to CO_2 gas. The CO_2 diffuses out of the solution and passes into a CO_2-free air stream where the concentration is measured by means of a Beckman infrared CO_2 gas analyzer. The output of the capnograph is measured with DC μV meters and continuously recorded on the polygraph. Calibration is carried out with sodium carbonate solutions, which permits monitoring of hemispheric respiratory quotient (RQ).

End-tidal P_{CO_2} is measured with a Beckman infrared gas analyzer and recorded continuously on the polygraph (see Fig. 8).

Glucose

The glucose content of arterial and cerebral venous blood is monitored with two Technicon AutoAnalyzers using a standard colorimetric method (Meyer *et al.*, 1967 a). Only a small amount of blood (0.32 ml/minute) is required, the principle being that glucose is dialyzed from blood into a potassium ferricyanide reagent. The ferricyanide is reduced by glucose to ferrocyanide in proportion to the amount of glucose and reducing substances present. Color changes are measured with a colorimeter using a 420-μ filter. Cerebral glucose consumption (CMR Gl) is calculated in mg/100 g brain/min. The cerebral glucose:oxygen utilization ratio (G/O) is derived as the ratio of cerebral to arteriovenous glucose differences over that of oxygen: (A–V)Gl:(A–V)O_2.

Lactate

Cerebral venous and arterial lactate differences and cerebrospinal concentration are

* Kipp and Zonen, Delft, Holland.
** Godart N.V., De Bilt, Holland.

measured in this laboratory using the enzymatic method of Hochella and Weinhouse (1965) with a microsample modification to reduce the amount of blood required (Meyer *et al.*, 1968 b). Arterial and cerebral venous blood samples are drawn from catheters placed in the femoral artery and the transverse sinus. In animals, cerebrospinal fluid is drawn from a catheter placed in the cisterna magna. Colorimeters are used to record the concurrent levels. Calibration solutions of known lactate content are employed at the beginning and the end of the recording, and the reproducibility of the method is 0.1 mg per 100 ml of blood.

Pyruvate

To measure pyruvate levels in man, blood is sampled from the femoral artery and the cerebral transverse sinus (Meyer *et al.*, 1968 b). Blood mixed with phosphate buffer, pH 7.4, is propelled to a dialyzer unit of the Technicon AutoAnalyzer apparatus, and pyruvate acid is then dialyzed across a thin cellophane membrane into a phosphate buffer with a pH of 7.4. An enzyme mixture of DPNH, lactic dehydrogenase of rabbit muscle, and 10% Triton X-100 is added at a flow rate of 0.10 ml/min. The Triton X-100 is a colloidal solution which makes the mixture homogeneous and prevents precipitation. This mixture is then propelled through a water bath of 37°C where pyruvic acid is reduced to lactic acid by coupling of DPNH to DPN by the addition of lactic dehydrogenase. The oxidation of DPNH is proportional to the pyruvate present and the quenching of DPNH is measured fluorometrically. Cerebral pyruvate production (CMR Pyr) is calculated from CBF in mg/100 g brain/min times mean cerebral venous arterial pyruvate (V–A Pyr) difference.

Ammonia

The method for monitoring arterial and cerebral venous blood ammonia is based upon the method of Logsdon (1960) modified for the Technicon AutoAnalyzer. Blood is made alkaline by sodium carbonate solution which converts ammonium ions into ammonia which is then dialyzed into an alkaline solution. When mixed with hypochlorite, a color reaction occurs which is recorded photometrically with a 620-μ filter and expressed as mg per 100 ml of blood. The error caused by any amino acids present is negligible. Arterial and cerebral venous samples are recorded continuously using the Technicon AutoAnalyzer.

Sodium and potassium

Sodium and potassium concentrations have been measured in the cerebrospinal fluid using a modification of the standard Technicon AutoAnalyzer technique (Technicon, 1963). Cerebrospinal fluid is withdrawn continuously from the cisterna magna by means of a catheter. Sodium and potassium are dialyzed from the cerebrospinal fluid into distilled water and analyzed with the flame photometer.

The reproducibility of this method is good. However, there are considerable difficulties associated with the low volume of cerebrospinal fluid that is found in the monkey. It is possible to perform continuous measurements of sodium and potassium from samples as small as 0.1 ml/min.

Section II: PHYSIOLOGICAL AND PATHOPHYSIOLOGICAL
STUDIES OF CEREBRAL BLOOD FLOW AND METABOLISM

PHYSIOLOGY

Regulation of cerebral blood flow

CBF is a function of the pressure of the blood perfusing the brain and the resistance
or capacitance of the intracranial vasculature, as expressed by the equation:

$$\text{Flow} = \frac{\text{Perfusion pressure}}{\text{Cerebrovascular resistance}}$$

The mechanisms which regulate CBF may be considered extrinsic and intrinsic in
nature. Extrinsic mechanisms, though important, will be mentioned only briefly
since they were reviewed in depth by Meyer and Gilroy in 1968. These mechanisms
include maintenance of systemic blood pressure by means of the baroreceptor system
and the efficiency of the cardiac output. Changes in blood viscosity greatly alter blood
flow; *e.g.*, CBF increases in patients in anemic states and decreases in those with
polycythemia. Blood flow is also dependent on the capacitance of the arterial system
and is reduced by narrowing of the vessels such as that which occurs with atherosclerosis. Work in this laboratory has been concerned primarily with the study of the
intrinsic regulation of the cerebral circulation.

Cerebral autoregulation

One of the fundamental mechanisms that controls CBF is autoregulation, which
is defined as the inherent property of the brain to maintain blood flow constant
despite changes in perfusion pressure (Zwetnow, 1968). Fog (1934), using a Forbes
window, observed pial artery constriction in response to increased systemic arterial
pressure and dilatation when the blood pressure was decreased. The pressure of the
blood perfusing the cerebrum is the difference between the mean arterial blood pressure
(MABP) and the intracranial (ICP) and intracerebral venous pressure (ICVP).

Autoregulation has been studied in our laboratory in the monkey employing
electromagnetic flowmeters (Meyer *et al.*, 1965 d). The ability of the cerebral arteriole
to compensate for reduction and elevation of blood pressure becomes limited only
during extremes of blood pressure change. During induced hypotension, a sharp
drop in CBF was not observed until the MABP was reduced to levels below 60 to
70 mm Hg. When the MABP was increased in excess of 120 mm Hg, severe vasoconstriction (vasospasm) occurred and blood flow decreased (Yoshida *et al.*, 1966).

Autoregulation appears to have two different phases. Immediately after the onset
of hypertension, cerebral vascular resistance (CVR) within the internal carotid and
vertebral arterial beds increases rapidly and significantly, followed by a slower,

progressive secondary increase during the next three minutes of sustained hypertension. This increase in CVR is due primarily to active cerebral vasoconstriction. The initial phase, or rapid response, is interpreted as being due to a primary myogenic reflex or "Bayliss effect" combined with a lesser effect apparently mediated via the sympathetic nervous system and probably affecting the major cerebral arteries (Meyer et al., 1960 b; Mchedlishvili, 1964).

The second, more delayed phase of vasoconstriction is probably produced by biochemical factors that regulate CBF, e.g., changes in CO_2 and metabolites and P_{O_2} (Roy and Sherrington, 1890). Meyer and Gotoh (1961 a) observed that reduction in blood pressure and blood flow results in decreased tissue P_{O_2} and increased tissue P_{CO_2}, which in turn lead to a decrease in CVR and an increase in blood flow due primarily to the sensitivity of smooth muscle to changes in P_{CO_2} and pH. Changes in tissue P_{CO_2} probably exert this effect on the smooth muscle in the cerebral arterial wall by reducing pH within smooth muscle cells.

Blood flow in the external carotid artery, unlike flow through the internal carotid artery, is passive and related directly to fluctuation in blood pressure. However, when the external carotid artery was made to act as collateral circulation to supply the internal carotid artery, autoregulation could be demonstrated (Meyer et al., 1965 d). Conversely, when the internal carotid artery was made to share a portion of its blood supply with the external carotid artery, autoregulatory mechanisms were lost or impaired, proving that autoregulation is a property of the intracranial vasculature.

Autoregulation can also be demonstrated within a range of intracranial pressures that correlate well with the range of blood pressure changes (Harper, 1966). When intracranial pressure increases higher than 100 mm Hg, further increase in intracranial pressure will cause a corresponding decrease in CBF.

In the early 1900s, Cushing (1901, 1902, 1903) in his classic experiments demonstrated that a rise in systemic arterial pressure regularly followed large induced increases in intracranial pressure accompanied by bradycardia and irregular respirations. He attributed the vasopressor response to an attempt by cerebral mechanisms to maintain cerebral circulation. The actual mechanism behind this homeostatic response is still a matter of conjecture. Langfitt et al. (1965) conducted an experiment supporting Cushing's early theory that intracranial hypertension produces medullary ischemia and causes an elevation in blood pressure. They were able to demonstrate a vasopressor threshold when the intracranial pressure was increased with an extradural balloon. When the intracranial pressure reached a threshold, arterial pressure increased causing increased CBF and a further increase in intracranial pressure. Successive waves of this sort eventually lead to a failure in the vasopressor mechanism, CBF becomes decreased, and death occurs. Investigations of these mechanisms in our laboratory have emphasized the importance of the site and vectors of force of an expanding intracranial mass in determining the pressure gradients between the different intracranial compartments. This study confirmed that the important factor which regulates blood flow following increased intracranial pressure appears to be ischemia of the vasomotor center caused either by direct pressure on or distortion of the brain stem (Huber et al., 1965).

References pp. 339–347

This same study emphasized the importance of regional changes of intracranial pressure in determining CBF. In recent unpublished investigations of HBF carried out in our laboratory in patients with edema due to cerebral infarction, small reductions in intracranial pressure, induced by intravenous glycerol or mannitol, caused large increases in blood flow in the infarcted hemisphere. Tissue pressure within the brain has an important influence on CBF in physiological states and a more pronounced effect in pathological states where intracranial pressure is increased, cerebral edema is present, and autoregulation may be impaired. The intracerebral venous pressure and the intracranial pressure may vary independently of each other under certain conditions, *e.g.*, abdominal compression or leakage of cerebrospinal fluid. Hence, the following equation is suggested to derive cerebral perfusion pressure to allow for this variation:

$$PP = MABP - \left(\frac{MICVP + MICP}{2} \right)$$

Neurogenic mechanisms

The nature of neurogenic control of CBF is subject to some debate and has been extensively investigated in this laboratory under physiological conditions. Sokoloff (1959) and Lassen (1959), from their own work on average CBF in man as well as from evidence gathered in the literature, concluded that neurogenic influences appeared to exert a minor effect on the control of CBF. From a purely morphological standpoint, it is not unreasonable to suppose that the rich sympathetic nerve supply that accompanies the arteries leaving the circle of Willis and extending to the smallest arterioles within the brain must have some important function (Falck *et al.*, 1968; Nelson and Rennels, 1968). Recent investigations from this laboratory have been directed toward clarification of the part played by the parasympathetic as well as the sympathetic system and the importance of central neurogenic factors that exert an important control on CBF (Meyer *et al.*, 1971, d).

1. Parasympathetic control of cerebral blood flow. Chorobski and Penfield (1932) first described vasodilator fibers in the facial nerve passing through the geniculate ganglion via the greater superficial petrosal nerve to the internal carotid plexus and to the intracerebral vessels. Vasodilation of the cerebral vessels with an increase in CBF was reported after stimulation of the vagus and seventh nerves (Forbes and Cobb, 1938; James *et al.*, 1969). In these studies, the increase in CBF was inferred by the degree of dilation observed in the pial vessels. Studies in this laboratory in which blood flow was measured directly by means of electromagnetic flowmeters have failed to show a significant increase when the third, seventh, ninth, and tenth cranial nerves were stimulated (Meyer *et al.*, 1971, d). Further investigation indicated that when increases in CBF do occur, they can be accounted for by increases in cerebral metabolism (Meyer and Toyoda, 1971).

2. Sympathetic control of cerebral blood flow. Since Donders reported his studies in 1859, other investigators have assumed that the sympathetic nerves have a vasoconstrictor function, and this early observation has been corroborated in many laboratories. Histologic studies of cerebral arteries have provided no structural evidence for an active vasodilatory function. Sympathetic effects are entirely of a constrictor nature; hence, stimulation of the sympathetic nervous system can only result in vasodilatation by inhibiting vasoconstrictor tone.

Experiments on monkeys using electromagnetic flowmeters have shown that when the cervical sympathetic chain is stimulated, CBF decreases in both the internal and external carotid circulation (Meyer *et al.*, 1967 g). However, the reduction of blood flow in the internal carotid distribution during sympathetic stimulation is only 25 to 50% of that which occurs in the external carotid distribution, an observation in keeping with the differences noted in adrenergic supply to the two systems. Sympathectomy is said to have no effect on CBF. Stimulation of the sympathetic system caused a consistent reduction in cerebral arterial inflow, the decrease in vertebral flow being significantly smaller than the carotid flow. This difference is probably due to the fact that the vertebral arteries have a smaller sympathetic innervation than the carotid vessels. Decreases in flow within both systems during sympathetic stimulation were much larger after 5% CO_2 inhalation than while breathing air. James *et al.* (1969) confirmed this observation and interpreted it as an interaction between CO_2 and sympathetic activity. However, since the percentage reduction of flow values which we observed during 5% inhalation was much the same as that during inhalation of air, it would seem that sympathetic activity is influenced by vasomotor tone.

3. Central neurogenic control. In recent years, increasing attention has been given to the role of the brain stem in controlling CBF. Molnár and Szántó (1964) electrically stimulated the brain stem of cats and concluded that neurogenically mediated centers exist in the brain stem which control vasoconstriction and vasodilatation. Langfitt and Kassell (1968) increased the internal carotid flow of monkeys by 40% after electrical stimulation of the brain stem. Shalit *et al.* (1969) studied the response of the cerebral vasculature to CO_2 after freezing areas of the brain stem and postulated the existence of neuromechanisms in the pons which respond to CO_2 stimulus by causing vasodilation. More recently, Fujishima *et al.* (1970) noted, in the dog, decreased CBF and metabolism following experimental basilar artery occlusion along with reduced responsiveness of the cerebral vessels to increased Pa_{CO_2}.

Studies in our laboratory, in general, have confirmed the presence of an important regulatory mechanism in the brain stem which controls CBF (Meyer *et al.*, 1954; Meyer *et al.*, 1966 a, 1966 b). Stimulation of the brain stem reticular formation in 6 monkeys was carried out while CBF was being measured by electromagnetic flowmeters and $CMRO_2$ by the use of the Guyton analyzer (Meyer *et al.*, 1969 a) (Fig. 10). Electroencephalograms at the time of stimulation showed desynchronization associated with a mean increase of 7.7% in $CMRO_2$ and 9.7% in CBF (Table 3). After discontinuation of stimulation, the EEG immediately reverted to the resting pattern and $CMRO_2$ returned to the steady state within three minutes. We concluded that the increase in CBF was mainly due to increased cerebral metabolism associated with the EEG desynchronization but that smaller increases which occurred after stimulation were probably due to a neurogenic factor. Ingvar and Söderberg (1958) reported similar results in an earlier study.

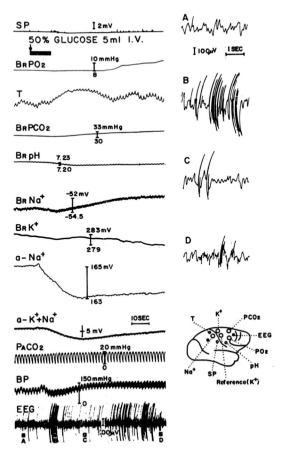

Fig. 10. Effect of intravenous injection of 5 ml 50% glucose during hypoglycemia. A, B, C, and D are samples of EEG made at conventional speed at the points marked with black squares on the polygraphic record. Note increase in brain and alveolar CO_2, increased cerebral blood flow and oxygen tension, and the rise in extracellular brain sodium and fall in extracellular brain potassium. The EEG shows increased fast activity with some spikes. (From Meyer *et al.* (1962) *Arch. Neurol.*, 7, 560–581).

More recently, we have measured changes in cerebral venous blood gases and pH during rapid eye movement (REM) sleep (Meyer and Toyoda, 1971). At the onset, rapid increases in cerebral venous P_{O_2} (CVP_{O_2}), CVS_{O_2}, and cerebral venous pH ($CVpH$) occurred in association with a decrease in cerebral venous P_{CO_2} (CVP_{CO_2}), followed in 20 seconds by decreased CVP_{O_2} and $CVpH$ with an increase in CVP_{CO_2}. The arterial blood gases, pressure, and respiration remained unchanged. Furthermore, concurrent recording of cerebral arterial and venous hydrogen curves during REM sleep after inhalation of hydrogen gas showed a marked decrease in the arteriovenous hydrogen difference due to a rapid increase in CBF. These factors indicate that a rapid increase in CBF takes place during REM sleep without metabolic changes. Changes in CBF during REM sleep were calculated from differences in cerebral

TABLE 3

CHANGES IN CEREBRAL BLOOD FLOW AND OXYGEN CONSUMPTION DURING EEG DESYN-
CHRONY INDUCED BY STIMULATION OF THE RETICULAR FORMATION OF THE MONKEY
(43 MEASUREMENTS IN SIX MONKEYS)

	MABP (mmHg)	CBF cc/min/100 g	A–VO$_2$ vol %	CMRO$_2$ cc/min/100 g	CVR mmHg/ cc/min/100 g
Steady state Mean ± S.D.	97.7 ±17.1	45.3 ±16.9	6.83 ±1.63	2.85 ±0.48	2.48 ±0.56
Stimulation Mean ± S.D.	109.9 ±20.1	49.7 ±16.7	6.64 ±1.60	3.07 ±0.53	2.53 ±0.58
Percentage change	+12.5	+ 9.7	−2.80	+7.70	+2.00
Level of significance	$0.001 > p^*$	$0.001 > p^*$	$0.001 > p^*$	$0.001 > p^*$	$0.1 > p > 0.05$

* Statistically significant.

A–V O$_2$, and our findings are in concord with those of Reivich *et al.* (1968). The increase in CBF observed during REM sleep was probably due to neurogenic cerebral vasodilation and was not secondary to any measurable metabolic change.

In recent experiments, we have measured CBF and CMRO$_2$ during electrical stimulation of other parts of the brain stem and diencephalon (Meyer *et al.*, 1971, d). Various points within the cortex, brain stem, and diencephalon were stimulated with a bipolar electrode having tips 1 mm apart. Stimulation was maintained for about 20 seconds at a frequency of 100 counts/sec for 2 msec at 15 V. Stimulation of the cerebral cortex produced no effect on CBF or metabolism, but when the diencephalon and brain stem were stimulated, large increases in CBF occurred both with and without EEG activation. The areas in which stimulation caused increases in CBF were the pontine and midbrain reticular formation, thalamus, and hypothalamus. Autoregulation was also investigated while these areas were stimulated, and when stimulation was continued for 20 seconds it was temporarily lost. It returned to normal when stimulation was discontinued. Prolongation of stimulation for two minutes abolished the rapid and slow responses of autoregulation. When autoregulation was impaired by anoxic anoxia, stimulation in the same areas of the brain stem and diencephalon resulted in an increase in CBF which was significantly less than that seen after stimulation in the physiological state. This indicates that cerebral vasodilatory mechanisms are intimately associated with autoregulation, require integrity of brain function to operate maximally, and are sensitive to anoxia. The finding that the rapid component of autoregulation is lost during stimulation supports the apparently neurogenic nature of the cerebral vasodilation. Neither inhalation of CO$_2$, lowering the CO$_2$ by hyperventilation, nor cervical sympathectomy qualitatively or quantitatively alters the CBF response during stimulation of these areas. It was concluded that large increases in CBF produced by electrical stimulation of the brain stem and diencephalon are due to rapidly occurring vasodilation of cerebral vessels and are later augmented by increases in cerebral metabolism.

It is apparent, therefore, that centers do exist within the brain which influence CBF and metabolism. The fact that these centers correlate closely with the central pathway of the sympathetic system seems to suggest that control may be mediated via this neurogenic pathway, probably by inhibition of sympathetic tone or some para-sympathetic influence. Central control may account for the rapidly occurring increases in CBF during REM sleep, seizures, and the observed loss of autoregulation which accompanies injury and infarction of the brain.

Metabolic control

Studies in animals and man during seizures, sensory stimulation, or arousal show that these conditions increase cerebral metabolism, causing a secondary or indirect increase in CBF (Meyer *et al.*, 1966 b). It became apparent that local increases in brain tissue P_{CO_2} caused by increased metabolism are responsible for the increase in flow and that local reduction of tissue P_{O_2} which accompanies increased metabolic activity may contribute in part to this process. Conversely, CBF is decreased during anesthesia and during states of reduced metabolism, such as drowsiness, when tissue P_{CO_2} production and oxygen utilization are reduced. A delicate homeostatic mechanism exists in animals and man whereby the cerebral circulation under normal physiologic conditions is able to adjust to small fluctuations in blood pressure. A slight increase in blood pressure is not only compensated for by autoregulation, but any increase in CBF decreases cerebral P_{CO_2} and increases cortical P_{O_2} resulting in reduced CBF due to vasoconstriction. The opposite situation applies to a reduction in blood flow following a drop in blood pressure.

Glucose and oxygen are the primary substrates metabolized to provide energy for neuronal mechanisms (Sacks, 1957). Normally, the cerebral arteriovenous difference for glucose averages 10 mg/100 ml blood (Gibbs *et al.*, 1942). Since normal CBF is around 45 to 50 ml/100 g brain/min, glucose utilization amounts to 16 μmoles of glucose/g brain/min or 4.5 to 5 mg/100 g brain/min.

Studies of induced hypoglycemia have provided additional information on the interrelationship between metabolism and CBF. Hypoglycemia produced in the monkey by fasting or intravenous injection of insulin causes reduced tissue P_{CO_2} due to depressed glucose metabolism (Meyer *et al.*, 1962 b). Both CBF and cerebral tissue P_{O_2} decrease, rendering the brain more susceptible to the effects of hyperventilation since the decrease of blood flow further limits the available glucose. Oxygen availability to the tissue also is reduced. Injection of glucose during hypoglycemia rapidly brings about an increased cortical P_{CO_2}, indicating that an increase in cerebral metabolism brought about by restoration of deficient substrate increases CBF (Fig. 10) (Meyer *et al.*, 1962 b).

1. Carbon dioxide. Many investigators have reported that CBF increases stepwise with stoichiometric increases in arterial carbon dioxide partial pressure (Pa_{CO_2}), and this has been confirmed repeatedly in our own laboratory in experiments in which a variety of methods for measurement of blood flow in man and animals have been used (Gotoh *et al.*, 1966 c; Meyer *et al.*, 1962 b, 1964 b, 1967 b; Meyer and Gotoh, 1964). Inhalation of CO_2 gas caused average blood flow increases with increasing percentages of CO_2. If the Pa_{CO_2} is increased to 70 mm Hg or above, the arterioles become dilated maximally. Autoregulation is abolished and CO_2 narcosis usually supervenes when Pa_{CO_2} increases above this level. The response to the inhalation of CO_2 mixtures is rapid, occurring within a few seconds. MABP increases slightly during inhalation of low CO_2 mixtures and accounts for the small percentage of the increase in CBF. After cessation of CO_2 inhalation, CBF continues to increase for one minute due to increased tissue P_{CO_2} within the brain despite falling alveolar CO_2 but returns thereafter to the steady state.

2. Hyperventilation and cerebral blood flow. Both alveolar CO_2 and Pa_{CO_2} decrease during hyperventilation, while Pa_{O_2} and Sa_{O_2} increase. In spite of increases of Pa_{O_2}, measurements of cerebral venous or jugular blood during hyperventilation indicate a significant decrease in CVP_{O_2} and cerebral venous oxygen saturation ($CVSO_2$). CBF starts to decrease almost immediately after the onset of hyperventilation and progressively decreases thereafter, but stabilizes at low levels if hyperventilation is continued. The slight drop in blood pressure which usually occurs may contribute to the reduction in CBF. The rate of flow begins to increase within 30 seconds after ceasing hyperventilation. The decrease in CVP_{O_2} is due to a combination of decreased CBF and the Bohr effect (Gotoh *et al.*, 1965). The latter can be defined as changes in the oxygen-combining power of hemoglobin as the blood pH is altered. When blood becomes increasingly alkaline, hemoglobin combines with oxygen more readily and plasma P_{O_2} is reduced. Thus, during hyperventilation the Bohr effect further reduces cerebral tissue and venous O_2 and intensifies the anoxia resulting from cerebral vaso-constriction. Cerebral metabolism does not increase significantly or contribute to the lowering of CVP_{O2}. The effects of hyperventilation in reducing CBF were observed to be greater in persons under 35 years of age than in the older age groups, indicating that cerebral vascular reactivity decreases with age. This also explains the greater susceptibility to EEG changes during hyperventilation in young individuals.

The P_{CO_2} of brain tissue is also important in controlling CBF. Measurements in this laboratory have shown increases in brain P_{CO_2} associated with increased cerebral metabolism produced by maneuvers such as arousal, photic stimulation, strychniniza-tion of the cortex, and induction of seizures (Meyer and Gotoh, 1961 a). The increase in P_{CO_2} was followed after a 60 to 90-second delay by an increase in CBF. Studies of the transport of gases through brain tissue have proved that CO_2 applied directly to the exposed cortex causes dilation of cerebral blood vessels (Gotoh *et al.*, 1961). The latency for vasodilation due to the *endovascular* effects of changes in P_{CO_2} brought about by inhalation of CO_2 is shorter (15 to 30 seconds) than the latency for blood flow increases brought about by *extravascular* changes in tissue P_{CO_2} (60 to 90 seconds). It was apparent that changes in endovascular CO_2 dominate extravascular effects. The dominance of endovascular P_{CO_2} changes in controlling CBF was established by increasing cerebral tissue P_{CO_2} by maneuvers such as occluding the superior vena cava and ligating the jugular vein. Intravenous injection of sodium bicarbonate also increases tissue P_{CO_2} and CBF. Progressive cerebral vasoconstriction was noted when hyperventilation was carried out simultaneously with these procedures.

Acetazolamide is a potent carbonic anhydrase inhibitor and blocks the reaction:

$$CO_2 + H_2O \rightleftharpoons H^+ + HCO_3^-$$

Intravenous injection of acetazolamide in monkeys causes no measurable increase in CBF after inhalation of CO_2 and blocks the extravascular effect of carbon dioxide (Meyer and Gotoh, 1961 a; Gotoh et al., 1961). The conclusion was reached that CO_2 must first enter into solution and become ionized to hydrogen and bicarbonate ions in order to affect vascular tone. Furthermore, injection of sodium bicarbonate after treatment with acetazolamide produced no change in CBF.

It seems evident from these experiments that vasomotor effects are caused by CO_2 entering into solution with plasma and tissue fluids, passing through cell membranes and blood–brain barriers, and entering smooth muscle where it is converted by carbonic anhydrase into hydrogen and bicarbonate ions. Changes in pH of the smooth muscle cells appear to be the principal cause of the control of vasomotion by CO_2, probably by altering calcium ion concentration (Fig. 11). Intravenous injection of acetazolamide alone causes an increase in CBF due to a remarkable increase in tissue

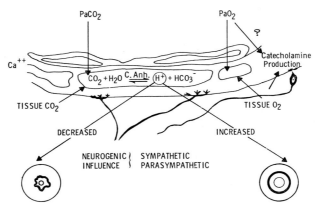

Fig. 11. Diagrammatic representation of the possible factors involved with the alteration of vaso-motor tone of the arteriolar wall and illustrating the intracellular H^+ content of the smooth muscle cell as the dominant factor.

CO_2 (Meyer et al., 1961 a), establishing the importance of P_{CO_2} in regulating rCBF.

   3. Oxygen. An increase in arterial or tissue P_{O_2} causes cerebral vasoconstriction and reduces CBF (Meyer and Gotoh, 1964). Like CO_2, the constrictor effect of oxygen may be produced extravascularly by increase in brain tissue P_{O_2} as well as endovascularly (Gotoh et al., 1961). Inhalation of 100% oxygen rapidly increases the Pa_{O_2} level to 400 or 500 mm Hg, at which point CBF decreases pro-gressively (Meyer et al., 1962 b). In spite of high arterial P_{O_2} levels, cerebral venous Pa_{O_2} increases slightly, rarely more than 20 mm Hg, due to cerebral vasoconstriction caused by the direct effect of oxygen. Nevertheless, brain tissue P_{O_2} increases during oxygen breathing, particularly in areas of ischemia.

In general, any reduction in arterial or tissue P_{O_2} produces cerebral vasodilation with an accompanying increase in CBF (Meyer and Gotoh, 1961 a, 1964), thereby serving as a protective mechanism to compensate for any reduction of oxygen supply to the brain.

Marked increases in CBF are caused by anoxic anoxia induced by apnea or breathing 100% nitrogen (Meyer et al., 1962 b). Pa_{O_2} falls rapidly, followed by a decrease in cortical P_{O_2} and jugular venous P_{O_2}. CBF increases due to the combined effects of a low P_{O_2} and increased Pa_{CO_2} and tissue P_{CO_2}. Increased Pa_{CO_2} and tissue P_{CO_2} are, of course, the result of CO_2 retention during apnea. An increase in blood pressure secondary to medullary anoxia also contributes to the increase in CBF. With prolonged apnea, cardiac failure occurs, blood pressure decreases, and CBF decreases. When oxygenation is resumed, blood pressure is restored and with it CBF and tissue P_{O_2} increase and tissue P_{CO_2} decreases.

The direct action of oxygen as a vasoconstrictor on the cerebral vessels is independent of lowered CO_2 levels during hyperventilation with 100% oxygen inhalation. Only during periods of severe hypoxia does the vasodilator effect of lowered P_{O_2} become greater than the vasoconstrictor effect of low P_{CO_2} caused by hyperventilation.

One theory for the action of oxygen on the cerebral circulation is a direct effect on chemoreceptors within the vessel walls (Gotoh and Meyer, 1965; Meyer et al., 1967 d). Recently, Hartman and Udenfriend (1970), in an elegant study utilizing an immunofluorescent technique, demonstrated large accumulations of dopamine β-hydroxylase adjacent to blood vessel walls. This finding indicates that the vessel wall has the capacity to produce large amounts of norepinephrine. Enzyme activity is sensitive to changes in tissue P_{O_2} which possibly exerts its effect on vasomotion by the alteration of norepinephrine levels in the vessel walls (see Fig. 11).

4. Cerebral tissue and venous pH changes. Sokoloff (1959), in an important review, concluded that acidosis produces increased CBF while alkalosis causes a decrease. In studies in experimental animals, Meyer et al. (1962 b) and Meyer and Gotoh (1961 a) showed that intravenous injection of small volumes of either 1 N HCl or 2% acetic acid causes an increase in cortical blood flow and a decrease in brain tissue pH. However, as a result of the pH changes, brain tissue P_{CO_2} also increases, and it was concluded that the P_{CO_2} increase was the prime factor causing cerebral vasodilation. The increase in tissue P_{O_2} is accounted for by both cerebral vasodilation and the Bohr effect, a phenomenon later termed the "luxury perfusion syndrome" (Lassen, 1966). Intravenous injection of sodium bicarbonate causes a rapid increase in tissue P_{CO_2}, and CBF increases in spite of an alkaline shift in extracellular pH. Intravenous injection of 9-trishydroxyaminomethane (THAM), a buffer base which combines with CO_2 in the blood, increases the extracellular tissue pH but reduces cortical tissue P_{CO_2}. Vasoconstriction occurs, followed by reduced CBF and a reduction of cerebral P_{O_2} as a consequence of this change and the Bohr effect. Wahl et al. (1970), in a recent publication, described a micropipette technique to induce local changes in pH of the cerebrospinal fluid surrounding the arterioles on the exposed cerebral cortex of experimental animals. These workers stressed the importance of extra-cellular pH change as the dominant factor in vasomotor control. However, it is apparent from our own experiments just described that intracellular pH change is the controlling factor.

In striated muscle, myoplasmic calcium activity may be affected by intracellular pH change (Briggs *et al.*, 1957), and it is possible that the effect of pH on vasomotor changes of the arterioles may be caused by changes in calcium activity of the muscle cell. Arteriolar dilation, for example, is produced by injection of EDTA into the perivascular space.

5. Hypothermia and hyperthermia. Circulation and metabolism of the body as a whole are affected by a temperature change. Few efforts have been made to study the effect of temperature change on CBF and metabolism. Field *et al.* (1944) demonstrated in rat brains that oxygen consumption increases with elevated temperature. The increase is stepwise but ceases above 44 °C (Himwich *et al.*, 1940). Sustained hyperpyrexia at high levels eventually reduces $CMRO_2$ (Himwich *et al.*, 1942). Heyman *et al.* (1950) found, in man, that cerebral A–V O_2 differences increase more than 2 vol.% during fever, and concluded that either metabolism in brain tissue must increase to a greater degree than in other organs or that CBF diminishes. The latter was considered unlikely. The effects of hyperthermia on CBF and metabolism were investigated in the monkey in our laboratory (Meyer and Handa, 1967), and CBF remained unchanged until temperatures reached 39 to 39.4 °C. It was established that at this point, CBF steadily increases to a maximum of 30 to 50% at 41.5 to 41.9 °C. $CMRO_2$ increases concomitantly with CBF and is believed to account for the increase in flow. When the body temperature rises above 42 °C, CBF and metabolism suddenly decrease and the EEG activity slows. When the temperature is stabilized at 41 °C, CBF and $CMRO_2$ progressively decrease. Reduction of CBF and metabolism at high body temperatures is presumably due to cerebral enzymatic damage.

Hypothermia also alters CBF and metabolism. Lowering of the body temperature produces reversible metabolic neuronal impairment, but this state is readily reversible by increasing the body temperature (Meyer and Hunter, 1957 a). Hypothermia is accompanied by a decrease in CBF due to cerebral vasoconstriction, and, since blood flow and oxygen demand decrease *pari passu*, there is a progressive decrease in $CMRO_2$ without a significant reduction of available oxygen to the brain parenchyma. The basic mechanism in hypothermia is assumed to be impairment of the neuronal enzymes since neither morphological nor functional neuronal damage occur. Reduction of cerebral metabolism during hypothermia affords protection against anoxic anoxia or ischemic anoxia and has proved to be therapeutically useful during some neurosurgical procedures.

Pharmacological control

Certain drugs have a direct effect on the cerebral circulation due to their vasoactive properties, a subject which Sokoloff reviewed extensively in 1959. The effects of many of these drugs have been studied in our laboratories (Handa *et al.*, 1965 b; Meyer *et al.*, 1964 b, 1964 c).

Epinephrine produces a small increase in CBF as a passive phenomenon secondary to the pressor effect of the drug, which is in agreement with the work of other investigators that this drug exerts no direct vasoconstrictor action on cerebral vessels.

Norepinephrine produces a marked increase in blood pressure and vasoconstriction of cerebral vessels. The increase in CVR is greater than that which would be expected secondary to an increase in the systemic blood pressure, resulting in a moderate reduction in blood flow to the brain.

Acetylcholine causes a decrease in systemic blood pressure and CVR; however, the decrease in CVR in the territory supplied by the vertebral system is greater than that in the carotid arterial system and serves to maintain flow constant in the vertebral system alone. Intravenous injection of histamine phosphate reduced both MABP and CVR in the carotid and vertebral territories with no change in rate of blood flow. Studies have shown that papaverine hydrochloride injected intravenously or administered orally has a significant cerebral vasodilator action in man and animals, resulting in an increase in CBF (Meyer *et al.*, 1964 b; McHenry *et al.*, 1970 b). Based on these observations, this drug has been utilized in treating patients with occlusive cerebrovascular disease (Meyer *et al.*, 1965 c; Gilroy and Meyer, 1966). Recent investigations in animals have proved that the new drug Hexobendine is a potent vasodilator (Meyer *et al.*, 1970 d) (Fig. 12). Acetazolamide, due to its action as a carbonic anhydrase inhibitor, also increases CBF by permitting the accumulation

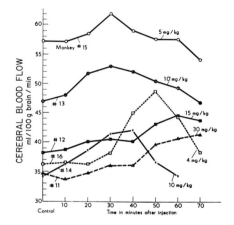

Fig. 12. Effect of Hexobendine in 6 monkeys administered intraduodenally in different doses. (From Meyer *et al.* (1970) *J. Neurol. Sci.*, **11**, 137–145).

of carbon dioxide in brain tissue (Gotoh *et al.*, 1966 b). Low molecular weight dextran is another drug which has been shown to increase CBF (Gilroy *et al.*, 1969; Gottstein and Held, 1969). Intravenous glycerol and mannitol increase CBF by decreasing cerebral tissue volume (Table 4).

Importance of cerebral ionic homeostasis

Measurements of sodium and potassium ionic movement between the intracerebral and extracerebral spaces have been accomplished with specially designed glass electrodes that are sensitive to changes in sodium and potassium concentrations. Changes in the cerebrospinal fluid have been correlated with concomitant changes in arterial and cerebral venous blood (Meyer et al., 1961 b). Sodium and potassium concentrations of extracellular fluid during steady state conditions appear remarkably constant. During cerebral ischemia or anoxic anoxia when CVP_{O_2} is reduced below 20 mm Hg, sodium moves out of the extracellular space and potassium into it. If blood flow is restored within a few minutes, the reverse process takes place. The recovery of ionic equilibrium depends on the duration of anoxia. If active sodium transport is interrupted for longer than eight minutes, ionic homeostasis may not be restored.

TABLE 4

CHANGES OF HEMISPHERIC BLOOD FLOW AND METABOLISM IN DISEASED HEMISPHERE AFTER INJECTION OF MANNITOL IN PATIENTS WITH UNILATERAL CEREBRAL INFARCTION

	HBF ml/100 g brain/min	HMIO₂ ml/100 g brain/min	HMIGl mg/100 g brain/min	HRQ	Central venous pressure mm H₂O	MABP mm Hg	Intracranial venous pressure mm H₂O
Control	32.6 ± 3.5	1.99 ± 0.36	2.40 ± 0.56	0.76 ± 0.13	56 ± 53	98 ± 18	100 ± 45
After Mannitol	35.8 ± 3.0	1.88 ± 0.48	2.29 ± 0.67	0.86 ± 0.21	61 ± 50	103 ± 20	115 ± 42
p Value	p < 0.02	N.S.	N.S.	N.S.	N.S.	N.S.	N.S.

Average dosage was 0.35 g/kg of body weight given in 25 % intravenous solution.
N.S. = no statistically significant change.

Cerebral acidosis also causes an increase of extracellular potassium levels usually accompanied by a decrease of extracellular sodium. Prolonged hyperventilation with cerebral anoxia also suppresses sodium transport, causing a decrease in extracellular sodium and an increase in extracellular potassium. The same pattern of change in electrolyte homeostasis was observed (1) during hypoglycemia, which could be reversed by glucose injection, and (2) during epileptic seizures when the change correlated with associated spike activity in the EEG. The conclusion was reached that extracellular sodium and potassium exist in a dynamic state which is influenced by the electrical activity of the cortex, the energy metabolism of the brain necessary to maintain an "ionic pump", and changes in the hydrogen ion concentration of cerebral tissue fluids. In experiments carried out recently in our laboratory, measurement of sodium and potassium activity in the CSF employing conventional flame photometry confirmed these findings (Meyer et al., 1970 a).

PATHOPHYSIOLOGY

Experimental cerebral ischemia and infarction

Experiments have been carried out since 1953 in animals in an effort to define the regional hemodynamic and metabolic alterations that take place following occlusion of the cerebral vessels. Measurements have been made of pial vessel flow, regional P_{O_2}, P_{CO_2}, pH, and rCBF. Hudgins and Garcia (1970), using the transorbital approach in the squirrel monkey, determined that occlusion of the middle cerebral artery is an excellent model for carrying out these studies. Infarction occurs only following severe ischemic anoxia and damages both the neural and vascular tissues supplied by the occluded vessel (Meyer, 1958 b). The extent of infarction depends also upon the blood pressure level and adequacy of the cerebral collateral circulation. If the latter two components are adequate, occlusion of the middle cerebral artery may cause only temporary reversible effects. Regional P_{O_2} decreases in the area of supply which accounts for the blue-black appearance of the veins. Reversed flow may occur in pial vessels and redirect collateral flow. Impaired circulation may persist for a few minutes to as long as eight hours, usually followed by hyperemia in the once ischemic zone due to increased flow via the collateral circulation and the veins become red. Collateral flow can be further increased at this stage by raising the blood pressure, indicating that autoregulation has been impaired (Meyer and Denny-Brown, 1957).

These early observations showed that collateral flow may be provided by vessels of all sizes – from the large vessels in the circle of Willis to the small pial vessels. The importance of pressure gradients whereby blood flows from areas of high pressure to areas of low pressure, and metabolic factors causing vasodilation, were shown to be the important factors regulating the collateral circulation (Ishikawa et al., 1965; Symon et al., 1963 a). The work of Handa et al. (1965 a) confirmed earlier observations that delayed circulatory adjustments occur for several weeks and that these are probably mediated by revascularization as well as metabolic changes (Fig. 13). This type of reversible ischemia or infarction may cause no neurologic deficit at all or only transient hemiparesis with complete or partial recovery (Meyer, 1958 c).

If collateral circulation should fail, e.g., following a fall in blood pressure below 60 mm Hg systolic, or by the application of multiple clips to the important collateral vessels after occlusion of the middle cerebral artery, the P_{O_2} in the ischemic zone may be reduced to zero and irreversible infarction will result. The duration of this regional anoxia determines the severity of the infarction. Endothelial damage occurs followed by extravasation of the fluid constituents of the blood, resulting in edema of the brain and further reduction of rCBF. Increased vascular permeability also causes diapedesis of red cells, and if the damage is severe enough the vessels will rupture and small perivascular hemorrhages develop.

The vessels involved are usually the small venules of 25 to 200 μ located in the terminal distribution of the middle cerebral artery, particularly in the watershed area between the occluded vessel and its main collateral channel. In this instance also,

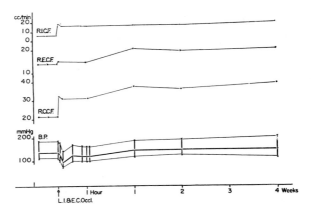

Fig. 13. Changes in right internal, external, and common carotid flow during the interval of four weeks after left internal and external carotid occlusion.

the sufficiency of collateral circulation and systemic arterial pressure are determining factors in the actual size of the infarct. The terminal arterioles are less consistently involved. Injury to the vascular endothelium and hemoconcentration and stasis cause clumping of erythrocytes and formation of mural thrombi by agglutinated platelets in the terminal vessels. The extent of these pathologic changes may vary with collateral circulation, which is in turn dependent on blood pressure. Increased collateral flow may cause movement of clumps of red cells to zones of normal flow where they disintegrate. Resumption of normal flow to infarcted areas, however, may incur perivascular hemorrhage and cause hemorrhagic infarction. Small hemorrhagic infarctions may be scattered throughout the total area of an otherwise pale infarct. The action of low molecular weight dextran, anticoagulant drugs and platelet inhibitors prevents stasis, thereby increasing the flow of blood to ischemic zones through the collateral channels. Transient failure of the collateral circulation, such as that which may occur during spontaneous hypotension, is difficult to induce in experimental animals in the heparinized state (Meyer, 1958 a, 1958 c; Denny-Brown and Meyer, 1957). Once infarction has occurred, recovery is more rapid than in the absence of heparin.

Histologic examination reveals patchy cortical infarction with polymorphonuclear leucocytes and histiocytes invading the necrotic area. Ischemic lesions of the neural tissue include edema of the stroma with neuronal and glial swelling, pallor of Nissl bodies, neuronal necrosis, and proliferation of astrocytes. The size and extent of these lesions is dependent upon the duration and level of reduction in P_{O_2}.

Metabolic studies and correlation with the EEG have shown that the area of infarction consists of three different zones (Fig. 14): (1) a central ischemic zone; (2) a bordering zone; and (3) a surrounding zone of collateral circulation (Meyer et al., 1962 a). In the central ischemic zone, slowing of venous capillary flow first

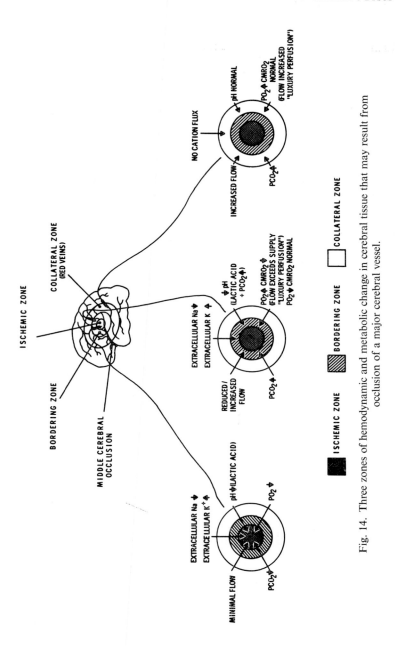

Fig. 14. Three zones of hemodynamic and metabolic change in cerebral tissue that may result from occlusion of a major cerebral vessel.

occurs, accompanied by increased P_{CO_2} and decreased tissue pH. A progressive fall in tissue P_{O_2} follows, and if it drops below 8 mm Hg a decrease in extracellular sodium and an increase in extracellular potassium take place. At this stage, EEG activity begins to slow and cortical pH becomes increasingly acidic. As cortical P_{O_2} decreases even further, the sodium influx increases and the EEG becomes flat. Cortical P_{CO_2} and pH decrease further as a result of anaerobic metabolism and the production of acid metabolites. CO_2 production ceases altogether and tissue CO_2 falls to even lower levels. If cortical blood flow is not quickly restored, these changes become irreversible and infarction results.

The zone bordering the infarct is subject to fluctuating hemodynamic and metabolic changes. Moderate ischemia results in accumulation of CO_2 and acid metabolites. The cortical P_{O_2} may be reduced to near zero levels, and a sodium and potassium flux occurs accompanied by slowing of EEG activity. The high CO_2 and low pH contribute to vasodilation and flow becomes maximal. As a consequence of the increased flow plus the reduced $CMRO_2$ and the low pH providing more oxygen to the tissue due to the Bohr effect, the zone may become hyperoxic; *i.e.* the "luxury perfusion syndrome" may occur. When $CMRO_2$ returns to normal, the tissue P_{O_2} may again become reduced.

In the collateral zone, arterial blood flow increases due to increased P_{CO_2} resulting from decreased capillary circulation. The blood flow in this area is in excess of tissue needs and hyperoxia becomes established.

Hyperoxia was first observed by Meyer and co-workers (1954) using the polarographic oxygen electrode. Quantitative evidence was obtained in a series of 11 monkeys in which the mean CBF was 57.3 ml/100 g brain/min and the $CMRO_2$ was 3.02 ml/100 g brain/min during the steady state. CBF decreased to 11.9 ml/100 g brain/min and $CMRO_2$ to 0.90 ml/100 g brain/min during occlusion of both the carotid and vertebral arterial systems. After flow was re-established, CBF increased to 67 and $CMRO_2$ to 2.41 (Meyer, 1968). To what extent hyperoxia occurs during the actual state of occlusion is uncertain, but evidence exists that as blood supply is restored by collateral circulation in formerly ischemic areas the brain may become hyperoxic.

Cerebrovascular disease in the clinical patient

At least two patterns of abnormal CBF and metabolism appear to exist in association with occlusive cerebrovascular disease. One form is associated with severe neurologic deficit plus severe vascular lesions, all demonstrated arteriographically. In this group, CBF, $CMRO_2$, and cerebral metabolic consumption of glucose (CMRGl) are all reduced. Patients with this pattern of metabolism may be assumed to have irreversible cerebral infarction. On the other hand, in patients with neurological deficits that are usually less severe than in the first group and are associated with little or no arteriographic abnormality, the CMRGl may be normal and there is less reduction in CBF and $CMRO_2$ than in the group with irreversible cerebral infarction. These patients have a good prognosis for recovery. Patients with irreversible damage are unable to respond metabolically to either an increase or a decrease in cerebral circulation and have the worst prognosis. In the second type of patient, ischemia leads to anaerobic glycolysis, and inhalation of 5 % CO_2 in air and oxygen rapidly reverses the metabolic deficit.

Cerebral blood flow

Numerous investigators in the last two decades have studied extensively the CBF in patients with cerebrovascular disease. Complete agreement has been reached that CBF is reduced following cerebral hemorrhage, occlusive cerebrovascular disease, and hypertensive cerebrovascular disease (Heyman *et al.*, 1953; Lindén, 1955; Aizawa *et al.*, 1961). Table 5 shows the results obtained from HBF measurements using

TABLE 5

HEMISPHERIC BLOOD FLOW AND METABOLISM IN PATIENTS WITH
CEREBROVASCULAR DISEASE

Clinical diagnosis	Number of cases	HBF ml/100 g brain/min	HMIO$_2$ ml/100 g brain/min
Unilateral cerebral infarction	40		
Diseased side		35.0 ± 3.5 } $p < 0.01$	2.13 ± 0.49 } $p < 0.05$
Healthy side		38.1 ± 4.2	2.44 ± 0.58
Diffuse cerebrovascular disease	4		
Left side		35.9 ± 5.0	2.09 ± 0.54
Right side		37.8 ± 2.7	2.35 ± 0.86
Bilateral cerebral infarction	3		
Left side		39.6	2.80
Right side		38.6	2.54
Brain stem infarction	1		
Left side		38.9	2.22
Right side		39.8	2.23
Arteriovenous malformation	1		
Diseased side		246.3	2.49
Healthy side		53.6	2.54
Transient ischemic attack	1		
Diseased side		43.1	1.72
Healthy side		42.9	2.36

HBF = hemispheric blood flow.
HMIO$_2$ = hemispheric metabolic index for oxygen.

hydrogen intracarotid injection techniques in a group of patients with cerebrovascular disease. The development of the method of intracarotid injection of hydrogen gas for measuring HBF made it possible to determine the hemodynamic changes that occur in the affected hemisphere. Not only is HBF reduced on the affected side but that on the contralateral side is reduced also, though to a lesser extent (Fig. 15) (Meyer *et al.*, 1969 c).

The patient with a localized neurogenic lesion may manifest diffuse depression of function in areas of the brain not involved in the primary pathological process. This phenomenon, known as diaschisis, was first described by Von Monakow (1914) and later confirmed by Høedt-Rasmussen and Skinhøj (1964) and by Skinhøj (1965). Blood flow and metabolism are depressed on the side contralateral to the involved

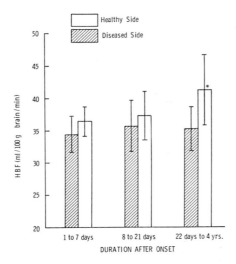

Fig. 15. HBF measurement in patients with unilateral cerebral infarction showing reduction of blood flow to the healthy cerebral hemisphere (diaschisis) as well as to the infarcted hemisphere. Blood flow to the healthy hemisphere is seen to recover to near normal levels in the weeks following infarction.

hemisphere and may persist as long as three weeks (Meyer *et al.*, 1969 c; Meyer *et al.*, 1970 e). The blood flow on the healthy side then increases while that on the diseased side remains depressed (see Fig. 15). It is known that local cerebral metabolism may regulate local blood supply and that the remote effects may be due in part to the depression of metabolism, which in itself reduces blood flow. However, experiments in monkeys recently carried out have shown that the effect of diaschisis is less pronounced on the healthy side than on the infarcted side (Shinohara *et al.*, 1969).

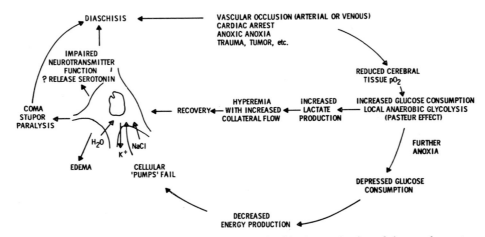

Fig. 16. Representation of the possible pathways involved in the production of signs and symptoms of certain neurological conditions and the mechanisms which may lead to recovery of neurological function.

This observation suggests, as Von Monakow (1914) pointed out, that diaschisis is enhanced by latent circulatory disorders in both the affected and unaffected areas of the brain. Nevertheless, the primary factor is probably metabolic depression of neuronal or neurohumoral origin (Fig. 16).

Metabolism

Paralleling the decrease in CBF in patients with cerebrovascular disease, a concomitant reduction in $CMRO_2$ occurs (see Table 5). Hemispheric oxygen consumption was decreased bilaterally but more so on the diseased side (Meyer *et al.*, 1970 e). In patients with severe occlusive cerebrovascular disease, the CMRGl was also reduced. In another series of patients with less severe cerebrovascular disease, CMRGl was normal or nearly normal despite reduced $CMRO_2$ and CBF (Meyer *et al.*, 1967 a, b). This metabolic pattern suggests that anaerobic glycolysis may exist in poorly perfused areas.

Theoretically, 1 vol. % of oxygen is required to oxidize 1.34 mg of glucose. The values obtained in *in vivo* studies have always exceeded the theoretical value (Gottstein *et al.*, 1964; Meyer *et al.*, 1967 a; Scheinberg and Stead, 1949). The results of these studies have been interpreted as an indication that some degree of anaerobic glycolysis must normally be present in the brain. This argument is strengthened by the fact that lactate and pyruvate are added to the cerebral venous blood by the brain in normal human subjects. Gurdjian *et al.* (1944 a) suggested some years ago that ionized lactate passes the blood–brain barrier. Gottstein *et al.* (1963), in a study of 45 normal subjects, observed that the mean arteriovenous difference for lactate (V–A Lact) was 0.8 mg/100 g brain/min and production of lactate by the brain was 0.42 mg/100 g brain/min. In a series of stroke patients studied in our laboratories, V–A Lact was 1.45 mg/100 ml and CMR Lact was 0.69 mg/100 g brain/min (Meyer *et al.*, 1968 b). Increased cerebral lactate production was accompanied by decreased $CMRO_2$ though CMRGl remained normal. The cerebral glucose : oxygen utilization (G/O) ratio was abnormally high at 1.87, and pyruvate metabolism was unchanged.

Metabolic changes of this nature, which may be associated with either reduced or increased CMRGl, are considered typical of anaerobic glycolysis. Hyperventilation produces a shift from aerobic cerebral metabolism to an increase in anaerobic glycolysis and increased lactate production. Conversely, inhalation of 100% oxygen decreases anaerobic glycolysis which proves that, in the brain, oxygen availability provides a balance between aerobic and anaerobic metabolism, a phenomenon known as the Pasteur effect (Meyer *et al.*, 1969 b). The claim by Gottstein *et al.* (1965) that insulin increases the uptake of glucose by cerebral tissue and thereby facilitates metabolism in stroke has not been substantiated in our laboratories (Meyer *et al.*, 1968 b).

The differences observed between the theoretical and practical G/O ratio values can be accounted for partly by oxidation of substances other than glucose in the brain, such as ketone bodies, lipids, and amino acids. The calculated average respiratory quotient (RQ) of human brain is 0.95; however, RQ at this level is not always an indication that carbohydrate only is oxidized by the brain. Under some circumstances, oxidation of a combination of other substances may produce the same results. The fact that pyruvate is the principal metabolite in the cerebral venous blood bears out the concept that normally carbohydrate is probably the chief fuel of the brain, although a small amount of noncarbohydrate substances may be utilized. Reduced CO_2 production may result from oxidation of these noncarbohydrate substances since fixation of CO_2 is required to supply intermediates to the metabolic cycles involved. It is possible, therefore, that during ischemia in addition to shifting of anaerobic glycolysis, the brain may metabolize substances such as ketone bodies, fatty acids, and amino acids in order to maintain the energy necessary for normal function (Meyer et al., 1971, a). In patients with cerebrovascular disease, the RQ is reduced in the steady state. Inhalation of 5% CO_2 causes a further decrease in RQ which was interpreted as being due, in part, to accelerated removal of CO_2 from the ischemic tissues caused by increased CBF, as well as increased rCBF in ischemic tissue causing an increase in metabolism of substances other than glucose with fixation of CO_2. Gottstein et al. (in press) recently reported evidence that the decrease in RQ in a group of patients with liver disease, some of whom had stroke, could be accounted for by the metabolism of ketone bodies. This has not been confirmed in our laboratories in initial measurements in 3 patients with stroke.

Oxygen and carbon dioxide inhalation and hyperventilation

Inhalation of 100% oxygen by patients who have suffered stroke decreases CBF about 12%, increases $CMRO_2$, and decreases the anaerobic glycolysis by the Pasteur effect (Meyer et al., 1969 b). Inhalation of 5% CO_2 in those with occlusive cerebro-

TABLE 6

CHANGES OF HBF AND METABOLISM IN DISEASED HEMISPHERE AFTER 5% CO_2
IN AIR AND HYPERVENTILATION

	HBF ml/100 g brain/min	HMIO₂ ml/100 g brain/min	HMICO₂ ml/100 g brain/min	HMIGl mg/100 g brain/min	HRQ	HG/O
CO₂ Inhalation						
Control	34.1 ± 3.2	2.08 ± 0.53	1.94 ± 0.50	4.02 ± 1.15	0.99 ± 0.16	1.79 ± 0.59
5% CO₂ + air						
inhalation	41.4 ± 7.6	2.00 ± 0.50	1.62 ± 0.41	3.87 ± 1.57	0.87 ± 0.17	1.93 ± 0.95
p Value	p < 0.02	N.S.	N.S.	N.S.	p < 0.05	N.S.
	(N = 9)	(N = 9)	(N = 7)	(N = 7)	(N = 7)	(N = 8)
Hyperventilation						
Control	35.0 ± 2.2	2.08 ± 0.50	1.72 ± 0.38	3.28 ± 1.04	0.86 ± 0.23	1.74 ± 0.85
Hyper-						
ventilation	30.8 ± 1.1	2.28 ± 0.57	1.94 ± 0.50	3.82 ± 1.19	0.88 ± 0.21	1.95 ± 0.94
p Value	p < 0.01	N.S.	N.S.	N.S.	N.S.	N.S.
	(N = 7)	(N = 7)	(N = 7)	(N = 6)	(N = 7)	(N = 6)

N.S. = not a statistically significant change.

vascular disease increases CBF but to a lesser extent than that which occurs in healthy subjects. This can be explained by the reduced cerebral vasodilatory capacitance in patients with cerebral arterial disease. Inhalation of a mixture of 5% CO_2 and 95% oxygen produced a remarkable increase in CBF and $CMRO_2$ as well as an increase in CMRGl (Meyer et al., 1968 a). Table 6 shows a similar effect on HBF and metabolism produced by inhalation of 5% CO_2 and air. Intermittent inhalation of 5% CO_2 and 95% oxygen is, under the majority of conditions, an effective form of therapy in patients with cerebrovascular disease. Conversely, hyperventilation in these patients reduces CBF, depresses $CMRO_2$, and causes a shift to anaerobic metabolism (see Table 6).

Control of blood flow

Brawley et al. (1967) and Lassen and Pálvölgyi (1968) proposed that vessels in an ischemic area of brain are maximally dilated due to accumulated CO_2 and acid metabolites. They stated, therefore, that these vessels are no longer able to dilate in response to increased arterial P_{CO_2} while vessels in the bordering zones of more normal brain remain vasoactive and dilate during hypercapnia. Proponents of this theory believe that the resultant reduction in arteriolar pressure in zones of infarction leads to shunting of blood from infarcted to normal areas of brain. This phenomenon was termed the "intracerebral steal". According to this theory, hypocapnia caused by hyperventilation would have the converse effect, producing vasoconstriction in the normal bordering zone vessels and diverting blood flow toward the ischemic area. This was named the "inverse steal" and, on the assumption that this hypothetical situation would occur in patients with stroke, treatment with hyperventilation was recommended.

This theory has been criticized on several counts. Brawley et al. (1967) utilized inhalation of 100% CO_2 to the point of apnea and observed steal in some experiments without the benefit of statistical analysis. Other workers who observed steal in some experiments (50% of Waltz' experiments) have also used unphysiological levels of CO_2 (Halsey and Clark, 1970; Waltz, 1968). The "steal phenomenon" was detected in only two of 32 electrode placements (6%) located in infarcted zones in monkeys following middle cerebral artery occlusion (Meyer et al., 1971, b). The so-called "steal" has not been observed in several different series of patients with stroke during treatment with either CO_2 inhalation or vasodilator drugs (Cooper et al., 1970; McHenry et al., 1970 a, b; Meyer et al., 1970 b, 1971, c).

High concentrations of CO_2 are known to cause brain swelling (Goldberg et al., 1963; Barlow et al., 1963). Brock et al., (1971) pointed out that in areas of brain ischemia any increase in blood flow during hyperventilation probably results from reduction of intracranial pressure occasioned by cerebral vasoconstriction. In our laboratories, HBF and metabolism have been measured in some patients and rCBF in others by the use of intracarotid injection of ^{133}Xe and the Anger camera. The so-called "intracerebral steal" has been observed only in patients with brain tumor and intracerebral hematoma. The majority of patients referred to by Lassen and Pálvölgyi suffered from brain tumor with increased intracranial pressure.

Another explanation for the phenomenon of decreased flow in the diseased areas in patients with intracerebral tumor, hematoma, or massive infarction caused by CO_2 inhalation is that the increased intracranial pressure in these zones is increased with passive displacement of blood from the tumor tissue or necrotic and swollen brain since intracranial pressure is further increased by CO_2 inhalation. A better term which has been suggested for this phenomenon is "intracerebral squeeze" (Welch and Meyer, 1970). Conversely, when intracranial pressure is decreased, such as occurs during hyperventilation, blood flow in the tumor tissue or necrotic zone is increased.

Cerebral blood flow and metabolism during epileptic seizures

The dramatic cerebral metabolic and circulatory changes accompanying epileptic seizures have interested investigators for many years. The exact mechanism of the epileptic seizure is still uncertain, but data have now been accumulated concerning blood flow and metabolic changes accompanying seizures in animals and man.

Gibbs et al. (1934) and Penfield et al. (1939) first demonstrated that increased CBF occurs during epileptic seizures in man. This was confirmed in animals and in man in our laboratory (Meyer et al., 1962 b; Meyer et al., 1966 a). In man, increases in CBF up to four times that during the steady state have been measured during seizure activity, and a reduction in blood flow was recorded during the postictal stage. The increase in CBF is due to the combined effect of increased blood pressure with accumulation of CO_2 and increased metabolite formation resulting from increased cerebral metabolism. The highest blood flows recorded in man, other than in patients with arteriovenous malformations, have been during seizures or 20% CO_2 inhalation.

Measurement of gas tensions in the cerebral venous blood during induced generalized seizures indicate reduction in CVP_{O_2} and $CVSO_2$ (Meyer et al., 1965 a), with a concomitant increase in CVP_{CO_2} and reduced pH. These metabolic changes are clearly indicative of increased $CMRO_2$ and CO_2 production and, therefore, increased cerebral metabolism. The decrease in CVP_{O_2} occurs in spite of increased CBF, which indicates that the demand of increased $CMRO_2$ is not met by increased CBF. Thus, the brain tissue is actually hypoxic during seizure activity. Plum et al. (1968) found no evidence of cerebral hypoxia in animals during induced seizure activity. However, the animals were anesthetized and artificially respired so that the physiological findings cannot be compared to those that occur during seizure activity in patients without assisted respiration or oxygen breathing.

Likewise, an increase in CVP_{CO_2} with a decrease in blood pH during seizures in our patients indicates that the production of acid metabolites is greater than the hyperemic brain can handle. CVP_{O_2} falls well below the threshold at which EEG activity and cerebral function become impaired (Meyer et al., 1965 b). Additional evidence for increased cerebral metabolism is gained from a study of electrodecremental seizures during which the conscious state is usually maintained and postictal paralysis is not apparent. Hyperoxia of the cerebral venous blood occurs with an increase in CVP_{CO_2}. The increased CO_2 is the product of active cerebral metabolism and, with a concomitant increase in blood pressure, contributes to a sufficient increase in CBF to overcome the increased $CMRO_2$.

When the generalized seizures terminate, P_{O_2} levels in the cerebral venous blood become extremely elevated. In our studies in man, decreased $CMRO_2$ following seizures has been observed (Meyer et al., 1966 a), which accounts for the state of postepileptic paralysis. The depression of $CMRO_2$ in association with increased CBF and accumulation of acid metabolites causes hyperoxia of brain tissue.

Cerebral venous pH continues to fall after termination of seizure activity due to accumulation of CO_2 and acid metabolites consequent upon increased cerebral metabolic activity as well as metabolic acidosis due to lactate release from the violent contractions of skeletal musculature. The EEG tends to slow in man because of metabolic acidosis after a pH of 7.09 has been reached, even though an abundant oxygen supply may be available to the brain tissue. When pH rises above 7.09, the EEG returns to its normal range and CVP_{O_2} begins to decrease. Recovery of pH and EEG is delayed for several minutes after a seizure, suggesting that cerebral acidosis is responsible in part for postepileptic suppression of electrical activity and postepileptic paralysis. Postepileptic suppression of electrical activity is believed to be initiated by cerebral anoxia and perpetuated by cerebral acidosis.

$CMRO_2$ was significantly increased during seizure activity in our experiments, and cerebral venous arterial and lactate levels increased. This pattern of change is compatible with an increase during seizure activity of both anaerobic and aerobic glycolysis (Meyer et al., 1966 a).

During induced seizures, a decrease of sodium and an increase of potassium occurred at the pial surface of the brain (Meyer et al., 1961 b). This was assumed to be an indication of sodium influx and potassium efflux from the brain. The same mechanisms are found in man. Cerebral venous potassium and arteriovenous difference for sodium also increase, indicating a sodium uptake into the brain and a potassium release during seizure activity. In a recent study, Teraura et al. (in preparation) observed movement of chloride as well as sodium ions into the brain during induced seizures in monkeys.

Attempts have been made to correlate inhibitory effect of seizures on neuronal electrical activity with metabolic changes during the postictal state. Anoxia and acidosis are believed to produce at least some of these effects, confirming the earlier work of other investigators (Jasper and Erickson, 1941). In two studies carried out in our laboratories, the observation was made that periodic seizures can be terminated intermittently by cerebral anoxia (Meyer and Portnoy, 1959; Meyer et al., 1961 b) and that severe cerebral anoxia is related to postictal suppression. Cerebral anoxia during minor seizures of the petit mal type is less severe and postictal paralysis does not occur. These data support the findings of Gurdjian et al. (1946) that cerebral anoxia is the initiating factor in epileptic paralysis. However, our studies have included the observation that seizure activity may be inhibited by cerebral acidosis resulting from CO_2 inhalation and this was confirmed by the intravenous injection of weak acids (Meyer and Gotoh, 1961 a). Acetazolamide has an inhibitory effect on seizure activity (Meyer et al., 1961 a).

References pp. 339–347

Brain injury and coma

The diverse etiology of coma and its metabolic concomitants were reviewed extensively by Meyer and Gotoh (1961 b). In general, any abnormal situation, *e.g.*, uremia or B12 deficiency, which impairs the delivery or utilization of substrates for production of energy in the brain or which disturbs the enzyme or coenzyme action needed to produce energy may bring about a comatose state. Coma is a common manifestation of acute traumatic cerebral injury causing neuronal paralysis of the reticular activating system of the brain stem or a more diffuse neuronal paralysis. The hemodynamics and metabolism underlying the comatose state have been investigated extensively in many laboratories with conflicting results (Gurdjian *et al.*, 1944 b; Lindquist and Leroy, 1944; German *et al.*, 1947; Brown and Brown, 1954). Studies of brain injury in the monkey in this laboratory (Meyer *et al.*, 1970 c) disclosed that following a *mild* concussive blow, temporary *excitation* of the central nervous system manifested by EEG desynchronization and a brief increase in $CMRO_2$ and CBF occurred. *Severe* concussive blows were followed by temporary slowing of EEG activity and a transient decrease in $CMRO_2$ and CBF, indicating the occurrence of reversible paralysis of the central nervous system. Severe contusion and laceration in experimental animals produced profound decrease in $CMRO_2$ but a smaller degree of reduction in CBF, causing temporary hyperoxia with masking of the EEG change. However, $CMRO_2$, CBF, and CVpH became increasingly reduced with slowing and flattening of the EEG and a fatal outcome.

The maximum degree of cerebral metabolic depression was caused by lesions to the brain stem with paralytic injury to the reticular formation resulting in inhibition of its normal excitatory drive and consequently a state of diaschisis. Nevertheless, metabolic depression was also noted as a result of diffuse neuronal paralysis resulting from cerebral injuries.

Analysis of data from studies of CBF and metabolism in humans shows that depression of $CMRO_2$ is the most common change to take place during all types of coma. Kety (1949) found in a group of comatose patients that $CMRO_2$ was reduced below 2.0 cc/100 g/min, while in a group who were semicomatose or mentally confused the level was between 2.5 and 3.0 cc. However, wide experience shows that not all patients in coma have such marked depression of $CMRO_2$. In such cases, regional injury to the brain stem or diencephalon with neuronal paralysis may be an explanation for this lack of comparison. Alternatively, uncoupling of oxidative phosphorylation may have occurred (Teraura *et al.*, in press, a). Fazekas *et al.* (1953) reported that many patients with cerebrovascular disease remained conscious in spite of marked depression of $CMRO_2$, and we have confirmed these observations. The depression of $CMRO_2$ in such cases can be explained by the fact that nonoxidative sources of energy metabolism are being utilized. In general, however, in states of coma energy metabolism is depressed and impairs neuronal membrane function, altering ionic distribution (Fig. 16) (Gotoh *et al.*, 1962; Meyer *et al.*, 1961 b). The alteration in ionic distribution is apparently the common factor in all types of coma, a conclusion supported by the fact that in virtually all cases of coma, the EEG shows either high voltage delta waves or an isoelectric recording. The rare exception to this rule includes some cases of barbiturate poisoning and regional brain stem lesions.

Hypertension

Considering the intimate relationship between blood pressure and CBF, it is not surprising that serious cerebral dysfunction may result from chronic hypertension and acute hypertensive crisis. For example, the sudden rises in MABP that occur with malignant hypertension are regularly accompanied by spasm of the retinal arteries, papilledema, headache, drowsiness, vomiting, scotomas, focal seizures, and mental obtundity. If the condition is untreated, more serious signs and symptoms such as generalized seizures, cerebral hemorrhage, transient or permanent hemiparesis or monoparesis, and visual field defects occur eventually followed by death, usually from a fatal cerebral hemorrhage. Intracerebral hemorrhage may also follow rupture of intracranial arterial aneurysms or malformations. If hypotensive therapy is instituted too late, the patient's life may be saved but dementia and bradykinesis persist.

Gowers (1876) was the first to comment on the spasm of the retinal arteries observed by the judicious use of the newly developed ophthalmoscope in patients during episodes of severe hypertension, and Fog (1939 b) was the first to show constriction of the cerebral arterioles with a rise in blood pressure. Byrom (1954) induced hypertension by placing a Goldblatt clamp about the renal artery in rats and observed narrowing or spasm of the pial vessels, both diffusely or in small segments, when the systolic blood pressure exceeded 200 mm Hg. As described earlier, autoregulation maintains constant CBF between well defined limits of blood pressure. If MABP exceeds 120 mm Hg, however, excessive autoregulation takes place and cerebral vasospasm occurs. Chronic as well as acute malignant hypertension is known to impair autoregulation due to pathological changes in the small cerebral arterioles, such as hyperplastic arteriolopathy, hyalinosis, and necrosis of the media.

Meyer *et al.* (1960 a) observed vasoconstriction of small cerebral arterioles, decreased CBF, and increased intracranial pressure in response to acute increases in blood pressure produced by clamping the thoracic aorta. Cerebral edema occurred since the metarteriolar pressure exceeded the colloid osmotic pressure when systolic pressure became higher than 180 mm Hg. The eventual outcome of prolonging such a degree of hypertension was compression of the capillary bed with progressive ischemia, brain herniation, and eventually compression of the vasomotor center with a greater increase in blood pressure due to the Cushing phenomenon. Brain herniation usually resulted in dealth unless the blood pressure was reduced.

Arterial constriction was not as great following hypertension induced by clamping the aorta as that caused by renal hypertension, suggesting that circulating agents such as angiotensin are responsible for additional spasm. In patients with occlusion of a large cerebral vessel, severe hypertension reduces the collateral circulation and further ischemia occurs in the territory supplied by that vessel. This is consonant with clinical observations of hypertension in patients with cerebral atherosclerosis. Reduction of blood pressure in such patients reduces cerebral vasoconstriction and improves the collateral circulation to the ischemic area. Trials of antihypertensive therapy carried out in hypertensive stroke patients showed improved CBF as well as clinical improvement (Meyer *et al.*, 1967 f).

Section III: THERAPEUTIC CONSIDERATIONS IN CEREBROVASCULAR DISEASE

The familiar aphorism that the best medicine is preventive medicine is pertinent in considering treatment of a patient with early warning signs of stroke, when the first thought should be the correction of commonly associated risk factors (Meyer and Ericsson, 1970). In patients with progressive stroke, the aim should be to reduce and minimize the neurologic deficit by increasing blood flow via the collateral circulation and decreasing cerebral edema. Any systemic changes in blood composition that might influence unfavorably the blood flow to the ischemic zone should be avoided. These changes include those caused by high lipid diet, polycythemia, hemoconcentration, dehydration, and high molecular weight substances sometimes used as plasma expanders, all which tend to increase the viscosity of the blood and further impede blood flow to the ischemic area (Waltz and Meyer, 1959; Meyer and Waltz, 1959; Meyer, 1970).

Medical treatment

In treating the stroke patient, maintenance of an adequate cardiac output is essential and, therefore, it is important to recognize myocardial infarction, congestive heart failure, and cardiac dysrhythmias and treat them appropriately.

Early studies showed that anticoagulant therapy or medication directed at preventing platelet aggregation may improve flow to the ischemic area of the brain by preventing hemostasis in the microcirculation (Meyer, 1958 a). However, the risk of hemorrhagic infarction should be borne in mind when anticoagulants, platelet inhibitors, and fibrinolytic agents are used in the patient with acute progressive stroke. Anticoagulant therapy has been found beneficial in association with both medical and surgical treatment of stroke patients (Bradshaw and Casey, 1967; McDowell and McDevitt, 1965). Such drugs are best indicated in patients with transient ischemic attacks, particularly of cardiac origin, in order to reduce the risk of embolization to the brain (Marshall, 1968). Surgical removal of ulcerative plaques in the extracranial vessels also reduces the risk of cerebral embolization (Fields et al., 1970). Dipyramidole, a drug which reduces platelet adhesiveness and aggregation, effectively decreases the incidence of emboli to the brain after cardiac valve replacement (Sullivan et al., 1968). Dissolution of intracranial cerebral emboli and thrombi by the use of streptokinase or streptokinin-activated plasmin proved disappointing because of the incidence of cerebral hemorrhage, but the use of urokinase appears more promising (Meyer et al., 1966 d).

Control of hypertension reduces the incidence of intracerebral hemorrhage and patients with primary hypertensive hemorrhage appear to fare better when treated with hypotensive drugs (Meyer and Bauer, 1962). Since regional autoregulation fails during and for a period after acute cerebral ischemia, attention should be directed toward the maintenance of systolic blood pressure between 140 and 160 mm Hg. Systolic pressures above this level are undesirable since they tend to cause cerebral vasospasm and increase intracranial pressure and cerebral edema, thus causing further reduction in blood flow. Control of moderate to severe hypertension has been found to decrease CVR and to increase CBF (Meyer et al., 1960 a, 1967 f, 1968 a). It is important that treatment with hypotensive drugs be initiated with caution since sudden, large decreases in blood pressure will cause further ischemia. When hypotension occurs for any reason, the cautious use of vasopressor drugs may be indicated. Adrenocortical steroid therapy has also been found beneficial in rare cases since the hypotensive episode may be the result of pituitary–adrenal insufficiency (Gilroy and Meyer, 1963).

Inhalation of oxygen for the first 24 hours following cerebral infarction is beneficial since delivery of oxygen to ischemic zones of the brain is enhanced. Prolonged oxygen therapy should be avoided because of the possibility of oxygen toxicity. Hyperbaric oxygenation may be more effective than inhalation of oxygen at normal pressures, but this method is neither practical nor a widely available form of treatment.

Based on the hypothesis that "intracerebral steal" and "inverse steal" frequently occur in infarcted areas of brain, prolonged moderate hyperventilation has been advocated in the treatment of focal cerebrovascular disease (Soloway et al., 1968). The validity of this hypothesis is questionable. Hyperventilation has not been found to be the appropriate treatment in studies of patients with stroke since the cerebral vasoconstriction that is produced further reduces tissue oxygenation with increased lactic acid production by enhanced anaerobic glycolysis. A rational approach to therapy in the majority of these patients should be directed toward increasing blood flow and oxygen availability to ischemic brain tissue by the intermittent inhalation of 5 % CO_2 and 95 % oxygen, vasodilator therapy such as administration of papaverine, and reduction of brain edema with mannitol, glycerol, or steroids.

The "intracerebral steal" or "squeeze" phenomenon may occur if vasodilator therapy is used in patients with increased intracranial pressure due to recent intracerebral hematoma or massive infarction. In cases such as this, intracranial pressure and brain edema should be reduced by the use of hyperosmolar agents and steroids, while CO_2 inhalation should be avoided.

Papaverine is a potent cerebral vasodilator, and controlled studies of patients with unilateral cerebral infarction and reduced CBF showed that its use brought about improved oxygen delivery to the brain and clinical improvement (Meyer et al., 1965 c; Gilroy and Meyer, 1966). More recent trials with the new drug Hexobendine, when administered either orally or intravenously, show that the drug is effective in increasing blood flow in ischemic areas of the brain (Meyer et al., 1971, c) and produces clinical improvement in some cases.

Intravenous administration of low molecular weight dextran in a randomized series of 100 patients with occlusive cerebrovascular disease, who were treated within the first 72 hours of stroke, lowered the mortality rate and improved the quality of survival in the treated group (Gilroy et al., 1969).

Surgical therapy

During the last two decades, surgical techniques for excision of occlusive lesions of the extracranial vessels and aortic arch have proved to be effective in reducing mortality and morbidity from this disease (Fields *et al.*, 1970; Meyer and Fields, in press). The first operations for the restoration of carotid artery flow were performed in the 1950s by vascular surgeons and neurosurgeons (DeBakey *et al.*, 1965; Cooley *et al.*, 1956; Fields *et al.*, 1958; Gurdjian *et al.*, 1960).

Ligation of the carotid artery for treatment of aneurysms arising from this vessel or from the posterior communicating artery is of established benefit (McKissock *et al.*, 1960). Clipping of readily accessible aneurysms of other cerebral vessels may also be beneficial.

CONCLUDING COMMENTS

This chapter is a review of investigations carried out in our laboratory and by other researchers into the relationship of cerebral blood flow and metabolism to neurological symptoms, particularly those associated with cerebrovascular disease. These studies constitute only a prelude to a full understanding of CBF and metabolism which should result from continued interest in this field of research in medical centers all over the world. Such understanding will contribute to improved medical and surgical management of patients with cerebrovascular disease.

REFERENCES

AIZAWA, T., TAZAKI, Y. AND GOTOH, F. (1961) Cerebral circulation in cerebrovascular disease. *World Neurol.*, **2**, 635–648.

ANGER, H. O. (1958) Scintillation camera. *Rev. Sci. Instr.*, **29**, 27–33.

AUKLAND, K., BOWER, B. F. AND BERLINER, R. W. (1964) Measurement of local blood flow with hydrogen gas. *Circulation Res.*, **14**, 164–187.

BARLOW, C. F., GOLDBERG, M. A. AND ROTH, L. J. (1963) The effect of carbon dioxide narcosis on S^{35} sulfate and C^{14} urea uptake in brain. *Trans. Amer. Neurol. Assoc.*, **88**, 65–68.

BRADSHAW, P. AND CASEY, E. (1967) Outcome of medically treated stroke associated with stenosis or occlusion of the internal carotid artery. *Brit. Med. J.*, **1**, 201–205.

BRAWLEY, B. W., STRANDNESS, D. E., JR. AND KELLY, W. A. (1967) The physiologic response to therapy in experimental cerebral ischemia. *Arch. Neurol.*, **17**, 180–187.

BRIGGS, F. N. AND PORTZEHL, H. (1957) The influence of relaxing factor on the pH dependent of the contraction of muscle models. *Biochim. Biophys. Acta*, **24**, 482–488.

BROCK, M., HADJIDIMOS, A. A., DERUAZ, J. P., FISCHER, F., DIETZ, H., KOHLMEYER, J., PÖLL, W. AND SCHÜRMANN, K. (1971) The effects of hyperventilation on regional cerebral blood flow. On the rule of changes in intracranial pressure and tissue perfusion pressure for shifts in rCBF distribution in cerebral vascular diseases. In: TOOLE, J. F., SIEKERT, R. G. AND WHISNANT, J. P. (Eds.), *Cerebral Vascular Diseases; Trans. Seventh Princeton Conference*, Grune & Stratton, New York, pp. 114–126.

BROWN, G. W. AND BROWN, M. L. (1954) Cardiovascular responses to experimental cerebral concussion in the rhesus monkey: discussion of similarity of responses to electroconvulsive shock and cerebral concussion in dogs, monkeys, and man. *Arch. Neurol. Psychiat.*, **71**, 701–713.

BYROM, F. B. (1954) The pathogenesis of hypertensive encephalopathy and its relation to the malignant phase of hypertension; experimental evidence from the hypertensive rat. *Lancet*, **ii**, 201–211.

CHOROBSKI, J. AND PENFIELD, W. (1932) Cerebral vasodilator nerves and their pathway from the medulla oblongata, with observations on the pial and intracerebral vascular plexus. *Arch. Neurol. Psychiat.*, **28**, 1257–1289.

COOLEY, D. A., YOUSIF, D. A. AND CARTON, C. A. (1956) Surgical treatment of arteriosclerotic occlusion of common carotid artery. *J. Neurosurg.*, **13**, 500–506.

COOPER, E. S., WEST, J. W., JAFFE, M. E., GOLDBERG, H. I., KAWAMURA, J. AND MCHENRY, L. C., JR. (1970) The relation between cardiac function and cerebral blood flow in stroke patients. 1. Effect of CO_2 inhalation. *Stroke*, **1**, 330–347.

CUSHING, H. (1901) Concerning a definite regulatory mechanism of the vaso-motor centre which controls blood pressure during cerebral compression. *Bull. Johns Hopkins Hosp.*, **12**, 290–292.

CUSHING, H. (1902) Some experimental and clinical observations concerning states of increased intracranial tension. *Amer. J. Med.*, **124**, 375–400.

CUSHING, H. (1903) The blood-pressure reaction of acute cerebral compression, illustrated by cases of intracranial hemorrhage. *Amer. J. Med.*, **125**, 1017–1045.

DAVIES, P. W. AND BRINK, F., JR. (1942) Direct measurement of brain oxygen concentrations with a platinum electrode. *Federation Proc.*, **1**, 19 (abstr.).

DEBAKEY, M. E., CRAWFORD, E. S., COOLEY, D. A., MORRIS, G. C., JR., GARRETT, H. E. AND FIELDS, W. S. (1965) Cerebral arterial insufficiency: one to 11-year results following arterial reconstructive operation. *Ann. Surg.*, **161**, 921–945.

DENNY-BROWN, D. AND MEYER, J. S. (1957) The cerebral collateral circulation. II. Production of cerebral infarction by ischemic anoxia and the reversibility of early stages. *Neurology*, **7**, 567–579.

DONDERS, F. C. (1850) Die Bewegungen des Gehirns und die Veränderungen der Gefässfüllung der Pia Mater auch bei geschlossenem unausdehnbarem Schädel unmittelbar beobachtet. *Lancet*, **5**, 521.

DONDERS, F. C. (1859) *Physiologie des Menschen*, S. Hertzel, Leipzig, p. 139.

FALCK, B., NIELSON, K. C. AND OWMAN, CH. (1968) Adrenergic innervation of the pial circulation. *Scand. J. Clin. Lab. Invest.*, *Suppl.* **102**, VI: B.

FAZEKAS, J. F., BESSMAN, A. N., COTSONAS, N. J., JR. AND ALMAN, R. W. (1953) Cerebral hemodynamics in cerebral arteriosclerosis. *J. Gerontol.*, **8**, 137–145.

FIELD, J., 2nd, FUHRMAN, F. A. AND MARTIN, A. W. (1944) Effect of temperature on the oxygen consumption of brain tissue. *J. Neurophysiol.*, **117**, 117–126.

FIELDS, W. S., CRAWFORD, E. S. AND DEBAKEY, M. E. (1958) Surgical considerations in cerebral arterial insufficiency. *Neurology*, **8**, 801–808.

FIELDS, W. S., MASLENIKOV, V., MEYER, J. S., HASS, W. K., REMINGTON, R. D. AND MACDONALD, M. (1970) Joint study of extracranial arterial occlusion. V. Progress report of prognosis following surgery or nonsurgical treatment for transient cerebral ischemic attacks and cervical carotid artery lesions. *J. Amer. Med. Assoc.*, **211**, 1993–2003.

FIESCHI, C., BOZZAO, L. AND AGNOLI, A. (1965) Regional clearance of hydrogen as a measure of cerebral blood flow. *Acta Neurol. Scand.*, **41**, *Suppl.* **14**, 46–52.

FOG, M. (1934) *Om Piaarterienes Vasomotoriske Reaktioner*, Munksgaard, Köpenhamn.

FOG, M. (1939a) Cerebral circulation. I. Reaction of pial arteries to epinephrine by direct application and by intravenous injection. *Arch. Neurol. Psychiat.*, **41**, 109–118.

FOG, M. (1939 b) Cerebral circulation. II. Reaction of pial arteries to increase in blood pressure. *Arch. Neurol. Psychiat.*, **41**, 260–268.

FORBES, H. S. (1928) The cerebral circulation. Observation and measurement of pial vessels. *Arch. Neurol. Psychiat.*, **19**, 751–761.

FORBES, H. S. AND COBB, S. (1966) Vasomotor control of cerebral vessels. In: COBB, S., FRANTZ, A. M., PENFIELD, W. AND RILEY, H. A. (Eds.), *The Circulation of the Brain and Spinal Cord; Proc. Assoc. Research in Nervous and Mental Disease, 1937*, Hafner Publishing Co., New York, p. 201.

FORSSMANN, W. (1929) Die Sondierung des rechten Herzens. *Wien. Klin. Wochschr.*, **8**, 2085.

FUJISHIMA, M., SCHEINBERG, P. AND REINMUTH, O. M. (1970) Effects of experimental occlusion of the basilar artery by magnetic localization of iron filings on cerebral blood flow and metabolism and cerebrovascular responses to CO_2 in the dog. *Neurology*, **20**, 925–932.

GERMAN, W. S., PAGE, W. R. AND NIMS, L. F. (1947) Cerebral blood flow and cerebral oxygen consumption in experimental intracranial injury. *Trans. Amer. Neurol. Assoc.*, **7**, 86–88.

GIBBS, E. L., LENNOX, W. G., NIMS, L. F. AND GIBBS, F. A. (1942) Arterial and cerebral venous blood: Arterial–venous differences in man. *J. Biol. Chem.*, **144**, 325–332.

GIBBS, F. A., LENNOX, W. G. AND GIBBS, E. L. (1934) Cerebral blood flow preceding and accompanying epileptic seizures in man. *Arch. Neurol. Psychiat.*, **32**, 257–272.

GILROY, J., BAUER, R. B., KRABBENHOFT, K. L. AND MEYER, J. S. (1963) Cerebral circulation time in cerebral vascular disease measured by serial angiography. *Amer. J. Roentgenol.*, **90**, 490–505.

GILROY, J. AND MEYER, J. S. (1963) Pituitary insufficiency with cerebrovascular symptoms. A new clinical syndrome. *New Engl. J. Med.*, **269**, 1115–1119.

GILROY, J. AND MEYER, J. S. (1966) Controlled evaluation of cerebral vasodilator drugs in the progressive stroke. In: MILLIKAN, C. H., SIEKERT, R. G. AND WHISNANT, J. P. (Eds.), *Cerebral Vascular Diseases*; *Proc. Fifth Princeton Conference*, Grune & Stratton, New York.

GILROY, J., BARNHART, M. I. AND MEYER, J. S. (1969) Treatment of acute stroke with dextran 40. *J. Amer. Med. Assoc.*, **210**, 293–298.

GOLDBERG, M. A., BARLOW, C. F. AND ROTH, L. J. (1963) Abnormal brain permeability in CO_2 narcosis. *Arch. Neurol.*, **9**. 498–507.

GOTOH, F., TAZAKI, Y. AND MEYER, J. S. (1961) Transport of gases through brain and their extra-vascular vasomotor action. *Exp. Neurol.*, **4**, 48–58.

GOTOH, F., TAZAKI, Y., HAMAGUCHI, K. AND MEYER, J. S. (1962) Continuous recording of sodium and potassium ionic activity of blood and brain in situ. *J. Neurochem.*, **9**, 81–97.

GOTOH, F. AND MEYER, J. S. (1965) Cerebral vascular reactivity in man: Influence of arterial gas tension on effective cerebral perfusion. *Neurology*, **15**, 268 (abstr.).

GOTOH, F., MEYER, J. S. AND TAKAGI, Y. (1965) Cerebral effects of hyperventilation in man. *Arch. Neurol.*, **12**, 410–423.

GOTOH, F., MEYER, J. S. AND EBIHARA, S. (1966 a) Continuous recording of human cerebral blood flow and metabolism: Methods for electronic monitoring of arterial and venous gases and electrolytes. *Med. Res. Eng.*, **5**, 13–19.

GOTOH, F., MEYER, J. S. AND TOMITA, M. (1966 b) Carbonic anhydrase inhibition and cerebral venous blood gases and ions in man. Demonstration of increased oxygen availability to ischemic brain. *Arch. Internal Med.*, **117**, 39–46.

GOTOH, F., MEYER, J. S. AND TOMITA, M. (1966 c) Hydrogen method for determining cerebral blood flow in man. *Arch. Neurol.*, **15**, 549–559.

GOTTSTEIN, U., BERNSMEIER, A. AND SEDLMEYER, I. (1963) Der Kohlenhydratstoffwechsel des menschlichen Gehirns: I. Untersuchungen mit substratspezifischen enzymatischen: Methoden bei normaler Hirndurchblutung. *Klin. Wochschr.*, **41**, 943–948.

GOTTSTEIN, U., BERNSMEIER, A. AND SEDLMEYER, I. (1964) Der Kohlenhydratstoffwechsel des menschlichen Gehirns: II. Untersuchungen mit substratspezifischen enzymatischen: Methoden bei Kranken mit verminderter Hirndurchblutung auf dem Boden einer Arteriosklerose der Hirngefässe. *Klin. Wochschr.*, **42**, 310–313.

GOTTSTEIN, U., HELD, K., SEBENNING, H. AND WALPURGER, G. (1965) Der Glucoseverbrauch des Menschlichen Gehirns unter dem Einfluss intravenöser Infusionen von Glucose, Glucogon und Glucose-Insulin. *Klin. Wochschr.*, **43**, 965.

GOTTSTEIN, U. AND HELD, K. (1969) Effekt der Hämodilution nach intravenöser Infusion von niedermolekularen Dextranen auf die Hirnzirkulation des Menschen. *Deut. Med. Wochschr.*, **94**, 522–526.

GOTTSTEIN, U., HELD, K., MÜLLER, W. AND BERGHOFF, W. (in press) Utilization of ketone bodies by the human brain. In: MEYER, J. S., REIVICH, M., LECHNER, H. AND EICHHORN, O. (Eds.), *Research on the Cerebral Circulation*; *Fifth Salzburg Conference*, Charles C. Thomas, Springfield.

GOWERS, W. R. (1876) The state of the arteries in Bright's disease. *Brit. Med. J.*, **2**, 743.

GURDJIAN, E. S., STONE, W. E. AND WEBSTER, J. E. (1944 a) Cerebral metabolism in hypoxia. *Arch. Neurol. Psychiat.*, **51**, 472–477.

GURDJIAN, E. S., WEBSTER, J. E. AND STONE, W. E. (1944 b) Experimental head injury with special reference to certain chemical factors in acute trauma. *Surg. Gynecol. Obstet.*, **78**, 618–626.

GURDJIAN, E. S., WEBSTER, J. E. AND STONE, W. E. (1946) Cerebral metabolism in metrazol convulsions in the dog. In: *Epilepsy*; *Proc. Assoc. Res. Nervous Mental Diseases*, Hafner Publishing Co., New York.

GURDJIAN, E. S., HARDY, W. G. AND LINDNER, D. W. (1960) The surgical consideration of 258 patients with carotid occlusion. *Surg. Gynecol. Obstet.*, **110**, 327–338.

HALSEY, J. H., JR. AND CLARK, L. D., JR. (1970) Some regional circulatory abnormalities following experimental cerebral infarction. *Neurology*, **20**, 238–246.

HANDA, J., MEYER, J. S., HUBER, P. AND YOSHIDA, K. (1965 a) Time course of development of cerebral collateral circulation. Experimental study of carotid occlusion in the monkey by electromagnetic flowmeters. *Vasc. Dis.*, **2**, 271–282.

HANDA, J., MEYER, J. S. AND YOSHIDA, K. (1965 b) Regional pharmacological responses of the vertebral and internal carotid arteries. *J. Pharmacol. Exp. Therap.*, **152**, 251–264.

HARPER, A. M. (1966) Autoregulation of cerebral blood flow; influence of the arterial blood pressure on the blood flow through the cerebral cortex. *J. Neurol. Neurosurg. Psychiat.*, **29**, 398–403.

HARTMAN, B. K. AND UDENFRIEND, S. (1970) Immunofluorescent localization of dopamine β-hydroxylase in tissues. *Mol. Pharmacol.*, **6**, 85–94.

HEISS, W. D., PROSENZ, P., ROSZUCZKY, A. AND TSCHABITSCHER, H. (1968 a) A quantitative gamma-camera technique. *Scand. J. Clin. Lab. Invest, Suppl.* **102**, XI: L.

HEISS, W. D., PROSENZ, P., ROSZUCZKY, A. AND TSCHABITSCHER, H. (1968 b) Die Verwendung von Gamma-Kamera und Vielkanalspeicher zur Messung der gesamten und regionalen Hirndurchblutung. *Nuclearmedizin*, **7**, 297–318.

HEISS, W. D. AND TSCHABITSCHER, H. (1969) Die Auswertung von Gamma-Kamera Szintigrammen durch Vielkanalspeicher Computer und Farbfernsehsystem. *Fortschr. Röntgenstr.*, **110**, 108–117.

HEYMAN, A., PATTERSON, J. L., JR. AND NICHOLS, F. T., JR. (1950) The effects of induced fever on cerebral functions in neurosyphilis. *J. Clin. Invest.*, **29**, 1335–1341.

HEYMAN, A., PATTERSON, J. L., JR., DUKE, T. W. AND BATTEY, L. L. (1953) The cerebral circulation and metabolism in arteriosclerotic and hypertensive cerebro-disease; with observations on effects of inhalation of different concentrations of oxygen. *New Engl. J. Med.*, **249**, 223–229.

HIMWICH, H. E., BOWMAN, K. M., FAZEKAS, J. F. AND GOLDFARB, W. (1940) Temperature and brain metabolism, *Amer. J. Med. Sci.*, **200**, 347–353.

HIMWICH, H. E., BOWMAN, K. M., GOLDFARB, W. AND FAZEKAS, J. F. (1942) Cerebral metabolism during fever. *Science*, **90**, 398–399.

HOCHELLA, N. J. AND WEINHOUSE, S. (1965) Automated lactic acid determination in serum and tissue extracts. *Ann. Biochem.*, **10**, 304–317.

HØEDT-RASMUSSEN, K. AND SKINHØJ, E. (1964) Transneural depression of the cerebral hemispheric metabolism in man. *Acta Neurol. Scand.*, **40**, 41–46.

HØEDT-RASMUSSEN, K., SKINHØJ, E., PAULSON, O., EWALD, J., BJERRUM, J. K., FAHRENKRUG, A. AND LASSEN, N. A. (1967) Regional cerebral blood flow in acute apoplexy. The "luxury perfusion" syndrome of brain tissue. *Arch. Neurol.*, **17**, 271–281.

HUBER, P., MEYER, J. S., HANDA, J. AND ISHIKAWA, S. (1965) Electromagnetic flowmeter study of carotid and vertebral blood flow during intracranial hypertension. *Acta Neurochir.*, **13**, 37–63.

HUDGINS, W. R. AND GARCIA, J. H. (1970) Transorbital approach to the middle cerebral artery of the squirrel monkey: a technique for experimental cerebral infarction applicable to ultrastructural studies. *Stroke*, **1**, 107–111.

INGVAR, D. H. AND SÖDERBERG, V. (1958) Cortical blood flow related to EEG patterns evoked by stimulation of the brain stem. *Acta Physiol. Scand.*, **42**, 130–143.

ISHIKAWA, S., HANDA, J., MEYER, J. S. AND HUBER, P. (1965) Haemodynamics of the circle of Willis and the leptomeningeal anastomoses. An electromagnetic flowmeter study of intracranial arterial occlusion in the monkey. *J. Neurol. Neurosurg. Psychiat.*, **28**, 124–136.

JAMES, I. M., MILLAR, R. A. AND PURVES, M. J. (1969) Observations on the extrinsic neural control of cerebral blood flow in the baboon. *Circulation Res.*, **25**, 77–93.

JASPER, H. AND ERICKSON, T. C. (1941) Cerebral blood flow and pH in excessive cortical discharge induced by metrazol and electrical stimulation. *J. Neurophysiol.*, **4**, 333–347.

JENKNER, F. L. (1966) *Rheoencephalography*, Moskow, Springfield, Ill.

JENKNER, F. L. (1968) Rheoencephalography: present status. In: LUYENDIJK, W. (Ed.), *Cerebral Circulation, Progress in Brain Research*, Vol. 30, Elsevier, Amsterdam, p. 127.

KETY, S. S. AND SCHMIDT, C. F. (1945) The determination of cerebral blood flow in man by the use of nitrous oxide in low concentrations. *Amer. J. Physiol.*, **143**, 53–66.

KETY, S. S. (1949) The physiology of the human cerebral circulation. *Anesthesiology*, **10**, 610–614.

LANDAU, W. M., FREYGANG, W. H., JR. AND ROLAND, L. P. (1955) The local circulation of the living brain; values in the unanesthetized and anesthetized cat. *Trans. Amer. Neurol. Assoc.*, **80**, 125–129.

LANGFITT, T. W. AND KASSELL, N. F. (1968) Cerebral vasodilatation produced by brain stem stimulation; neurogenic control vs. autoregulation. *Amer. J. Physiol.*, **215**, 90–97.

LANGFITT, T. W., WEINSTEIN, J. D. AND KASSELL, N. F. (1965) Cerebral vasomotor paralysis produced by intracranial hypertension. *Neurology*, **15**, 622–641.

LASSEN, N. A. (1959) Cerebral blood flow and oxygen consumption in man. *Physiol. Rev.*, **39**, 183–238.

LASSEN, N. A. AND INGVAR, D. H. (1961) The blood flow of the cerebral cortex determined by radio-active krypton. *Experientia*, **17**, 42–43.

LASSEN, N. A., HØEDT-RASMUSSEN, K., SØRENSEN, S. C., SKINHØJ, E., CRONQUIST, S., BODFORSS, B., ENG, E. AND INGVAR, D. H. (1963) Regional cerebral blood flow in man determined by Krypton[85]. *Neurology*, **13**, 719–727.

LASSEN, N. A. (1966) The luxury-perfusion syndrome and its possible relation to acute metabolic acidosis localized within the brain. *Lancet*, **ii**, 1113–1115.

LASSEN, N. A. AND PÁLVÖLGYI, R. (1968) Cerebral steal during hypercapnia and the inverse reaction during hypocapnia observed by the [133]Xenon technique in man. *Scand. J. Clin. Lab. Invest.*, *Suppl.* **102**, XIII: D.

LINDÉN, L. (1955) The effect of stellate ganglion block on cerebral circulation in cerebrovascular accidents. *Acta Med. Scand.*, *Suppl.* **301**, 7–110.

LINDQUIST, J. L. AND LEROY, G. V. (1944) Studies of cerebral oxygen consumption following experimental head injury. *Surg. Gynecol. Obstet.*, **75**, 28–33.

LOGSDON, E. E. (1960) A method for determination of ammonia in biological materials on the autoanalyzer. *Ann. N.Y. Acad. Sci.*, **87**, 801–807.

LORENZ, W. J. AND ADAM, W. E. (1967) Digitale und analoge Auswertung von Aufnahmen mit der Szintillationskamera. *Nuclearmedizin*, **6**, 367–377.

McDOWELL, F. AND McDEVITT, E. (1965) Treatment of completed stroke with longterm anticoagulation: six and one-half years experience. In: MILLIKAN, C. H., SIEKERT, R. G. AND WHISNANT, J. (Eds.), *Cerebral Vascular Diseases*; *Proc. Fourth Princeton Conference*, Grune & Stratton, New York.

McHENRY, L. C., JR., JAFFE, M. E. AND GOLDBERG, H. I. (1969) Evaluation of the rCBF method of Lassen and Ingvar. In: BROCK, M., FIESCHI, C., INGVAR, D. H., LASSEN, N. A. AND SHÜRMANN, K. (Eds.), *Cerebral Blood Flow*, Springer-Verlag, Berlin, p. 11.

McHENRY, L. C., JR., JAFFE, M. E., KAWAMURA, J. AND GOLDBERG, H. I. (1970 a) The effect of Hexobendine on regional cerebral blood flow in stroke patients. *Neurology*, **20**, 375 (abstr.).

McHENRY, L. C., JR., JAFFE, M. E., KAWAMURA, J. AND GOLDBERG, H. I. (1970 b) Effect of papaverine on regional blood flow in focal vascular disease of the brain. *New Engl. J. Med.*, **282**, 1167–1170.

McKISSOCK, W., RICHARDSON, A. AND WALSH, L. (1960) "Posterior-communicating" aneurysms. A controlled trial of the conservative and surgical treatment of ruptured aneurysms of the internal carotid artery at or near the point of origin of the posterior communicating artery. *Lancet*, **i**, 1203–1206.

MARSHALL, J. (1968) *The Management of Cerebrovascular Disease*, 2nd ed., Little, Brown and Co., Boston,

MARX, P., TERAURA, T., HASHI, K. AND MEYER, J. S. (in press) The movement of chloride ions during cerebral ischemia. In: MEYER, J. S., REIVICH, M., LECHNER, H. AND EICHHORN, O. (Eds.), *Research on the Cerebral Circulation*; *Fifth Intern. Salzburg Conference*, Charles C. Thomas, Springfield, Ill.

MATHEW, N., MEYER, J. S., BELL, R. L., AND ERICSSON, A. D. (1971) New method for measuring. regional cerebral blood flow and blood volume in man using the gamma camera. *Trans. Amer. Neurol. Ass.*, in press.

MCHEDLISHVILI, G. I. (1964) Vascular mechanisms pertaining to the intrinsic regulation of the cerebral circulation. *Circulation*, **30**, 597–610.

MEYER, J. S., FANG, H. C. AND DENNY-BROWN, D. (1954) Polarographic study of cerebral collateral circulation. *Arch. Neurol. Psychiat.*, **72**, 296–312.

MEYER, J. S. AND DENNY-BROWN, D. (1955) Studies of cerebral circulation in brain injury. I. Validity of combined local cerebral electropolarography, thermometry and steady potentials as an indicator of local circulatory and functional changes. *Electroencephalog. Clin. Neurophysiol.*, **7**, 511–528.

MEYER, J. S. AND DENNY-BROWN, D. (1957) The cerebral collateral circulation. I. Factors influencing collateral blood flow. *Neurology*, **7**, 447–458.

MEYER, J. S. AND HUNTER, J. (1957 a) Effects of hypothermia on local blood flow and metabolism during cerebral ischemia and hypoxia. *J. Neurosurg.*, **24**, 210–227.

MEYER, J. S. AND HUNTER, J. (1957 b) Polarographic study of cortical blood flow in man. *J. Neurosurg.*, **14**, 382–399.

MEYER, J. S. (1958 a) Localized changes in properties of the blood and effects of anticoagulant drugs in experimental cerebral infarction. *New Engl. J. Med.*, **278**, 151–159.

MEYER, J. S. (1958 b) Importance of ischemic damage to small vessels in experimental cerebral infarction. *J. Neuropathol. Exp. Neurol.*, **17**, 571–585.

MEYER, J. S. (1958 c) Circulatory changes following occlusion of the middle cerebral artery and their relation to function. *J. Neurosurg.*, **15**, 653–673.

MEYER, J. S. AND PORTNOY, H. D. (1958) Localized cerebral hypoglycemia simulating stroke. A clinical and experimental study. *Neurology*, **8**, 601–614.

MEYER, J. S. AND PORTNOY, H. D. (1959) Post-epileptic paralysis. *Brain*, **82**, 162–185.

MEYER, J. S. AND WALTZ, A. G. (1959) Effects of changes in composition of plasma on pial blood flow. 1. Lipid and lipid fractions. *Neurology*, **9**, 728–740.

MEYER, J. S., WALTZ, A. G. AND GOTOH, F. (1960 a) Pathogenesis of cerebral vasospasm in hypertensive encephalopathy: I. Effects of acute increases in intraluminal blood pressure on pial blood flow. *Neurology*, **10**, 735–744.

MEYER, J. S., WALTZ, A. G. AND GOTOH, F. (1960 b) Pathogenesis of cerebral vasospasm in hypertensive encephalopathy. 2. The nature of increased irritability of smooth muscle of pial arterioles in renal hypertension. *Neurology*, **10**, 859–867.

MEYER, J. S. AND GOTOH, F. (1961 a) Interaction of cerebral hemodynamics and metabolism, *Neurology*, **11**, (pt. 2) 46–65.

MEYER, J. S. AND GOTOH, F. (1961 b) Pathogenesis of coma. Clinical and metabolic considerations. *Intern. J. Neurol.*, **2**, 281–298.

MEYER, J. S., GOTOH, F. AND TAZAKI, Y. (1961 a) Inhibitory action of carbon dioxide and acetazolamide in seizure activity. *Electroencephalog. Clin. Neurophysiol.*, **13**, 762–775.

MEYER, J. S., GOTOH, F., TAZAKI, Y. AND HAMAGUCHI, K. (1961 b) Sodium and potassium activity of living brain. Relation to EEG and active sodium transport. *Trans. Amer. Neurol. Assoc.*, **86**, 17–22.

MEYER, J. S. AND BAUER, R. (1962) Medical treatment of spontaneous intracranial hemorrhage by the use of hypotensive drugs. *Neurology*, **12**, 36–47.

MEYER, J. S., GOTOH, F. AND TAZAKI, Y. (1962 a) Circulation and metabolism following experimental cerebral embolism. *J. Neuropathol. Exp. Neurol.*, **21**, 4–24.

MEYER, J. S., GOTOH, F., TAZAKI, Y., HAMAGUCHI, K., ISHIKAWA, S., NOUAILHAT, F. AND SYMON, L. (1962 b) Regional cerebral blood flow and metabolism in vivo. Effects of anoxia, hypoglycemia, ischemia, acidosis, alkalosis, and alterations of blood pCO_2. *Arch. Neurol.*, **7**, 560–581.

MEYER, J. S. AND GOTOH, F. (1964) Continuous recording of cerebral metabolism, internal jugular flow and EEG in man. *Trans. Amer. Neurol. Assoc.*, **89**, 151–156.

MEYER, J. S., GOTOH, F., NARA, M. AND HANDA, J. (1964 a) Recording cerebral blood flow and metabolism by electromagnetic, thermovelocity, local dilution, and arterio-venous difference methods. In: EICHHORN, O., LECHNER, H. AND AUELL, K. H. (Eds.), *Scientific and Clinical Research of the Cerebral Circulation*; *Proc. Salzburg Conference*, Verlag Brüder Hollinek, Wien.

MEYER, J. S., ISHIKAWA, S. AND LEE, T. K. (1964 b) Electromagnetic measurements of internal jugular venous flow in the monkey. Effect of epilepsy and other procedures. *J. Neurosurg.*, **21**, 524–529.

MEYER, J. S., LAVY, S., ISHIKAWA, S. AND SYMON, L. (1964 c) Effects of drugs and brain metabolism on internal carotid flow. An electromagnetic flow meter study in the monkey. *Amer. J. Med. Electron.*, **3**, 169–180.

MEYER, J. S., GOTOH, F. AND FAVALE, E. (1965 a) Cerebral metabolism during epileptic seizures in man. *Trans. Amer. Neurol. Assoc.*, **90**, 23–29.

MEYER, J. S., GOTOH, F. AND FAVALE, E. (1965 b) Effects of carotid compression on cerebral metabolism and electroencephalogram. *Electroencephalog. Clin. Neurophysiol.*, **19**, 362–376.

MEYER, J. S., GOTOH, F., GILROY, J. AND NARA, M. (1965 c) Improvement in brain oxygenation and clinical improvement in patients with strokes treated with papaverine hydrochloride. *J. Amer. Med. Assoc.*, **194**, 957–961.

MEYER, J. S., HANDA, J., HUBER, P. AND YOSHIDA, K. (1965 d) Effect of hypotension on internal and external carotid blood flow. Demonstration of a homeostatic mechanism peculiar to cerebral vessels and its importance in cerebrovascular occlusion. *J. Neurosurg.*, **23**, 191–198.

MEYER, J. S., GOTOH, F. AND FAVALE, E. (1966 a) Cerebral metabolism during epileptic seizures in man. *Electroencephalog. Clin. Neurophysiol.*, **21**, 10–22.

MEYER, J. S., GOTOH, F. AND TOMITA, M. (1966 b) Cerebral metabolism during arousal and mental activity in stroke patients. *J. Amer. Geriat. Soc.*, **14**, 986–1012.

MEYER, J. S., GOTOH, F., TOMITA, M. AND AKIYAMA, M. (1966 c) New techniques for recording cerebral blood flow and metabolism in subjects with cerebrovascular disease. In: MILLIKAN, C. H., SIEKERT, R. G. AND WHISNANT, J. P. (Eds.), *Cerebral Vascular Diseases*; *Proc. Fifth Princeton Conference*, Grune & Stratton, New York, p. 197.

MEYER, J. S., HERNDON, R. M., JOHNSON, J. F. AND BARNHART, M. (1966 d) Treatment of cerebrovascular thrombosis with plasmin and plasminogen activators. In: MILLIKAN, C. H. (Ed.), *Cerebrovascular Disease*, *Proc. Assoc. Res. Nervous Mental Disease*, Williams and Wilkins, Baltimore, p. 373.

MEYER, J. S. AND HANDA, J. (1967) Cerebral blood flow and metabolism during experimental hyperthermia. *Minn. Med.*, **50**, 37–44.

MEYER, J. S., GOTOH, F., AKIYAMA, M. AND YOSHITAKE, S. (1967 a) Monitoring cerebral blood flow, oxygen and glucose metabolism. Analysis of cerebral metabolic disorder in stroke and some therapeutic trials in human volunteers. *Circulation*, **36**, 197–211.

MEYER, J. S., GOTOH, F., AKIYAMA, M. AND YOSHITAKE, S. (1967 b) Monitoring cerebral blood flow, oxygen, glucose, lactate and ammonia metabolism. Experimental trials in animals. *Circulation Res.*, **21**, 649–660.

MEYER, J. S., GOTOH, F., AKIYAMA, M. AND YOSHITAKE, S. (1967 c) Automatic recording of cerebral blood flow by nitrous oxide inhalation without blood loss. *Neurology*, **17**, 838–853.

MEYER, J. S., GOTOH, F. AND TAKAGI, Y. (1967 d) Inhalation of oxygen and carbon dioxide. Effect on composition of cerebral venous blood. *Arch. Internal Med.*, **119**, 4–15.

MEYER, J. S., SAKAMOTO, K., AKIYAMA, M., YOSHIDA, K. AND YOSHITAKE, S. (1967 e) Monitoring cerebral blood flow, metabolism, and EEG. *Electroencephalog. Clin. Neurophysiol.*, **23**, 497–508.

MEYER, J. S., SAWADA, T., KITAMURA, A. AND TOYODA, M. (1967 f) Improved cerebral blood flow after control of hypertension in stroke. *Trans. Amer. Neurol. Assoc.*, **92**, 79–84.

MEYER, J. S., YOSHIDA, K. AND SAKAMOTO, K. (1967 g) Autonomic control of cerebral blood flow measured by electromagnetic flowmeters. *Neurology*, **17**, 638–648.

MEYER, J. S. (1968) The nature of high oxygen tensions in bordering zones of cerebral ischemia. *Scand. J. Clin. Lab. Invest.*, *Suppl.* **102**, XVI: A.

MEYER, J. S. AND GILROY, J. (1968) Regulation and adjustment of the cerebral circulation. *Diseases Chest*, **53**, 30–40.

MEYER, J. S., SAWADA, T., KITAMURA, A. AND TOYODA, M. (1968 a) Cerebral blood flow after control of hypertension in stroke. *Neurology*, **18**, 772–781.

MEYER, J. S., SAWADA, T., KITAMURA, A. AND TOYODA, M. (1968 b) Cerebral oxygen, glucose, lactate, and pyruvate metabolism in stroke. Therapeutic considerations. *Circulation*, **37**, 1036–1048.

MEYER, J. S., TOYODA, M., SHINOHARA, Y., KITAMURA, A., RYU, T., WIEDERHOLT, I. AND GUIRAUD, B. (1968 c) Regional cerebral blood flow (carotid perfusion) measured by clearance of hydrogen from cerebral venous blood. *Trans. Amer. Neurol. Assoc.*, **93**, 246–248.

MEYER, J. S., NOMURA, F., SAKAMOTO, K. AND KONDO, A. (1969 a) Effect of stimulation of the brainstem reticular formation on cerebral blood flow and oxygen consumption. *Electroencephalog. Clin. Neurophysiol.*, **26**, 125–132.

MEYER, J. S., RYU, T., TOYODA, M., SHINOHARA, Y., WIEDERHOLT, I. AND GUIRAUD, B. (1969 b) Evidence for a Pasteur effect regulating cerebral oxygen and carbohydrate metabolism in man. *Neurology*, **19**, 954–962.

MEYER, J. S., SHINOHARA, Y., KANDA, T., FUKUUCHI, Y., ERICSSON, A. AND RODPRASERT, P. (1969 c) Hemispheric blood flow and metabolism in neurological disease – a note on the metabolic accompaniments of diaschisis. *Trans. Amer. Neurol. Assoc.*, **94**, 304–307.

MEYER, J. S., WIEDERHOLT, I. C., TOYODA, M., RYU, T., SHINOHARA, Y. AND GUIRAUD, B. (1969 d) A new method for continuous sampling of cerebral venous blood without extracranial contamination in man. Bilateral transbrachial catheterization of the cerebral venous sinuses, *Neurology*, **19**, 353–358.

MEYER, J. S. (1970) Newer concepts of cerebral vascular disease. *Med. Clin. N. Amer.*, **54**, 349–360.

MEYER, J. S. AND ERICSSON, A. D. (1970) Diagnosis and prevention of acute stroke. *Sandoz Panorama*, 4–8.

MEYER, J. S., KANDA, T., SHINOHARA, Y. AND FUKUUCHI, Y. (1970 a) Changes in cerebrospinal fluid sodium and potassium concentrations during seizure activity. *Neurology*, **20**, 1179–1184.

MEYER, J. S., KANDA, T., SHINOHARA, Y., FUKUUCHI, Y., ERICSSON, A. D. AND KOK, N. (1970 b) Effects of Hexobendine on cerebral blood flow and metabolism in cerebrovascular disease. *Neurology*, **20**, 375 (abstr.).

MEYER, J. S., KONDO, A.. NOMURA, F., SAKAMOTO, K. AND TERAURA, T. (1970 c) Cerebral hemo-dynamics and metabolism following experimental head injury. *J. Neurosurg.*, **32**, 304–319.

MEYER, J. S., KONDO, A., SZEWCZYKOWSKI, J., NOMURA, F. AND TERAURA, T. (1970 d) The effects of a new drug (Hexobendine) on cerebral hemodynamics and oxygen consumption. *J. Neurol. Sci.*, **11**, 137–145.

MEYER, J. S., SHINOHARA, Y., KANDA, T., FUKUUCHI, Y., ERICSSON, A. D. AND KOK, N. K. (1970 e) Diaschisis resulting from acute unilateral cerebral infarction. Quantitative evidence for man. *Arch. Neurol.*, **23**, 241–247.

MEYER, J. S. AND SHINOHARA, Y. (1970) A method for measuring cerebral hemispheric blood flow and metabolism. *Stroke*, **1**, 419–431.

MEYER, J. S. AND TOYODA, M. (1971) Studies of rapid changes in cerebral circulation and metabolism during arousal and rapid eye movement sleep in human subjects with cerebrovascular disease. In: ZÜLCH, K. J. (Ed.), *Cerebral Circulation and Stroke*, Springer-Verlag, Heidelberg.

MEYER, J. S., FUKUUCHI, Y., KANDA, T. AND SHIMAZU, K. (1971, a) Interactions between cerebral metabolism and blood flow. In *Symposium on Regulation of CBF, London, 1970*.

MEYER, J. S., FUKUUCHI, Y., KANDA, T. AND SHIMAZU, K. (1971, b) Regional measurements of cerebral blood flow and metabolism using intracarotid injection of hydrogen, with comments on intracerebral steal. In: *Symposium on Regulation of CBF, London, 1970*.

MEYER, J. S., KANDA, T., SHINOHARA, Y., FUKUUCHI, Y., SHIMAZU, K., ERICSSON, A. D. AND GORDON, W. H., JR. (1971, c) Effect of Hexobendine on cerebral hemispheric blood flow and metabolism. Preliminary clinical observations concerning its use in ischemic cerebrovascular disease. *Neurology.* **21**, 691–702.

MEYER, J. S., TERAURA, T., SAKAMOTO, K. AND KONDO, A. (1971, d) Central neurogenic control, of cerebral blood flow. *Neurology.* **21**, 247–262.

MEYER, J. S. AND FIELDS, W. S. (in press) A controlled therapeutic trial of carotid endarterectomy versus nonsurgical treatment in occlusive cerebrovascular disease. Five-year follow-up of patients with transient neurologic deficit. In: MEYER, J. S., REIVICH, M., LECHNER, H. AND EICHHORN, O. (Eds.), *Research on the Cerebral Circulation*; *Fifth Intern. Salzburg Conference*, Charles C. Thomas, Springfield, Ill.

MOLNÁR, L. AND SZÁNTÓ, J. (1964) The effect of electrical stimulation of the bulbar vasomotor centre on the cerebral blood flow. *Quart. J. Exp. Physiol.*, **49**, 184–193.

MYERSON, A., HALLORAN, R. O. AND HIRSCH, H. L. (1927) Technique for obtaining blood from the internal jugular vein and internal carotid artery. *Arch. Neurol. Psychiat.*, **17**, 807.

NELSON, E. AND RENNELS, M. (1968) Electron microscopic studies on intracranial vascular nerves in the cat. *Scand. J. Clin. Lab. Invest.*, *Suppl.* **102**, VI: A.

PENFIELD, W., VONSANTHA, K. AND CIPRIANI, A. (1939) Cerebral blood flow during induced epilepti-form seizures in animals and man. *J. Neurophysiol.*, **2**, 257–267.

PEREZ-BORJA, C. AND MEYER, J. S. (1964) A critical evaluation of rheoencephalography in control subjects in proven cases of cerebrovascular disease. *J. Neurol. Neurosurg. Psychiat.*, **27**, 66–72.

PLUM, F., POSNER, J. B. AND TROY, B. (1968) Cerebral metabolic and circulatory responses to induced convulsions in animals. *Arch. Neurol.*, **18**, 1–13.

REIVICH, M., ISAACS, G., EVARTS, D. AND KETY, S. S. (1968) The effect of slow wave sleep and REM sleep on regional cerebral blood flow in cats. *J. Neurochem.*, **15**, 301–306.

REIVICH, M., JEHLE, J., SOKOLOFF, L. AND KETY, S. S. (1969) Measurement of regional cerebral blood flow with antipyrine-^{14}C in awake cats. *J. Appl. Physiol.*, **27**, 296–300.

ROY, C. S. AND SHERRINGTON, C. S. (1890) On the regulation of the blood-supply of the brain. *J. Physiol.*, **11**, 85–108.

SACKS, W. (1957) Cerebral metabolism of isotopic glucose in normal human subjects. *J. Appl. Physiol.*, **10**, 37–44.

SCHEINBERG, P. AND STEAD, E. A., JR. (1949) Cerebral blood flow in male subjects as measured by the nitrous oxide technique. Normal values for blood flow, oxygen utilization, glucose utilization and peripheral resistance, with observations on effect of tilting and anxiety. *J. Clin. Invest.*, **28**, 1163–1171.

SELDINGER, S. I. (1953) Catheter replacement of needle in percutaneous arteriography; new technique. *Acta Radiol.*, **39**, 368–376.

SHALIT, M. N., REINMUTH, O. M., SHIMOJYO, S. AND SCHEINBERG, P. (1969) A mechanism by which carbon dioxide influences cerebral circulation independent of a direct effect on vascular smooth muscle. In: MEYER, J. S., LECHNER, H. AND EICHHORN, O. (Eds.), *Research on the Cerebral Circula-*

tion; *Third Intern. Salzburg Conference*, Charles C. Thomas, Springfield, Ill., p. 173.

SHINOHARA. Y., MEYER, J. S., KITAMURA, A., TOYODA, M. AND RYU, T. (1969) Measurement of cerebral hemispheric blood flow by intracarotid injection of hydrogen gas. Validation of the method in the monkey. *Circulation Res.*, **25**, 735–745.

SKINHØJ, E. (1965) Bilateral depression of CBF in unilateral cerebral diseases. *Acta Neurol. Scand.*, **41**, *Suppl.* **14**, 161–163.

SOHLER, T. P., LOTHROP, G. N. AND FORBES, H. S. (1941) Pial circulation of normal, non-anesthetized animals; description of a method of observation. *J. Pharmacol. Exp. Therap.*, **71**, 325–330.

SOKOLOFF, L. (1959) The action of drugs on the cerebral circulation. *Pharmacol. Rev.*, **11**, 1–85.

SOLOWAY, M., NADEL, W., ALBIN, M. S. AND WHITE, R. S. (1968) The effect of hyperventilation on subsequent cerebral infarction. *Anesthesiology*, **29**, 975–980.

SPENCER, G. O., JR., CLARK, L. C. AND LYONS, C. (1961) Continuous analysis of blood nitrous oxide content. *Surg. Forum*, **12**, 138–142.

SULLIVAN, J. M., HARKEN, D. E. AND GORLIN, R. (1968) Pharmacologic control of thromboembolic complications of cardiac-valve replacement. *New Engl. J. Med.*, **279**, 576–580.

SYMON, L., ISHIKAWA, S. AND MEYER, J. S. (1963 a) Cerebral arterial pressure changes and development of leptomeningeal collateral circulation. *Neurology*, **13**, 237–250.

SYMON, L., ISHIKAWA, S., LAVY, S. AND MEYER, J. S. (1963 b) Quantitative measurement of cephalic blood flow in the monkey. A study of vascular occlusion in the neck using electromagnetic flowmeters. *J. Neurosurg.*, **20**, 199–218.

TECHNICON INSTRUMENT CORPORATION (1963) Technicon AutoAnalyzer Methodology: New Method File, N-206, Chauncey, New York.

TECHNICON INSTRUMENT CORPORATION (1968) Technicon AutoAnalyzer Methodology: New Method, N-20b, Chauncey, New York.

TOMITA, M., MEYER, J. S. AND GOTOH, F. (1949) Desaturation of hydrogen gas from human brain after inhalation. In: MEYER, J. S., LECHNER, H. AND EICHHORN, O. (Eds.), *Research on the Cerebral Circulation*; *Third Intern. Salzburg Conference*, Charles C. Thomas, Springfield, Ill., p. 145.

TERAURA, T., MEYER, J. S., SAKAMOTO, K., HASHI, K., MARX, P., STERMAN-MARINCHESCU, C. AND SHINMARU, S. (in press, a) Brain swelling due to experimental cerebral infarction. I. Hemodynamic and metabolic concomitants. *J. Neurosurg.*

TERAURA, T., MEYER, J. S., SAKAMOTO, K., HASHI, K., MARX, P., STERMAN-MARINCHESCU, C. AND SHINMARU, S. (in preparation, b) Brain swelling due to experimental cerebral infarction. II. Continuous measurements of chloride, DC potential, and a change in cerebral vessels to CO_2 inhalation and loss of autoregulation.

VON MONAKOW, C. (1914) *Die Lokalisation im Grosshirn und der Abbau der Funktion durch korticale Herde*, J. F. Bergmann, Wiesbaden, Germany, p. 26.

WAHL, M., DEETJEN, P., THURAU, K., INGVAR, D. H. AND LASSEN, N. A. (1970) Micropuncture evaluation of the importance of perivascular pH for the arteriolar diameter on the brain surface. *Pflügers Arch.*, **316**, 152–163.

WALTZ, A. G. AND MEYER, J. S. (1959) Effects of changes in composition of plasma on pial blood flow. II. High molecular weight substances, blood constituents, and tonicity. *Neurology*, **8**, 815–825.

WALTZ, A. G. (1968) Regional cerebral blood flow: responses to changes in arterial blood pressure and CO_2 tension. In: TOOLE, J. F., SIEKERT, R. G. AND WHISNANT, J. P. (Eds.), *Cerebral Vascular Diseases*; *Proc. Sixth Princeton Conference*, Grune & Stratton, New York.

WELCH, K. M. A. AND MEYER, J. S. (1970) Control of cerebral blood flow (letter to the editor). *Lancet*, **ii**, 1316.

WESTERMAN, B. R. AND GLASS, H. I. (1968) Physical specification of gamma camera. *J. Nuclear Med.*, **9**, 24–30.

WOLFF, H. G. AND LENNOX, W. G. (1930) Cerebral circulation; effect on pial vessels of variations in oxygen and carbon dioxide content of blood. *Arch. Neurol. Psychiat.*, **23**, 1097–1120.

YOSHIDA, K., MEYER, J. S., SAKAMOTO, K. AND HANDA, J. (1966) Autoregulation of cerebral blood flow. Electromagnetic flow measurements during acute hypertension in the monkey. *Circulation Res.*, **19**, 726–738.

ZWETNOW, N. (1968) CBF autoregulation in blood pressure and intracranial pressure variations. *Scand. J. Clin. Lab. Invest.*, *Suppl.* **102**, V: A.

The Effects of Prolonged Anesthesia on the Cerebral Blood Flow in the Rabbit

J. C. DE VALOIS AND J. P. C. PEPERKAMP

Central Institute for Brain Research, Amsterdam (The Netherlands)

INTRODUCTION

General anesthetics exert their action on the central nervous system. The dependence of cerebral function on its blood supply makes an understanding of the influence of general anesthetics on cerebral blood flow (CBF) necessary. Although various reports on this subject have been published since 1960, some of the published results are at variance. As regards the barbiturates a generally accepted opinion has been reached. Barbiturate anesthesia depresses cerebral metabolism in proportion to the depth of anesthesia. The cerebral blood flow follows these changes in metabolic rate, so that the greatest reduction in CBF occurs along with the deepest anesthesia (McDowall, 1965). The time course of CBF changes during barbiturate anesthesia has not been the subject of many investigations. Most authors confine themselves to one or two CBF determinations during anesthesia. By using manifold CBF determinations over periods of 5–6 hours we have studied the effects of a single dose of barbiturates on CBF. In this way we may be able to determine the relationship between depth of anesthesia and reduction of CBF.

Data on the effect of neuroleptanalgesia on the cerebral circulation are sparse. A thorough investigation has been performed by Kreuscher (1967), who found a reduction of CBF and cerebral metabolism after the simultaneous intravenous injection of droperidol (0.28 mg/kg) and fentanyl (0.007 mg/kg) in the dog. Long term changes in these conditions were not studied. Whether the reduction in CBF was caused by droperidol or by fentanyl is not clear.

Freeman and Ingvar (1967) showed that fentanyl increased cortical blood flow in the unanesthetized cat depending on the dosage (0.005–0.02 mg/kg). As a contribution to this problem we studied the effect of fluonisone and fentanyl (10 mg and 0.2 mg/kg resp.) on the central circulation by repetitive CBF measurements.

Also concerning the effect of halothane on CBF some conflicting reports have been published. There is a tendency to attribute vasodilatory influence to halothane in respect to the cerebral circulation (Christensen *et al.*, 1967; McDowall, 1967 a).

In reviewing the current literature on this subject it became evident that marked differences exists in the experimental procedures. Most investigators use some kind of premedication or supplementary drugs, and halothane is frequently vaporized in

References pp. 362–363

a nitrous oxide–oxygen mixture. The number of CBF determinations is usually limited. We performed our CBF studies under standardized conditions with two purposes in mind, firstly to determine the effect of halothane on cerebral haemodynamics and secondly to study the effect of a combination of nitrous oxide and halothane on cerebral blood flow. A control series of experiments was performed to detect long term changes in CBF in unanesthetized animals.

MATERIAL AND METHODS

The experiments were performed on adult rabbits (Alaska F_1 bastards) weighing about 2500 g. The animals were obtained from "TNO Centraal Proefdierenbedrijf" at Zeist.

In order to minimize the effects of surgery on the cerebral circulation, a thin polyethylene catheter (outer diameter 0.6 mm) was implanted into one of the internal carotid arteries, one day prior to the CBF measurements. This implantation was performed under neuroleptanalgesia using Hypnorm[R] i.m. (Philips Duphar), containing 10 mg fluonisone and 0.2 mg fentanyl per ml. The right internal carotid artery was exposed and canulated. The canula was guided subcutaneously towards the skin of the neck of the animal, where the skin was perforated leaving the canula 1–2 cm outside. In this way, displacements of the canula by movements of the animal were prevented and an easy access to the cerebral circulatory system was obtained. The canula was filled with saline containing 500 I.U. of heparin per ml, and sealed with a stainless steel plug. The whole procedure lasted about 20 min, and the animals could then recover for about 18 h. Although the right internal carotid artery was occluded by this procedure no motor disturbances were observed during the recovery period and also the EEG of the animals showed no signs of cerebral ischaemia. A quantitative histological investigation of the diameter of the internal carotid artery and the vertebral artery showed that in the rabbit the former is about twice as small as the latter. Occlusion of one of the internal carotid arteries is therefore assumed to have little or no effect on CBF in this species.

CBF was measured by the intra-arterial isotope clearance technique of Ingvar and Lassen (1962). The isotope employed was [85]Krypton (obtained from Philips Duphar), the gamma emissions of which were counted by a scintillation detector mounted above the intact skull of the animal. 0.1–0.4 ml of saline containing 1 mC [85]Kr/ml was injected into the internal carotid artery. Injection time was less than 10 sec. The total counting time was 15 min. The measured γ activity was fed into a pulse height analyser and thereafter into an integrator in which the count rate per 10 sec was stored and punched on paper tape. Analysis of the experimental curve was performed with an IBM-1130 computer using a two-compartmental least squares best fit method (De Valois et al., 1970). In this way the mean CBF and the flow through a fast ("fast flow") and a slow ("slow flow") perfused compartment was calculated in ml/100 g/min. The relative weights of the fast and slow perfused compartments were also determined. Cerebral vascular resistance (CVR) was calculated for whole brain and the two respective compartments as the ratio of mean arterial pressure and cerebral blood flow as expressed in peripheral resistance units (PRU).

The following series of experiments were performed. (The number of animals used for each series is placed between brackets).

A. Control group. No anesthesia is given, in order to detect changes in CBF that might occur spontaneously over a long period of time ($n = 9$).

B. Barbiturate anesthesia. After two control measurements Kemithal[R] (100 mg/kg, ICI) ($n = 8$) or Nembutal[R] (25 mg/kg, Abott) ($n = 9$) were given intravenously.

C. Neuroleptanalgesia. After two control measurements Hypnorm[R] (Philips Duphar) was given intramuscularly (1 ml/kg). Hypnorm contains 10 mg fluonison and 0.2 mg fentanyl per ml ($n = 8$).

D. Volatile anesthetics. This series included unsupplemented halothane ($\frac{1}{2}\%$) anesthesia ($n = 10$), a series in which halothane ($\frac{1}{2}\%$) was added to a nitrous oxide–oxygen mixture (70% N_2O and 30% O_2) (Vol I series, $n = 9$), and a series in which halothane ($\frac{1}{2}\%$) was added to a nitrous oxide–oxygen mixture in the course of anesthesia at the end of which nitrous oxide was withdrawn from the anesthetic mixture (Vol II series, $n = 9$). Halothane was delivered from a calibrated halothane vaporizer (Vapor-Dräger).

In the series A, B and C, all animals were breathing spontaneously. To prevent undesired movement they were kept in a special animal holder. In the series D all animals were intubated using the technique of Hoge *et al.* (1969) and after muscle relaxation with Muscuryl[R] (Povite, containing 20 mg of succinyl choline per ml) connected to an electronic respirator based on intermittent positive pressure in a non-return circuit. End tidal P_{CO_2} was measured with an infrared gas analyser (Beckman LB1) in order to adjust the respirator to obtain normocapnia.

In all experiments the femoral artery was canulated under local anesthesia using Xylocaine 2%. In this way blood pressure could be measured and arterial blood samples could be obtained. Blood samples were analysed for pH, P_{CO_2}, standard bicarbonate, buffer base and base excess with the Astrup apparatus (Radiometer). The EEG was continuously monitored from 2-pin electrodes placed over the sensori-motor cortex. Rectal temperature was monitored continuously and heating was supplied if necessary to maintain constant body temperature. After these initial procedures followed by a rest period of about $\frac{1}{2}$ hour, the first control measurement was performed. Fig. 1 shows the time relationship of the individual CBF determina-

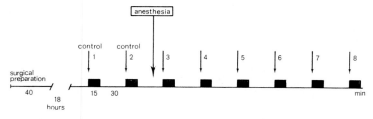

Fig. 1. Schematic representation of the experimental set up. 18 h before the CBF determinations the internal carotid artery was canulated. After two control measurements anesthesia was induced. In general 8 CBF measurements were performed in each animal. The time between two determinations is 30 min, while the determination lasts 15 min.

References pp. 362–363

tions. During each CBF measurement mean arterial blood pressure was registered and an arterial sample was taken. In total 62 animals were used for this study in which more than 500 CBF determinations were performed.

Statistical procedures

The data for each anesthetic were tested for normality by determining skewness and kurtosis.

Outlying observations were omitted when the values differed more than 2.88 times the standard deviation from the total population mean. For each variable a two-level

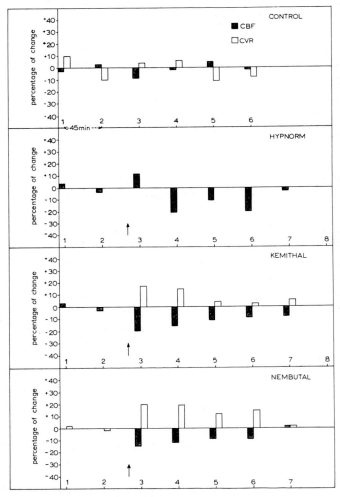

Fig. 2. CBF and CVR changes during anesthesia. CBF and CVR are expressed as the percentage of the mean values of the control values. The results are shown for the neuroleptic agent hypnorm and for the barbiturates kemithal and nembutal. The arrow indicates the onset of anesthesia.

nested analysis of variance was performed and for each variable in each group averages were calculated and plotted as a function of time. The averages were tested for homogeneity ($p < 0.05$) by means of a sum of squares simultaneous test procedure (Gabriel, 1964). All computations were carried out on an IBM-1130 computer. Mean values are given $\pm$ standard error of the mean.

RESULTS

The mean cerebral blood flow in response to various anesthetics as a function of time is demonstrated in Figs. 2 and 3. Absolute flow values, cerebrovascular resistance and

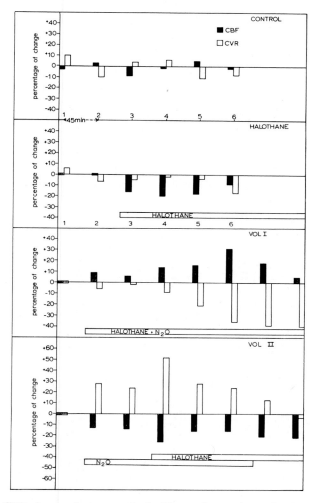

Fig. 3. CBF and CVR changes during anesthesia. The results are shown for the volatile anesthetics halothane and nitrous oxide. The horizontal bar indicates the onset of anesthesia and the anesthetic mixture used.

References pp. 362–363

TABLE 1

ABSOLUTE FLOW VALUES, CEREBROVASCULAR RESISTANCE AND CO_2 PRESSURE DURING PROLONGED ANESTHESIA

Series		1	2	3	4	5	6	7	8
Control (n = 9)	CBF	48.7 ± 4.7	52.2 ± 2.9	45.7 ± 2.1*	49.2 ± 2.3	53.0 ± 3.3	49.1 ± 3.7		
	CVR	2.23 ± 0.24	1.87 ± 0.09	2.13 ± 0.08	2.17 ± 0.09	1.80 ± 0.16	1.89 ± 0.18		
	P_{CO_2}	28.8 ± 1.46	27.6 ± 1.08	23.2 ± 1.59	21.6 ± 1.01	20.7 ± 1.70	23.0 ± 1.67		
Kemital[R] (n = 8)	CBF	52.0 ± 4.3	49.0 ± 4.3	40.4 ± 1.6*	42.1 ± 2.8*	44.4 ± 2.5	45.5 ± 4.3	46.1 ± 3.4	
	CVR	1.98 ± 0.19	1.99 ± 0.13	2.32 ± 0.12	2.28 ± 0.18	2.06 ± 0.09	2.14 ± 0.17	2.10 ± 0.15	
	P_{CO_2}	33.9 ± 2.6	34.1 ± 2.6	34.7 ± 2.7	29.4 ± 1.4	31.8 ± 1.8	33.6 ± 2.8	32.2 ± 3.1	
Nembutal[R] (n = 9)	CBF	44.8 ± 2.5	45.6 ± 2.9	38.3 ± 2.1*	39.7 ± 1.7*	41.0 ± 1.9	40.8 ± 3.1	45.8 ± 3.8	
	CVR	2.22 ± 0.16	2.14 ± 0.15	2.62 ± 0.14	2.59 ± 0.12	2.44 ± 0.14	2.51 ± 0.24	2.23 ± 0.28	
	P_{CO_2}	32.9 ± 2.2	33.6 ± 2.0	38.6 ± 2.1	37.8 ± 3.1	35.7 ± 1.6	38.3 ± 1.7	33.4 ± 2.2	
Hypnorm[R] (n = 8)	CBF	48.8 ± 4.3	45.7 ± 1.8	52.7 ± 4.2*	40.9 ± 2.3*	42.0 ± 2.7*	41.0 ± 4.0*	45.9 ± 4.6	
	CVR								
	P_{CO_2}	33.2 ± 2.1	33.1 ± 2.1	41.6 ± 2.0	38.4 ± 1.8	37.2 ± 1.9	37.9 ± 1.6	36.3 ± 1.9	
Halothane[R] (n = 10)	CBF	50.4 ± 7.0	50.5 ± 3.4	42.1 ± 2.7*	40.0 ± 1.5*	40.8 ± 2.7*	45.6 ± 2.7		
	CVR	2.40 ± 0.44	2.11 ± 0.13	2.15 ± 0.16	2.21 ± 0.08	2.17 ± 0.16	1.87 ± 0.12		
	P_{CO_2}	30.4 ± 1.7	34.0 ± 1.6	32.2 ± 1.6	35.6 ± 2.7	35.4 ± 2.2	35.9 ± 2.4		
Vol I (n = 9)	CBF	43.4 ± 3.6	47.4 ± 3.5	45.8 ± 3.3	49.2 ± 5.3	50.5 ± 4.5*	56.3 ± 2.8*	51.8 ± 3.2*	45.1 ± 4.3
	CVR	2.40 ± 0.20	2.26 ± 0.15	2.35 ± 0.15	2.17 ± 0.22	1.91 ± 0.19	1.54 ± 0.07	1.46 ± 0.07	1.44 ± 0.12
	P_{CO_2}	32.8 ± 2.6	34.9 ± 3.3	33.4 ± 3.2	34.6 ± 2.9	36.4 ± 1.4	38.2 ± 1.5	37.4 ± 1.4	37.8 ± 2.5
Vol II (n = 9)	CBF	56.5 ± 4.1	49.0 ± 3.2	48.6 ± 2.0	41.9 ± 4.1*	47.5 ± 6.0	47.4 ± 4.6	44.8 ± 3.6	44.4 ± 2.4
	CVR	1.76 ± 0.11	2.09 ± 0.28	2.18 ± 0.12	2.67 ± 0.31	2.25 ± 0.32	2.16 ± 0.32	1.99 ± 0.32	1.70 ± 0.24
	P_{CO_2}	36.7 ± 2.0	41.1 ± 4.6	40.4 ± 4.2	44.1 ± 3.9	42.2 ± 3.2	39.2 ± 3.7	43.0 ± 2.4	44.6 ± 4.8

* $p < 0.05$

P_{CO_2} during prolonged anesthesia are shown in Table 1. The mean arterial blood pressure never fell below 70 mm Hg except for the kemithal series.

After the intravenous injection of 100 mg kemithal a sharp decline in blood pressure was observed to values around 30 mm Hg, which lasted about 1 min. By the time of the CBF determinations the mean arterial blood pressure had always reached the preanesthetic level. The temperature of all animals was kept within fairly narrow limits, the average being $39.1 \pm 0.1\,°C$.

A. Changes in blood flow in unanesthetized animals

Within a period of about 5 h the CBF remained fairly constant despite marked variations in arterial CO_2 tension. The changes in CBF and CVR observed in the control series were less than 10% of the control value. The mean value of the first and second CBF determination was arbitrarily taken as the 100% level. The third CBF value was the lowest and reached statistical significance ($p = 0.05$), without any demonstrable cause. The P_{CO_2} values of the control group were significantly lower than any of the P_{CO_2} values of the other series ($p < 0.01$). This is probably due to profound hyperventilation of unanesthetized but obviously restrained animals. In a comparison of CBF values and P_{CO_2} values of the control group with a group consisting of the first (preanesthetic) control values of the series B, C, and D the mean

TABLE 2

COMPARATIVE VALUES IN THE VARIOUS GROUPS

	CBF	MABP	CVR	P_{CO_2}
Control values series A	50 ± 1.4	98 ± 1.4	2.0 ± 0.03	24.4 ± 9.7
Control values of series B, C and D	49 ± 1.8	99 ± 1.3	2.15 ± 0.11	33.4 ± 0.6

values shown in Table 2 were obtained. There are no significant differences between these two groups for any of the parameters reported in Table 2 except P_{CO_2} ($p < 0.01$). We must conclude that the stress of the experimental condition increases CBF, in this way counteracting the vasoconstrictor effect of low P_{CO_2}.

B, C. Changes in blood flow in anesthetized animals (non-volatile anesthetics)

In these groups kemithal, nembutal and hypnorm were used as representatives of barbiturates and neuroleptanalgetics respectively. Although the clinical picture is quite different for each of these drugs in relation to the depth and duration of anesthesia, the CBF and CVR patterns are quite similar.

After induction of anesthesia CBF decreased by 15–20%; the decrease was the least with nembutal. During anesthesia CBF gradually increases to reach the pre-

self evident that anesthesia in general goes along with a reduction in CBF and also with a reduction in the relative weight of the fast perfused compartment. In the control series no significant changes were observed in the relative weights while in the Vol. I series the increase in CBF was coupled to an increase in the relative weight of the fast perfused compartment. This relationship (see Fig. 6) between CBF and relative weight has already been described in another series of experiments (De Valois and Peperkamp, 1971). These observations make it very difficult to draw conclusions from the flow values from any of these compartments alone.

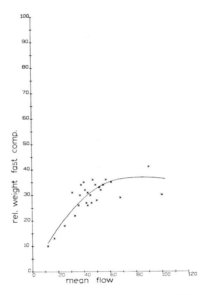

Fig. 6. Relative weight of the "fast" compartment as a function of the mean blood flow. Up to values of 30–40 ml/100 g/min the relative weight of the "fast" compartment increases proportionally with flow, at higher flow values the relative weights remain rather constant.

DISCUSSION

The measurement of CBF with the inert radioactive isotopes like [85]Krypton and [133]Xenon according to the technique of Ingvar and Lassen (1962) has many advantages. One of the disadvantages, however, is the discontinuity of CBF measurements! The determinations last about 15 min requiring a steady state during this period. In general, individual CBF measurements must be spaced at least 30 min to obtain reasonably low background activity. For these reasons it is impossible to detect fast changes in CBF.

The control experiments were carried out in unanesthetized non-curarized rabbits. It turns out to be very difficult to immobilize rabbits for long periods of time without undue stress. This is also reflected in a very low arterial P_{CO_2} value attributable to severe hyperventilation. Low P_{CO_2} values do not cause the cerebral blood flow to approach minimal values in the rabbit as could be expected (Wollman et al., 1965).

It is obvious that stress plays an important role in the regulation of CBF. In the other experiments much of this stress was relieved by the use of anesthetics. Another important factor in establishing the influence of CO_2 on CBF is the unfamiliarity with the normal P_{CO_2} in the rabbit. In a series of 30 animals we found a value of 31.3 ± 0.96 mm Hg. Arterial blood flow was sampled from the central ear arteries within 5 min after the animals were taken from their cage. Evidently even this type of handling leads to hyperventilation. The factors mentioned above made us decide that a correction of CBF for P_{CO_2} is not justifiable in this species. (Notwithstanding all this we have also corrected our CBF data to a standard P_{CO_2} of 36 mm Hg. These "standard" CBF values did not change our conclusions significantly.) The control series give above all an insight in the stability of CBF over a period of several hours. In these experiments spontaneous fluctuations of 5–10% were observed, without any trend or tendency to decrease in the course of the study.

The barbiturates

Thialbarbitone and pentobarbitone cause a reduction of CBF of about 20% for a period of at least 3 h duration. There were no significant differences between the two barbiturates in either decrease of CBF or duration of this effect. It is a well known fact, however, that thialbarbitone is a short-acting anesthetic drug in comparison to pentobarbitone. This divergence between anesthetic effect and the reduction of CBF is an interesting phenomenon not yet reported in the literature. It must be stressed that this observation has clinical importance.

Any premedication with barbiturates might very well give rise to a prolonged reduction of cerebral blood flow. Most investigators are not aware of the prolonged effects of additional drugs (see also Table 3). The decrease in CBF after a single dose of these barbiturates is in accordance with the literature (Sokoloff, 1963; Pierce *et al.*, 1962; McDowall, 1965). The absolute value of the reduction is not very relevant. It is dependent on the amount given, the time of CBF measurements and the variations in CBF under normal conscious conditions.

Neuroleptanalgesia

Hypnorm is composed of fentanyl (0.2 mg/ml) and fluonisone (10 mg/ml). Fluonisone belongs to the *butyrophenon* group like haloperidol and dehydrobenzperidol. In our experiments the cerebral blood flow decreased by about 20% for a duration of several hours, which is about the same as observed during barbiturate anesthesia. The initial increase in CBF after the intramuscular injection of hypnorm (1 ml/kg) can easily be explained by the concomitant hypoventilation resulting in an increase in arterial P_{CO_2} from 33 to 41 mm Hg. Defective blood pressure transducers were the reason that no blood pressure readings and subsequent CVR calculations could be performed. The changes in CBF after injection of this neuroleptanalgetic agent are in accordance with the observations of Kreuscher (1967) and Fitch *et al.* (1969) with the combination of droperidol and fentanyl.

References pp. 362–363

TABLE 3

RESULTS OBTAINED BY VARIOUS AUTHORS AND METHODS

Literature	Technique	Species	Anesthesia	% Change of CBF	Statistical significance
Galindo and Baldwin (1963)	Electromagnetic flow meter	dog	Premedication: Thiobarbitone Anesthesia: Halothane	+ 26.8	$p < 0.20$
Wollman et al. (1964)	85Krypton Inhalation method	man	No premedication: Anesthesia: Halothane 1.2%	+ 15%	$p < 0.10$
Schmahl (1965)	Local heat clearance	cat	Premedication: ? Anesthesia: Halothane 1.9%	+	?
Christensen et al. (1965)	85Krypton or 133Xenon injection method	man	No premedication Anesthesia: Halothane 1%	− 21%	$p < 0.05$
Christensen et al. (1967)	85Krypton inhalation and 133Xenon injection method	man	No premedication Anesthesia: Halothane 1%	+ 27%	$p < 0.02$
McHenry et al. (1965)	85Krypton inhalation method	man	Premedication: Thiobarbitone Anesthesia: $N_2O + O_2$ + Halothane 1%	+ 55%	
McDowall and Harper (1965)	85Krypton injection method	dog	Premedication: Thiobarbitone Anesthesia: $N_2O + O_2$ + Halotane ½%	− 20%	$p < 0.05$
McDowall (1967 a, b)	85Krypton injection method	dog	Premedication: Thiobarbitone Anesthesia: $N_2O + O_2$ + Halothane ½% (2%, 4%)	+ 20%	$p < 0.05$
Kreuscher and Grote (1969	Cardiogreen dye dilution method	dog	Premedication: Epontal Anesthesia: $N_2O + O_2$ + Halothane	− 45%	?
Pichlmayr et al. (1970)	133Xenon injection method	dog	Premedication: Methohexital Anesthesia: $N_2O + O_2$ + Halothane ½%	no change	—
De Valois and Peperkamp (present study)	85Krypton injection method	rabbit	No premedication Anesthesia: Halothane ½%	− 20%	< 0.05
De Valois and Peperkamp (present study)	85Krypton injection method	rabbit	No premedication Anesthesia: $N_2O + O_2$ + Halothane ½%	+ 15%	< 0.05

The analgetic effect of hypnorm, mediated by fentanyl, lasts for about 30 min while the neuroleptic action of fluonisone can be observed for several hours. None of the afore-mentioned authors are conclusive in attributing the CBF depression to either fentanyl or droperidol, although Fitch *et al.* (1969) refer to the paper of Freeman and Ingvar (1967) in which only fentanyl is studied in the cat. In these experiments fentanyl was given in a dose of 0.005–0.01 mg/kg thus in much lower concentrations than used in neuroleptanalgesia. Freeman and Ingvar found an increase in cortical blood flow with increasing dosage of fentanyl in animals under local anesthesia. These contradictory results might be explained by assuming that the butyrophenons (droperidol, fluonisone) have a depressing action on CBF, which might be demonstrated by the long duration of the CBF depression in our experiments. Species differences might also play a role, since it is a well known fact that the cat reacts to morphine and morphine-like compounds in an excitatory way. More work will be required to elucidate the effect of both drugs mentioned.

The volatile agents

In our experiments nitrous oxide and halothane were used, both separately and in combination. As regards their influence on CBF the reports in the literature are at variance. Table 3 shows the results of several investigators on the effect of halothane.

McDowall (1967 b) gives an excellent survey of the literature up to 1965. He came to the conclusion that "halothane is a cerebral vasodilator, the effect being small and short lived with 0.5% halothane but well marked with higher concentrations". From Table 3 it is obvious that the experimental conditions vary widely as does the anesthetic regime. In a few cases the effect of halothane alone was studied (Wollman *et al.*, 1964; Christensen *et al.*, 1965, 1967). In all other studies some kind of premedication was given or halothane was vaporized in a nitrous oxide–oxygen mixture.

In our experiments the individual variations of the animals have been minimised by always comparing observations in the same animal. Our results indicate that halothane even in a concentration of $\frac{1}{2}$% decreases cerebral blood flow at least in the normocapnic rabbit, although cerebral vascular resistance does not change significantly. In these experiments the blood pressure was allowed to fall (20%). Wollman *et al.* (1964) found an *increase* of 14% in normocapnic young man, anesthetized with 1.2% halothane, while Christensen *et al.* (1967) found an increase of 27% in *normotensive* and normocapnic young adults during halothane anesthesia (1%). McDowall (1967 b) formulated the following criticism on the publication of Wollman: "One further reservation that one might have about this carefully conducted study is some misgiving about the use of control values from a different group of subjects not studied at the same time, especially since there was in this study as in most others a considerable variation in cerebral blood flow under identical conditions".

About the same criticism can be put forward on the study of Christensen *et al.* (1967). Another important point in this study is the infusion of large amounts (approximately 1 l) of dextrose solutions in some cases to maintain normotension. Gottstein and Held (1969) have shown that the lowering of total blood viscosity leads to an increase in CBF in man. To our opinion a carefully guided clinical evaluation of the effect of unsupplemented halothane anesthesia remains necessary to decide whether halothane changes CBF, under conditions of normocapnia and normotension. In studying the combination of halothane and nitrous oxide we found an increase in CBF of 10-20% combined with a still greater decrease of CVR (up to 40%). These results agree well with the data shown in Table 3. Therefore we are inclined to conclude that the combination of halothane and nitrous oxide has vasodilating properties even when relatively low concentrations of halothane are employed. Whether this increase in flow is attributable to halothane, to nitrous oxide or to the combination of the two remains obscure. Wollman *et al.* (1965) have shown that CBF during nitrous oxide with oxygen anesthesia and normocapnia is very close to values obtained in unanesthetized man. In this study, however, barbiturates were used for the induction of anesthesia. McDowall and Harper (1965) have shown that nitrous oxide exhibits a slight vasodilatory action during steady light halothane anesthesia in the dog. We have tried to simulate these experiments of McDowall and Harper in the rabbit by adding and withdrawal of nitrous oxide or halothane from the anesthetic mixture (Vol. II series). Although these results are not conclusive they indicate an increase in CBF when halothane is added to nitrous oxide–oxygen anesthesia, and a fall in CBF when nitrous oxide is withdrawn from the anesthetic mixture. These experiments indicate that the combination of halothane and nitrous oxide has cerebral vasodilator properties. It is very difficult to detect how this potentiation of vasodilation by nitrous oxide and halothane is brought about. One explanation might be the so called "second gas" effect. When an anesthetic such as halothane (second gas) is administered with nitrous oxide (first gas) the rate of rise of the alveolar halothane is more rapid than when it is given alone (Stoelting and Eger, 1969). This effect explains our observation that halothane in low concentration (0.5%) without nitrous oxide does not show cerebrovasodilation until the sixth CBF determination. At the end of these experiments the alveolar halothane concentration was obviously high enough to cause some vasodilation and consequent increase in CBF. When halothane is added to nitrous oxide the alveolar halothane concentration rises much more rapidly, resulting in a more profound vasodilation.

In conclusion, we can endorse the view that halothane is a cerebral vasodilator. The effect is proportional to the concentration used. When hypotension can be avoided the decrease in CVR goes along with an increase in CBF. With very high concentrations (4%), however, mean arterial pressure decreases to levels which prevent any rise in CBF despite decreased CVR.

REFERENCES

CHRISTENSEN, M. S., HØEDT-RASMUSSEN, K. AND LASSEN, N. A. (1965) The cerebral blood flow during halothane anesthesia. Regional cerebral blood flow. *Acta Neurol. Scand., Suppl.* **14**, 152–155.

CHRISTENSEN, M. S., HØEDT-RASMUSSEN, K. AND LASSEN, N. A. (1967) Cerebral vasodilatation by halothane anesthesia in man and its potentiation by hypotension and hypercapnia. *Brit. J. Anaesthesia*, **39**, 927–933.

FITCH, W., BARKER, J., JENNETT, W. B. AND McDOWALL, D. G. (1969) The influence of neurolept analgesic drugs on cerebro spinal fluid pressure. *Brit. J. Anaesthesia*, **41**, 800–806.

FREEMAN, J. AND INGVAR, D. H. (1967) Effects of fentanyl on cerebral cortical blood flow and EEG in the cat. *Acta Anaesthesiol. Scand.*, 381–391.

GABRIEL, K. R. (1964) A procedure for testing the homogeneity of all sets of means in analysis of variance. *Biometrics*, **20**, 459–477.

GALINDO, A. AND BALDWIN, M. (1963) Intracranial pressure and internal carotid blood flow during halothane anesthesia in the dog. *Anesthesiology*, **24**, 318–326.

GOTTSTEIN, U. AND HELD, K. (1969) The effects of hemodilution caused by low molecular weight dextran on human cerebral blood flow and metabolism. In: BROCK, M., FIESCHI, C., INGVAR, D. H., LASSEN, N. A. AND SCHÜRMANN, L. (Eds.), *Cerebral Blood Flow*, Springer, Berlin, p. 104.

HOGE, R. S., HODESSON, S., SNOW, I. B. AND WOOD, A. I. (1969) Intubation technique and methoxyflurane administration in rabbits. *Lab. Animals Care*, **19**, 593–595.

INGVAR, D. H. AND LASSEN, N. A. (1962) Regional blood flow of the cerebral cortex determined by Krypton-85. *Acta Physiol. Scand.*, **54**, 325–338.

KREUSCHER, H. (1967) *Die Hirndurchblutung unter Neuroleptanaesthesie*, Springer-Verlag Berlin, Heidelberg, New York.

KREUSCHER, H. AND GROTE, J. (1969) Die Hirndurchblutung und cerebrale Sauerstoff-Aufnahme in Narkose. In: BETZ, E. AND WÜLLENWEBER, R. (Eds.), *Pharmakologie der lokalen Gehirndurchblutung*, p. 120–125.

MCDOWALL, D. G. (1965) The effects of general anesthetics on cerebral blood flow and cerebral metabolism. *Brit. J. Anaesthesia*, **37**, 236–245.

MCDOWALL, D. G. (1967 a) The effects of clinical concentrations of halothane on the blood flow and oxygen uptake of the cerebral cortex. *Brit. J. Anaesthesia*, **39**, 186–196.

MCDOWALL, D. G. (1967 b) The influence of volatile anesthetic drugs on the blood flow and oxygen uptake of the cerebral cortex and on cerebrospinal fluid pressure. *Thesis, University of Edinburgh*, pp. 327.

MCDOWALL, D. G. AND HARPER, A. M. (1965) Blood flow and oxygen uptake of the cerebral cortex of the dog during anesthesia with different volatile agents. Regional cerebral blood flow. *Acta Neurol. Scand., Suppl.* **14**, 146–151.

MCHENRY, L. C., SLOCUM, H. C., BIVENS, H. E., MAYES, H. A. AND HAYES, G. J. (1965) Hyperventilation in awake and anesthetized man. *Arch. Neurology*, **12**, 270–277.

PICHLMAYR, I., EICHENLAUB, D., KEIL-KURI, E. AND KLEMM, J. (1970) Veränderungen der Hirnrindedurchblutung unter Thiopental, Halothan und Fentanyl-Droperidol. *Der Anaesthesist*, **19**, 202–204.

PIERCE, E. C., LAMBERTSEN, C. J., DEUTSCH, S., CHASE, P. E., LINDE, H. W., DRIPPS, R. D. AND PRICE, H. L. (1962) Cerebral circulation and metabolism during thiopental anesthesia and hyperventilation in man. *J. Clin. Invest.*, **41**, 1664.

SCHMAHL, F. W. (1965) Effects of anesthetics on regional cerebral blood flow and the regional content of some metabolites of the brain cortex of the cat. Regional cerebral blood flow. *Acta Neurol. Scand., Suppl.* **14**, 156–159.

SOKOLOFF, L. (1963) Control of cerebral blood flow: The effects of anesthetic agents. In: PAPPER, E. M. AND KITZ, R. J. (Eds.), *Uptake and Distribution of Anesthetic Agents*, p. 140–157.

STOELTING, R. K. AND EGER, E. I. (1969) An additional explanation for the Second Gas effect: A concentrating effect. *Anesthesiology*, **30**, 273–277.

DE VALOIS, J. C., SMITH, J. AND PEPERKAMP, J. P. C. (1970) A computer program for the determination of cerebral blood flow using the Kr-85 or Xe-133 intra-arterial injection method. In: SCHADÉ, J. P. AND SMITH, J. (Eds.), *Progress in Brain Research*, Vol. **33**, Elsevier, Amsterdam.

DE VALOIS, J. C. AND PEPERKAMP, J. P. C. (1971) The influence of some drugs upon the regulation of cerebral blood flow in the rabbit. In: ROSS RUSSELL, R. W. (Ed.), *Proc. 4th Intern. Symp. on the regulation of CBF*, London, 1970. Pitman, London.

WOLLMAN, H., ALEXANDER, S. C., COHEN, P. J., CHASE, P. E., MELMAN, E. AND BEHAR, M. G. (1964) Cerebral circulation of man during halothane anesthesia. *Anesthesiology*, **25**, 180–184.

WOLLMAN, H., ALEXANDER, S. C., COHEN, P. J., SMITH, TH. C., CHASE, P. E. AND VAN DER MOLEN, R. A. (1965) Cerebral circulation during general anesthesia and hyperventilation in man. *Anesthesiology*, **26**, 329–334.

heart and lung before it reaches the brain (and only 10–20% of it will be distributed to the head) it has been found that it arrives there in a more compact form if the injectate is suddenly released into the circulation; this is achieved by having an arm cuff obstructing venous return during the injection, and then suddenly releasing it. Even using this method the indicator is streamed out, and enters the brain over a 10–14 second period, which is considerably longer than the normal circulation time; as a consequence not all of the indicator is in the brain at any one time, some having already left before the last of it has arrived.

The changing amount of radioactivity in the head is measured using one or more gamma ray detectors which consist of sodium iodide crystal photomultiplier systems suitably collimated. The count rate begins to rise some 7–9 seconds after release of the indicator into the arm vein, and as the most concentrated part of the bolus enters the counting field the maximum rate of rise will be recorded. As isotope leaves the head the count rate falls, but less crisply than it rose on entry; indeed it does not fall to the previous baseline because further indicator is arriving after circulation round the rest of the body. If the primary curve obtained (by processing through amplifier, pulse height analyser, rate meter and chart recorder) is electronically differentiated a curve is produced which shows the rate of change of radioactivity. The mode transit time is the interval between the maximum rate of increase and the maximum rate of decline of radioactivity on this secondary curve. The positive peak (arrival) can usually be defined to an accuracy of < 0.5 seconds, but the negative peak is broader and an error of 1–2 seconds is possible: when transit time is prolonged the peaks are less clear, particularly the negative (dispersal) one.

PATIENT SERIES REPORTED

The results of Oldendorf, a neurologist, and of Taylor, a neurosurgeon, will be reviewed; each used 50 μC to 500 μC of [^{131}I]hippuran and detectors which essentially "looked at" the whole head.

Oldendorf

In 65 normal subjects MCT tended to increase with age: all 14 > 60 had MCT > 9.5 seconds, 9 > 10.5 seconds. But < 65, 5/51 were > 10.5, and 12 were < 9.5 seconds. Hyperventilation increased MCT in 10 out of 12 normal subjects. MCT could also be prolonged in normal subjects by a 30 mm Hg cuff round the neck or by the Valsalva manoeuvre, each of which obstructs venous return from the head.

In 450 patients with neurological disease the MCT was shorter than normal with AV malformation or HA, and markedly prolonged with post-traumatic encephalopathy, "degenerative disease" and cerebral infarction associated with normal blood pressure (hypertensive infarction had a more normal MCT). A direct relationship was found between MCT and arm-to-head circulation time in a wide variety of conditions, indicating that a systemic circulatory inadequacy usually exists when brain circulation is slowed.

Taylor

In 50 patients studied soon after subarachnoid haemorrhage the MCT was longer in those with angiographic evidence of spasm than in those without spasm (Kak and Taylor, 1967 a). No such correlation was found when operative survivors with and without complications were compared. In another study 70 patients with symptoms after head injury associated with loss of consciousness were compared with 70 patients without head injury: most of the head injury cases had post-concussional type of subjective disorders, and were examined 4–8 weeks after injury. MCT was significantly longer in the post-concussional group of patients, but only means for each group are quoted, without standard deviation or standard errors.

This paper refers also to other measurements made on the primary curve, *e.g.* appearance to peak, peak to clearance, ascending and descending angles and amplitude (maximum count rate); and he records differences between the two groups of patients for each of these parameters. However, Oldendorf (1962) has stressed that the shape of the primary curve depends on so many variables that it is unwise to analyse it in this kind of detail: among these are the length of the bolus, the proportion which is distributed to the brain, the state of the cerebral vessels and the neck veins and so on. Furthermore Taylor refers in each of these papers to "cerebral blood flow" and even specifically to "volume flow"; this evoked criticism (James, 1967) and the comment that theoretically volume flow could alter without any change in MCT. It is note-worthy to compare statements made by these two investigators in summing up their view of the method. Taylor states: "the assumption that cerebral blood-flow (C.B.F.) is a reciprocal function of mean circulation-time (M.C.T.) will not lead to error at a clinical level." (Kak and Taylor, 1967 b). Oldendorf (1962) had stated five years previously: "Attempts at estimating flow rate by defining the linear rate of progress of the blood stream have, I believe, little place in absolute flow measurements unless there is some way of knowing the effective cross-sectional areas of the lumen at the point of measurement. This condition will seldom be met."

THEORETICAL AND PRACTICAL PROBLEMS

As a result of this controversy two questions about this method seemed to require answering, one theoretical and one practical. Is the velocity of the circulation, which this method measures, a reliable index of cerebral blood flow (or perfusion) which is the parameter of the circulation believed to be of most biological importance? And, whatever the theoretical implications, is the MCT in normal individuals sufficiently consistent to make it possible to identify abnormal states of the circulation from measurement of the MCT?

As Oldendorf has stressed, the assumption that transit time bears an inverse relationship to (volume) flow rate is valid only in the presence of a fixed blood pool volume, which in turn implies a fixed total cross-sectional area of the cerebral vasculature. However, all the evidence about the control of the cerebral circulation points to a frequently changing vessel calibre, as autoregulation to changing blood pressure, Pa_{CO_2} and cerebral metabolism operates to maintain adequate tissue per-

References pp. 373–374

Patient investigation

In these studies technetium-99m was used; its half-life is only 6 hours (compared with 8 days for ^{131}I) and better counting statistics can therefore be obtained without increasing the radiation hazard to the patient. Only 1.3 mc are required, a fraction of the dose normally employed for brain scanning; repeated studies can therefore be made.

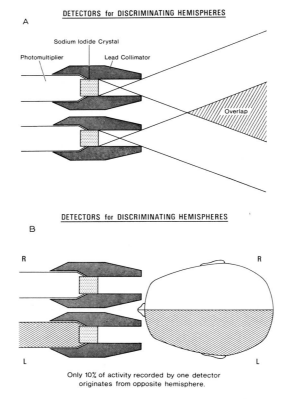

Fig. 3. Collimation to optimize discrimination between hemispheres. A. Some degree of overlap in volumes counted from is inevitable. B. In counting from the head, only 10% are cross counts.

With these higher count rates it has become possible to use smaller detectors, which are capable of discriminating between the two sides of the brain (Fig. 3). As many clinical conditions affect only one cerebral hemisphere it was hoped that this would improve the discrimination of the method. Only the MCT itself was measured, from the secondary (differentiated) curve.

Normal adults

Measurements on 21 members of staff showed a mean MCT of 9.5 sec which corresponds well with Oldendorf's figure; for right–left difference the mean was 1 sec $\pm$ 0.6.

On this basis the abnormalities shown by patients could be categorised according to the number of standard deviations away from this normal mean.

Patients

These 205 patients were mostly studied in the course of routine brain scanning the MCT being measured at the time of isotope injection prior to scanning. The mean MCT (in the affected hemisphere) was calculated for groups of patients in each of five diagnostic categories, and compared with the normal group. The group MCT's for cerebral ischaemia, intracranial haematoma and subarachnoid haemorrhage were all significantly prolonged (Table 1). In the subarachnoid haemorrhage group patients with spasm had significantly longer MCT than those without, and in the ischemic group more severe hemiparesis was associated with more prolonged MCT. But even so some 40% of the patients in these groups had an MCT within one S.D. of the normal

TABLE 1

ABSOLUTE MCT (seconds) IN AFFECTED HEMISPHERES

(mean for all patients in groups indicated)

Diagnostic group	n	Mean	S.D.	p
Total patient series				
Cerebral ischaemia	40	11.8	2.6	< 0.01
Intracranial haematoma	38	11.0	2.3	< 0.01
Subarachnoid haemorrhage	47	10.3	1.5	< 0.05
Intracranial tumour	36	10.2	1.4	ns
Head injury	29	10.1	2.2	ns
Patients with subarachnoid haemorrhage				
With spasm	16	11.2	2.1	< 0.05
Without spasm	31	9.9	1.5	
Patients with ischaemia				
Hemiparesis Grade 1	5	11.2	1.6	< 0.05
Hemiparesis Grade 2	9	13.6	3.0	

TABLE 2

PERCENTAGE OF PATIENTS WITH MCT WITHIN VARIOUS RANGES OF NORMAL. TOTAL PATIENT SERIES BY DIAGNOSTIC GROUPS

Diagnostic group	n	Within 1 S.D. $9.5 \pm (< 1.8)$
Ischaemia	40	40%
Haematoma	38	55%
Subarachnoid haemorrhage	47	68%
Tumour	36	78%
Head injury	29	58%

(Table 2). When all diagnostic groups are considered together more than half the patients with hemiparesis, no matter how severe, have an MCT within one S.D. of normal; for conscious state grades 1 and 2 the same holds, but only 32% of patients with severely impaired consciousness had an MCT within one SD of normal (Table 3).

Asymmetry between the hemispheres occurred significantly more often than normal in the same diagnostic groups that showed prolonged MCT (Table 4). But again, more than half the patients in each group had asymmetry within one S.D. of the normal group (Table 5).

TABLE 3

PATIENT SERIES BY CLINICAL STATES

Hemiparesis	n	Within 1 S.D. 9.5 ± (< 1.8)
Grade 1	42	60%
Grade 2	62	50%
Grade 3	22	59%
Conscious state		
Grade 1	83	55%
Grade 2	52	50%
Grade 3	22	32%

TABLE 4

ASYMMETRY OF MCT (seconds) BETWEEN HEMISPHERES

Diagnostic group	n	Mean	S.D.	p
Ischaemia	46	1.6	1.5	< 0.05
Haematoma	38	2.0	1.8	< 0.01
Subarachnoid haemorrhage	52	1.5	1.3	< 0.05
Tumour	37	1.2	1.2	ns
Head injury	32	1.3	1.4	ns

Serial MCT measurements were carried out in 45 patients; in the 40 pairs of results which differed by more than one second no correlation could be found between the direction or degree of change of the MCT and the clinical state. Not only did improving patients often have a slower MCT when they were better, but deteriorating patients frequently had a faster circulation when they were worse. Some patients who improved showed no change in MCT.

TABLE 5

PERCENTAGE OF PATIENTS WITH ASYMMETRY WITHIN VARIOUS RANGES OF NORMAL.
TOTAL PATIENT SERIES BY DIAGNOSTIC GROUPS

Diagnostic group	n	$1 \pm (< 0.6)$
Ischaemia	46	59%
Haematoma	38	53%
Subarachnoid haemorrhage	52	64%
Tumour	37	78%
Head Injury	32	72%

TOTAL PATIENT SERIES BY CLINICAL STATES

Hemiparesis	n	$1 \pm (< 0.6)$	$1 \pm (0.6–1.2)$	$1 \pm (> 1.2)$
Grade 1	43	58%	19%	23%
Grade 2	57	56%	16%	28%
Grade 3	22	45%	23%	32%
Conscious State				
Grade 1	84	70%	13%	17%
Grade 2	51	49%	27%	24%
Grade 3	24	58%	4%	38%

CONCLUSION

Although this investigation shows a trend towards a slower circulation in a group of patients with conditions in which circulatory disturbance is likely it does not yield information of much diagnostic or prognostic significance in the individual case. This standard deviation for the normal MCT (and for asymmetry between the hemispheres) is such that some 60% of patients prove to have measurements within *one* standard deviation of the normal mean. Even serial measurements do not yield consistent trends in accord with clinical progress. There are two reasons why these results are not unexpected. One is that the method "looks at" large areas of brain, and is likely to be insensitive to the local disorders of flow which multichannel rCBF methods have revealed. The other is that considerable changes in volume flow occur without a marked alteration in velocity, as our baboon experiments have shown. This method would seem to have a restricted application either as a screening test, or in the investigation of individual patients.

REFERENCES

GREITZ, T. (1956) Radiologic study of brain circulation by rapid angiography of the carotid artery. *Acta Radiol.*, Suppl. **140**, 123.
JAMES, I. M. (1967) Blood-flow in subarachnoid haemorrhage. *Lancet*, **i**, 956.
KAK, V. K. AND TAYLOR, A. R. (1967 a) Cerebral blood-flow in subarachnoid haemorrhage. *Lancet*, **i**, 875.

KAK, V. K. AND TAYLOR, A. R. (1967 b) Blood-flow in subarachnoid haemorrhage. *Lancet*, **i**, 1061.

NYLIN, G., SILVERSKIOLD, B. P., LOFSTEDT, S., REGNSTROM, O. AND HEDLUND, S. (1960) Studies on cerebral blood flow in man using radioactive-labelled erythrocytes. *Brain*, **83**, 293.

OLDENDORF, W. H. (1962) Measurement of the mean transit time of cerebral circulation by external detection of an intravenously injected radioisotope. *J. Nucl. Med.*, **3**, 382.

OLDENDORF, W. H. AND KITANO, M. (1963) Clinical measurement of brain uptake of radioisotope. *Arch. Neurol.*, **9**, 574.

OLDENDORF, W. H., KITANO, M., SHIMIZU, S. AND OLDENDORF, S. Z. (1965) Hematocrit of the cranial blood pool. *Circulation Res.*, **17**, 532.

Study of the Cerebral Circulation by Means of Inert Diffusible Tracers

SEYMOUR S. KETY

Harvard Medical School – Massachusetts General Hospital, Boston, Mass. (U.S.A.)

The decade that began in 1940 witnessed an expanding interest in clinical physiology, stimulated, perhaps, by the application of mathematical and physical sciences in the development of indirect approaches to hitherto inaccessible areas of human function and disease. Measurement of peripheral blood flow, of cardiac output, of renal circulation and glomerular filtration rate were successfully achieved in man at a time when quantitative information on the cerebral circulation had not been obtained even in lower animals. It was not until 1943 that such measurements were made in the rhesus monkey, a species whose cerebral circulation resembles that of man in being readily isolated from the extra-cerebral blood supply to the head. An ingenious bubble flow meter interposed in the arterial supply to the brain yielded quantitative estimates of total cerebral blood flow (Dumke and Schmidt, 1943).

In man so direct a procedure was out of the question. It was thought possible, however, that the Fick Principle which forms the basis of cardiac output and renal blood flow measurement, could be modified and successfully applied to the cerebral circulation.

Fick stated his important principle in two paragraphs of the Proceedings of the Würzberg Physikalische-medizinische Gesellschaft in 1870 (Fick, 1870). It was the simple and, in the wisdom of hindsight, the quite self-evident statement that the quantity of oxygen absorbed per minute must be equivalent to the pulmonary blood flow multiplied by the arteriovenous difference for oxygen across the lungs. In animals, and more recently in man, it is possible to measure with considerable precision the necessary components of that equation and to compute the pulmonary blood flow with few assumptions or approximations.

Unfortunately, the brain, unlike the kidney, does not specifically and selectively remove foreign substances from the blood and excrete them for accurate measurement. Furthermore, although it does consume large quantities of oxygen, that consumption cannot independently be measured or even assumed to be constant since it would be expected to vary with activity and disease. The brain does, however, absorb by physical solution an inert gas such as nitrous oxide, which reaches it by way of the arterial blood. It was hoped that the quantity of this gas absorbed by the brain would be independent of the state of mental activity and susceptible of measure-

References pp. 383–385

blood for nitrous oxide tension since calculation shows that it could result in an overestimation of the cerebral blood flow by 5 % under normal circumstances and by 10–12 % in those cases where the flow in white matter is reduced by one-half. Extending the equilibration time to 15 or 20 min has been suggested as one way of minimizing this error.

Another possible source of error is represented by the small fraction of blood in the internal jugular vein which is derived from extracerebral tissues. To the small contamination measured by dye injection into the external carotid, must be added the blood derived from the internal carotid but which drains the orbital tissues and the meninges. This admixture of blood from slowly perfused areas together with the slow equilibration of the cerebrospinal fluid with the inert gas results in the addition of several slowly equilibrating components of small magnitude to the more rapid equilibrium occurring in the brain itself. This may result in underestimating the cerebral blood flow in the average case by approximately 10 % when the calculation is made at 10 min, the error increasing nearly linearly as that time is extended.

Thus, the original nitrous oxide technique is probably subject to two relatively small errors of opposite sign and, at 10 min of equilibration, nearly equal in magnitude. If that is so, extending the equilibration time does not necessarily improve the accuracy.

Certain modifications in the nitrous oxide technique which Lassen and Munck (1955) have made would tend to reduce both of these errors. On the assumption that the rapidly perfused gray matter becomes equilibrated with the foreign gas during the first few minutes of its inhalation, the curve in mixed cerebral venous blood from 5 to 10 min represents predominantly the equilibration of white matter with a variable but relatively small admixture of slower, extracerebral components. These assumptions have been validated by recent measurements of regional perfusion rates within the brain. By appropriate extrapolation of the latter portion of the curve to infinity, it may be possible to obtain a reasonable approximation to that curve which would be described by the whole brain as it proceeds to complete equilibrium with arterial and venous blood with the effect of extracerebral contamination minimized. Use of the less soluble krypton permits the arterial concentration curve to approach a square wave in form and makes this extrapolation more reliable. Although computations based upon such a procedure in normal individuals may not necessarily improve the accuracy, their validity could be considerably greater in pathological states where the proportion of white matter is greater or its perfusion slower than normal and in the occasional case where extracerebral contamination is more than minimal.

Aukland (1964) demonstrated the feasibility of measuring molecular hydrogen in blood and tissues by a polarographic technique. The considerations outlined earlier would suggest that if such measurements were applied during a 10 to 20-min period of desaturation immediately following a similar period of saturation with a low tension of gaseous hydrogen, it would be possible to minimize the error due to incomplete equilibration of white matter and that resulting from extracerebral contamination. In addition, the continuous arterial and cerebral venous curves which would be obtained should permit more extensive and accurate computations.

The nitrous oxide technique has two important limitations. Since it requires a period of 10 min for the determination of a single value for cerebral blood flow, it is not applicable to the study of rapid changes in this function as are likely to occur in syncope or in convulsions. Further, since no generally applicable technique is at hand for obtaining venous blood from localized areas, the method yields only an average for the brain as a whole.

Lewis and collaborators (1960) demonstrated the feasibility of estimating total cerebral blood flow from equation (1) throughout the period of equilibration without assuming any relationship between cerebral tissue and venous blood. The use of a gamma-emitting inert gas (^{79}Kr) made it possible to estimate directly the accumulation of the gas in brain.

Considerations of the exchange of inert, diffusible substances between capillary and tissue (Kety, 1951) permitted the development of equations which have been useful in the measurement of regional blood flow in the brain. Here, in contrast to measurement of total blood flow, it is possible to measure arterial and tissue concentrations of the tracer but not the appropriate venous concentration.

As in the nitrous oxide technique, however, a relationship between tissue and venous concentrations was predicted on the basis of testable assumptions.

If the region in question is homogeneously perfused, if there are no arteriovenous shunts, and if diffusion of the tracer is sufficiently rapid that it is not limiting, then equilibrium between the tissue and its blood should be achieved during the transit of the latter through the tissue. A relationship was derived between a tissue concentration at any time, $C_i(T)$, the variable arterial concentration, A, and a constant, k_i, representing rate of perfusion per solubility-equivalent unit of tissue, $F/\lambda W$:

$$C_i(T) = k_i \lambda_i \exp\left(-k_i T\right) \int_0^T A \exp\left(k_i t\right) \mathrm{d}t \tag{2}$$

Where the arterial concentration rises abruptly at $t = 0$ and remains constant:

$$C_i(T) = \lambda_i A \left[(1 - \exp\left(-k_i t\right)\right] \tag{3}$$

and where the tissue is being cleared of the tracer in the presence of a negligible arterial concentration:

$$C_i(T) = A_0 \exp\left(-k_i T\right) \tag{4}$$

The general equation (2) permitted the development of an autoradiographic technique for measurement of local cerebral blood flow using $[^{131}\mathrm{I}]\mathrm{CF}_3$ (Landau et al., 1955) or $[^{14}\mathrm{C}]$antipyrine (Reivich et al., 1969) while equation (4) is the basis of the clearance methods developed by Ingvar and Lassen (1962) using radioactive gases.

Three assumptions have been made in the derivation of these equations which invite further examination. Arteriovenous shunts have not been found in the brain, and even if they were present, this would merely limit the measurement to capillary blood flow, a more valid physiological function for most purposes. Substantial support is found for the assumption that diffusion between cerebral capillary and tissue is not a limiting factor in the exchange of the tracers which have been used. Copperman (in Kety, 1951) computed the time of virtual equilibrium for diffusion from a central capillary radially through tissue; these computations indicate that for the intercapillary distances which exist in the brain, equilibrium with blood would be nearly complete in one second. Fieschi and coll. (1964) found a single exponential decay for the clearance of hydrogen from white matter (which has an intercapillary distance twice that of the cortex); in addition, the values for blood flow obtained by them with hydrogen are in agreement with those obtained using substances of considerably higher molecular weight which would be expected to have diffusion coefficients one-tenth as large.

The assumption that all the small tissue regions in which measurements have been made are homogeneously perfused, however, is open to serious question. Both Ingvar and Lassen (1962) and Fieschi and coll. (1964) found that in gray matter the clearance of the tracers used deviates from a single exponential function but may be approximated by the sum of at least two such functions. This suggests that the assumption of homogeneity may not be tenable for a number of regions, although alternative explanations may have to be ruled out. However, Ingvar and Lassen (1962) showed mathematically that under appropriate conditions the initial slope of a compound exponential curve, such as is obtained from a heterogeneous tissue, is determined by the average flow and the average partition coefficient of the region in question. This has permitted them to compute average flows for heterogeneous regions under local observation which are compatible with values obtained in the brain as a whole.

Significant heterogeneity of the small regions examined by means of the autoradiographic technique, if it occurred, would compromise the accuracy of the values which have been obtained. On the other hand, these measurements made at the end of only one minute of equilibration are probably sufficiently close to the initial slope to yield a satisfactory average perfusion value on the basis of Ingvar and Lassen's derivation. It is interesting that the weighted average for cerebral blood flow as a whole obtained from such regional measurements agrees well with values obtained by the nitrous oxide method which requires no assumptions regarding the absence of arteriovenous shunts or extremely rapid capillary–tissue equilibrium.

Measurement of cerebral blood flow also permitted the evaluation of two other cerebral functions. One of these is cerebrovascular resistance, a measure of all the factors opposing the cerebral blood flow, most prominent of which is the tone of the vessels themselves. Most important of all, however, is the ability to calculate the rate of cerebral metabolism in terms of oxygen or glucose consumption or, in fact, the utilization or production by the brain of any substance which can accurately be detected in arterial and venous blood. Normal values for these functions were obtained in a series of healthy young men (Kety and Schmidt, 1948 a). The blood flow of the brain was found to represent about one-sixth of the cardiac output and its oxygen consumption nearly one quarter of that of the entire body at rest.

The first application of the new method was to the problem of the effects on cerebral circulation of alterations in the oxygen and carbon dioxide tensions of arterial blood (Kety and Schmidt, 1948 b). The results confirmed classical experiments on animals which demonstrated that carbon dioxide was a potent cerebral vasodilator as was anoxia, whereas high oxygen tensions and low carbon dioxide pressures produced mild and severe vasoconstriction respectively. Evidence was acquired in these studies to suggest that the dominant control of cerebral vessels in man was a chemical one, activated by levels of carbon dioxide, oxygen and hydrogen ion. A study on the role of the cervical sympathetic supply to the brain (Harmel et al., 1949) cast further light on this question of the normal control of the cerebral circulation. It was found that procaine block of both stellate ganglia produced no change in cerebral circulation or resistance, suggesting that the known sympathetic channels to the brain do not exert an appreciable tonic effect on cerebral vessels.

One of the unique values of methods applicable to man is the opportunity thus afforded for studying the pathogenesis of human disease. Several diseases were found to be associated with significant disturbances in cerebrovascular resistance or cerebral blood flow. Increase in intracranial pressure as a result of brain tumor (Kety, Shenkin and Schmidt, 1948) was found to produce a progressive rise in cerebrovascular resistance undoubtedly as a result of external compression of the thin-walled vessels of the brain. The cerebral blood flow, however, was not significantly compromised until cerebrospinal fluid pressure exceeded 400 mm of water, a homeostasis achieved by a compensatory increase in blood pressure. Thus, Cushing's classical experiments on dogs were completely confirmed by observations on man.

The method was applied to essential hypertension with findings of some interest (Kety et al., 1948 b). There was practically a two-fold increase in cerebrovascular resistance which in the absence of significant changes in intracranial pressure or blood viscosity had to be attributed to vasoconstriction. This change, however, is in exact proportion to the elevation in blood pressure with the result that cerebral blood flow is practically normal. These observations on cerebral vessels were similar to those of other investigators who had studied the vascular beds of the kidneys, extremities, and splanchnic viscera in this disease. The effects of a reduction in the high blood pressure to more normal values (Kety et al., 1950) are of importance in understanding the nature of the increased cerebrovascular tone and in determining the wisdom of reducing the blood pressure of hypertensive patients. After interruption of the sympathetic outflow to the trunk and lower extremities achieved either by procaine or surgical sympathectomy (Shenkin et al., 1950), evidence was found of a relaxation of the abnormally increased cerebrovascular tone and a tendency to preserve a normal cerebral blood flow. These findings clearly demonstrated the remarkable autoregulatory properties of the cerebral circulation, and contradicted an earlier notion of the dependence of this circulation on arterial blood pressure.

A number of disturbances in cerebral metabolism were studied by means of this method. Among the earliest of these was that on diabetic acidosis and coma (Kety et al., 1948 c). It was learned that the state of coma, contrary to the prevailing theory, was not the result of a deficient cerebral blood flow – in fact, this function was actually somewhat greater than normal – but, rather, was associated with a significant reduction in cerebral oxygen utilization. This occurred in spite of an adequate supply of

References pp. 383–385

blood and oxygen to the brain and an oxyhemoglobin dissociation curve which favored the uptake of oxygen by the tissues. The evidence found suggested an intracellular defect possibly on the basis of acidosis or ketosis. The increased cerebral perfusion in the face of a markedly reduced carbon dioxide tension but a low pH was early evidence of the importance of hydrogen ion in the regulation of cerebral blood flow.

In the hypoglycemia and coma of insulin shock therapy were seen the results of a fairly acute reduction in glucose available for cerebral utilization (Kety et al., 1948 d). There was a progressive decrease in cerebral oxygen and glucose consumption as the blood glucose concentration fell. Blood pressure and cerebral blood flow were maintained within normal limits. In deep insulin coma, there was evidence that the brain utilizes its own carbohydrate stores at a rate which would exhaust them in approximately 90 min, corresponding to the length of time during which insulin coma may be maintained without the production of irreversible cerebral damage.

In surgical anesthesia produced by thiopental, there was found a marked reduction in oxygen consumption by the brain in spite of adequate blood oxygen saturation and a somewhat elevated cerebral blood flow (Wechsler et al., 1951).

A surprising result was obtained by Sokoloff and associates (1953) when it was learned that cerebral oxygen utilization in hyperthyroidism was not increased above the normal level in spite of a marked increase in oxygen consumption by the body as a whole. That interesting finding was the first suggestion that thyrotoxicosis may not represent a generalized acceleration in metabolism of all body cells. It was on the basis of that finding that Sokoloff went on to develop his concept of the major physiological action of thyroid hormone on protein synthesis and demonstrated, early on, an important hormonal control of this process (Sokoloff et al., 1963).

In the mental changes associated with increased intracranial pressure, diabetic or hypoglycemic coma, or anesthesia, it is not difficult to discern a cause–effect relationship between a gross defect in cerebral nutrition or metabolism and the alteration in mental activity. In one of the important mental illnesses such a relationship is still tenable. Studies in the psychoses of senility (Freyhan et al., 1951) showed a significant reduction in cerebral blood flow and oxygen consumption, presumably on the basis of an increased cerebrovascular resistance – a physiological confirmation of the well-known sclerosis of cerebral vessels often associated with this disorder. A systematic study of the cerebral circulation in various aging populations (Dastur et al., 1963) supported the thesis that a primary reduction in perfusion was responsible for an important component of senile dementia. Considerations of the dependence of brain tissue oxygen tension on perfusion and arterial oxygen content (Kety, 1957) provide a basis for the beneficial effects of hyperbaric oxygen administration in this condition.

In schizophrenia, on the other hand, similar studies revealed no detectable change in the total circulation or oxygen consumption of the brain even in severely affected patients (Kety et al., 1948 d). Performance of mental arithmetic was found not to affect cerebral energy metabolism appreciably (Sokoloff et al., 1955).

There were other examples of profound changes in mental function which show no correlation with overall blood flow or oxygen consumption of the brain. A study on normal sleep (Mangold *et al.*, 1955) showed a slight increase in cerebral blood flow and no significant change in cerebral oxygen consumption in this condition. These findings were incompatible with those theories of sleep which were predicated upon an ischemia or a narcosis of the brain and indicated that sleep was a phenomenon quite different from coma. They challenged the prevailing notion of the time of a generalized neuronal inactivity during sleep and anticipated the findings of electrophysiologists that sleep was a highly active neuronal state (Kety, 1967).

Studies in man yielded important insights into the pharmacology of the cerebral circulation (Sokoloff, 1959). This is understandable since only in human subjects or clinical disorders can relevant dosages of drugs be used, therapeutic effects studied and possible species differences circumvented. These studies have served to reinforce the characterization of a few of the cerebral dilator drugs but to question the efficacy of many more. They may be expected to play a significant role in the evaluation of new drugs and therapeutic procedures.

The nitrous oxide technique and its various modifications has been of value in elucidating the physiology of the circulation in the normally functioning human brain freed of such constraints as anesthesia or surgical intervention. It has provided information on human cerebral disease, which was previously unavailable, and on the effects of drugs under therapeutic conditions. In the clinical study of the individual patient, more convenient techniques, especially those which can examine specific regions within the brain, are desirable for diagnosis, localization and evaluation of progress. Here the regional clearance of radioactive gases, as developed by Lassen and Ingvar, or non-invasive techniques which require only external counting of gamma ray-emitting isotopes such as those developed by Veall or by Obrist are specially useful. The successful application of radioactive oxygen ($^{15}O_2$) by Ter-Pogossian and his associates (1969) to measurement of both oxygen consumption and blood flow within the brain is extremely promising. One may predict with considerable assurance that future developments such as these will continue to find important applications in the clinic while enriching our fundamental knowledge of the cerebral circulation and its regulation.

REFERENCES

AUKLAND, K. (1964) Measurement of local blood flow with hydrogen gas. *Circulation Res.*, **14**, 164.

DASTUR, D. K., LANE, M. H., HANSEN, D. B., KETY, S. S., BUTLER, R. N., PERLIN, S. AND SOKOLOFF, L. (1963) Effects of aging on cerebral circulation and metabolism in man. In: *Human Aging: A Biological and Behavioral Study*, Public Health Service Publication No. 986, U.S. Government Printing Office, Washington, D.C., pp. 59–76.

DUMKE, P. R. AND SCHMIDT, C. F. (1943) Quantitative measurements of cerebral blood flow in the macacque monkey. *Amer. J. Physiol.*, **138**, 421.

FICK, A. (1870) Ueber die Messung des Blutquantums in den Herzventrikeln. *S.-B. Phys.-Med. Ges. Würzburg*, July 9.

FIESCHI, C., AGNOLI, A. AND BOZZAO, L. (1964) Blood flow measurements in the brain of cats by analysis of the clearance curves of hydrogen gas with implanted electrodes, and of ^{85}Kr with external counting of gamma activity. In: EICHHORN, O., LECHNER, H. AND AUELL, K.-H. (Eds.), *Scientific and Clinical Research of the Cerebral Circulation*, Verlag Bruder Hollinek, Vienna, pp. 180–186.

FREYHAN, F. A., WOODFORD, R. B. AND KETY, S. S. (1951) The blood flow, vascular resistance and oxygen consumption of the brain in the psychoses of senility. *J. Nervous Mental Disease*, **113**, 449.

HARMEL, M. H., HAFKENSCHIEL, J. H., AUSTIN, G. M., CRUMPTON, C. W. AND KETY, S. S. (1949) The effect of bilateral stellate ganglion block on the cerebral circulation in normotensive and hypertensive patients. *J. Clin. Invest.*, **28**, 415.

INGVAR, D. H. AND LASSEN, N. A. (1962) Regional blood flow of the cerebral cortex determined by krypton[85]. *Acta Physiol. Scand.*, **54**, 325.

KETY, S. S. (1948) The quantitative determination of cerebral blood flow in man. In: POTTER, V. R. (Ed.), *Methods in Medical Research*, Vol. I, Year Book Publishers, Chicago, pp. 204–217.

KETY, S. S. (1951) The theory and applications of the exchange of inert gas at the lungs and tissues. *Pharmacol. Rev.*, **3**, 1.

KETY, S. S. (1957) Determinants of tissue oxygen tension. *Federation Proc.*, **16**, 666–670.

KETY, S. S. (1960) Measurement of local blood flow by the exchange of an inert, diffusible substance. In: BRUNER, H. D. (Ed.), *Methods in Medical Research*, Vol. VII, Year Book Publishers, Chicago, p. 228.

KETY, S. S. (1967) Relationship between energy metabolism of the brain and functional activity. In: KETY, S. S., EVARTS, E. V. AND WILLIAMS, H. L. (Eds.), *Sleep and Altered States of Consciousness*, *Res. Publ. Assoc. Nervous Mental Dis.*, Vol. XLV, Williams and Wilkins, Baltimore, pp. 39–45.

KETY, S. S. AND SCHMIDT, C. F. (1948 a) Nitrous oxide method for the quantitative determination of cerebral blood flow in man: theory, procedure, and normal values. *J. Clin. Invest.*, **27**, 476.

KETY, S. S. AND SCHMIDT, C. F. (1948 b) Effects of altered arterial tensions of carbon dioxide and oxygen on cerebral blood flow and cerebral oxygen consumption of normal young men. *J. Clin. Invest.*, **27**, 484.

KETY, S. S., SHENKIN, H. A. AND SCHMIDT, C. F. (1948) Effects of increased intracranial pressure on cerebral circulatory functions in man. *J. Clin. Invest.*, **27**, 493.

KETY, S. S., HARMEL, M. H., BROOMELL, H. T. AND RHODE, C. B. (1948 a) The solubility of nitrous oxide in blood and brain. *J. Biol. Chem.*, **173**, 487.

KETY, S. S., HAFKENSCHIEL, J. H., JEFFERS, W. A., LEOPOLD, I. H. AND SHENKIN, H. A. (1948 b) Blood flow, vascular resistance, and oxygen consumption of the brain in essential hypertension. *J. Clin. Invest.*, **27**, 511.

KETY, S. S., KING, B. D., HORVATH, S. M., JEFFERS, W. A. AND HAFKENSCHIEL, J. H. (1950) Effects of an acute reduction in blood pressure by means of differential spinal sympathetic block on the cerebral circulation of hypertensive patients. *J. Clin. Invest.*, **29**, 402.

KETY, S. S., POLIS, B. D., NADLER, C. S. AND SCHMIDT, C. F. (1948 c) Blood flow and oxygen consumption of the human brain in diabetic acidosis and coma. *J. Clin. Invest.*, **27**, 500.

KETY, S. S., WOODFORD, R. B., HARMEL, M. H., FREYHAN, F. A., APPEL, K. E. AND SCHMIDT, C. F. (1948 d) Cerebral blood flow and metabolism in schizophrenia. The effects of barbiturate semi-narcosis, insulin coma and electroshock. *Amer. J. Psychiat.*, **104**, 765.

LANDAU, W. M., FREYGANG, W. H., ROWLAND, L. P., SOKOLOFF, L. AND KETY, S. S. (1955) The local circulation of the living brain; values in the unanesthetized and anesthetized cat. *Trans. Amer. Neurol. Assoc.*, **80**, 125.

LASSEN, N. A. AND MUNCK, O. (1955) The cerebral blood flow in man determined by the use of radioactive krypton. *Acta Physiol. Scand.*, **33**, 30.

LASSEN, N. A., FEINBERG, I. AND LANE, M. H. (1960) Bilateral studies of cerebral oxygen uptake in young and aged normal subjects and in patients with organic dementia, *J. Clin. Invest.*, **39**, 491.

LEWIS, B. M., SOKOLOFF, L., WECHSLER, R. L., WENTZ, W. B. AND KETY, S. S. (1960) A method for the continuous measurement of cerebral blood flow in man by means of radioactive krypton (Kr[79]), *J. Clin. Invest.*, **39**, 707.

MANGOLD, R., SOKOLOFF, L., CONNER, E., KLEINERMAN, J., THERMAN, P. G. AND KETY, S. S. (1955) The effects of sleep and lack of sleep on the cerebral circulation and metabolism of normal young men. *J. Clin. Invest.*, **34**, 1092–1100.

MUNCK, O. AND LASSEN, N. A. (1957) Bilateral cerebral blood flow and oxygen consumption in man by use of krypton[85]. *Circulation Res.*, **5**, 163.

MYERSON, A., HALLORAN, R. D. AND HIRSCH, H. L. (1927) Technique for obtaining blood from the internal jugular vein and internal carotid artery. *Arch. Neurol. Psychiat.*, **17**, 807.

REIVICH, M., JEHLE, J., SOKOLOFF, L. AND KETY, S. S. (1969) Measurement of regional cerebral blood flow with antipyrine-^{14}C in awake cats. *J. Appl. Physiol.*, **27**, 296–300.

SHENKIN, H. A., HAFKENSCHIEL, J. H. AND KETY, S. S. (1950) Effects of sympathectomy on the cerebral circulation of hypertensive patients. *Arch. Surg.*, **61**, 319.

SHENKIN, H. A., HARMEL, M. H. AND KETY, S. S. (1948) Dynamic anatomy of the cerebral circulation. *Arch. Neurol. Psychiat.*, **60**, 240.

SOKOLOFF, L. (1959) The action of drugs on the cerebral circulation. *Pharmacol. Rev.*, **11**, 1–85.

SOKOLOFF, L., MANGOLD, R., WECHSLER, R. L., KENNEDY, C. AND KETY, S. S. (1955) The effect of mental arithmetic on cerebral circulation and metabolism. *J. Clin. Invest.*, **34**, 1101–1108.

SOKOLOFF, L., KAUFMAN, S., CAMPBELL, P. L., FRANCIS, C. M. AND GELBOIN, H. V. (1963) Thyroxine stimulation of amino acid incorporation into protein. Localization of stimulated step. *J. Biol. Chem.*, **238**, 1432–1437.

SOKOLOFF, L., WECHSLER, R. L., MANGOLD, R., BALLS, K. AND KETY, S. S. (1953) Cerebral blood flow and oxygen consumption in hyperthyroidism before and after treatment. *J. Clin. Invest.*, **32**, 202–208.

TER-POGOSSIAN, M. M., EICHLING, J. O., DAVIS, D. O. AND WELCH, M. J. (1969) The simultaneous measure *in vivo* of regional cerebral blood flow and regional cerebral oxygen utilization by means of oxyhemoglobin labelled with radioactive oxygen[15]. In: BROCK, M., FIESCHI, C., INGVAR, D. H., LASSEN, N. A. AND SCHURMANN, K. (Eds.), *Cerebral Blood Flow: Clinical and Experimental Results*, Springer-Verlag, Berlin, pp. 66–69.

WECHSLER, R. L., DRIPPS, R. D. AND KETY, S. S. (1951) Blood flow and oxygen consumption of the human brain during anesthesia produced by thiopental. *Anesthesiology*, **12**, 308–314.

Clinical Aspects of Regional Cerebral Blood Flow

CESARE FIESCHI AND LUIGI BOZZAO

Department of Neurology and Psychiatry, University of Rome and University of Siena (Italy)

The studies on CBF reported in this chapter have been performed using the technique developed by Lassen and co-workers in 1963; the method requires the injection of a bolus of a radioactive inert gas solution (^{85}Kr or ^{133}Xe) into the internal carotid artery. The clearance curves of the diffusible indicator from the brain are fitted to a double exponential function. Compartmental analysis of the curve is not the only approach used to calculate the regional blood flow. However, it offers the advantage of giving the clearance rate and relative weight of the two components of the curve that have been assumed to represent two separate tissue compartments; the gray and white matter of the brain. The transposition in biological terms of these data has been questioned, although Høedt-Rasmussen and Skinhøj (1966) have shown that the weights of gray and white matter may be actually estimated in vivo by this technique.

In clinical studies, analysis of the compartmental data has not been thoroughly exploited. Most authors rely either on the average rCBF (obtained with stochastic, non–compartmental analysis) or on the initial slope, "two-minutes flow index".

A completely computerized compartmental analysis with fitting obtained through a series of iterations is a time consuming process (about 4 min for each curve) that makes the data not available in real time.

A second type of compartmental analysis may be performed, with a best-fit obtained by the computer in first approximation called "automatic curve-peeling" in Table 1 (Fieschi *et al.*, 1970). This method is much shorter and almost as reliable.

Under special circumstances, recording of the curves, therefore analysis, must be limited to a few minutes. This is the case for example when temporary clamping the internal carotid artery for testing the tolerance of the brain to the ischemia during endarterectomy (Agnoli *et al.*, 1970).

In such circumstances, the "two minute flow index" is the best approximation we can obtain to measure the rCBF. The size of the error involved in this simplified procedure is apparent for the analysis of Table 1: the main problem with this procedure is the underestimation of high flows.

In control groups, average regional cerebral blood flow is 50 ml/100 g/min for young normals (Ingvar, 1967) and 45 ml/100 g/min for elderly normals (Fieschi *et al.*, 1966). (Table 2).

Flow of the fast component is 80 ml/100 g/min (78 in elderly normals), and its

References pp. 408–410

TABLE 1

MEAN rCBF IN 56 REGIONS (22 STUDIES) COMPUTED BY MEANS OF DIFFERENT
APPROACHES INDICATED IN THE TEXT. CASES ARE DIVIDED INTO THREE GROUPS:
LOW FLOWS, NORMAL FLOWS, HIGH FLOWS

	$ml/100\ g/min$	$ml/100\ g/min$	$ml/100\ g/min$
Compartmental Iterative	29.2	42.9	81.4
Compartmental Automatic: curve peeling	31.6	43.4	83.9
Non compartmental: stochastic	32.2	44.3	78.7
Non compartmental: 2-min-slope	31.7	42.9	69.3

TABLE 2

AVERAGE VALUES FOR REGIONAL CBF IN CONTROL SUBJECTS AND IN PATIENTS
WITH CEREBRAL ISCHEMIC LESIONS

		Compartmental analysis				Arterial Pa_{CO_2}
		f1	f2	W1	$\overline{f}$	
Normal	$\overline{X}$	78.2	20.8	43.0	44.7	41.6
	S.D.	18.3	2.7	6.3	6.2	
Cerebral lesions	$\overline{X}$	51.4	15.8	40.8	30.2	44.8
	S.D.	14.4	4.3	9.0	8.4	
% reduction from controls		34.0	24.0	5.0	32.0	

weight 49% (43% in elderly normals). Flow of the slow component is 20 ml/100 g/min (20.8 in elderly normals) and its weight 51% (57%).

The distribution of regional blood flow in the various regions of the brain is rather uniform, with a coefficient of variation of 9.3% ± 2.5% according to Høedt-Rasmussen and co-workers (1967). This implies that interregional variations above 15% are probably abnormal, although in clinical studies safer limits of 35% interregional variations have been chosen (30% according to Cronquist, 1967). Actually the error of the method becomes relatively higher at lower values of blood flow.

Another reason for accepting as abnormal only interregional variations higher than 35% is that the blood flow is not really homogeneous throughout the cerebral hemisphere according to Wilkinson et al. (1969). These authors found perfusion of the gray matter to be significantly lower in the temporal region and higher in the precentral region than through the rest of the hemisphere.

In cerebral disturbances that affect the circulation, the regional cerebral blood flow may be diffusely or regionally increased, diffusely or regionally decreased. This is particularly true in the acute stage of cerebro–vascular lesions.

Measurements of rCBF by intravenous injection of [133]*Xe*

Veal and Mallet (1966) and subsequently Obrist *et al.* (1967) have investigated ^{133}Xe inhalation techniques for measuring rCBF. Advantages of such methods are obvious, since they do not require direct puncture of the carotid artery, and can be repeated in the same subject over several days.

We have assayed a similar technique, with intravenous injection of a bolus of ^{133}Xe solution (Agnoli *et al.*, 1969). Our main purpose was to develop a technique suitable for studying with such repeatable methods diseased subjects, who—because uncooperative, and because of altered lung function— are unsuitable for the inhalation technique.

For the same reason we attempted a direct monitoring of the arterial blood for the recirculation of the isotope, which in the inhalation technique is derived from the end-tidal ^{133}Xe concentration (Fig. 1).

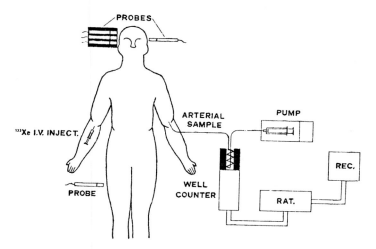

Fig. 1. Determination of the cerebral blood flow by the intravenous injection technique.

The results presented and obtained thus far indicate that accuracy and reproducibility of this technique is not yet acceptable for significant clinical studies of rCBF. Therefore, data reported below is based on the intra-arterial injection technique.

However, future development and application of rCBF studies as clinical tools largely depend on this and similar technological advancements.

Regional blood flow in cerebro-vascular disorders

In 50 patients with cerebral ischemic disease, whose mean age is 61 years, the rCBF is greatly reduced (Table 2): 30 ml/100 g/min. The main differences from control subjects were a 32% reduction of the average rCBF and 34% reduction of the blood flow of the fast component. The blood flow of the slow component is less decreased (24%); these differences are statistically significant. The relative weights of the two tissue phases are but little changed (5%). Other results from our case material have

References pp. 408–410

shown that: (a) time elapsed from the acute ischemic attack to the CBF measurement does not seem to influence average CBF; (b) the functional prognosis, i.e. the more or less favourable outcome of the neurological signs (motor and phasic), is not related to the rCBF measured in the acute stage of the disease: only the compartmental analysis shows that in cases with transient neurological impairment the relative weight of the fast component is significantly higher than in patients with permanent defects; (c) an impairment of the state of consciousness (which in our case material never reached the stage of coma) brings about a significant reduction of rCBF which is mainly due to a diminution of flow rate of the fast component (Table 3).

TABLE 3

REGIONAL BLOOD FLOW IN 37 PATIENTS WITH CEREBRAL ISCHEMIC LESIONS
(EXCLUDING CAROTID THROMBOSIS) EXAMINED WITHIN ONE MONTH OF THE STROKE

	Number of patients	Compartmental analysis			
		Mean flow	f2 Flow grey	f2 Flow white	W1 Weight grey
No occlusion:		31.9	54.2	16.5	42.1
Normal consciousness	24	28.4	44.8	14.4	44.3
Impaired consciousness	6				
Middle cerebral occlusion:					
Normal consciousness	4	21.7	39.7	12.1	34.5
Impaired consciousness	3	17.6	36.8	11.0	28.7

Twenty one patients were studied during the acute phase. They were 18 patients with ischemic and 3 with hemorrhagic lesions, examined the same day (4 cases), at one day (7 cases), two days (6 cases) three days (3 cases) and four days (1 case) after the stroke. The blood flow measurement was carried out on the same side as the diseased hemisphere, with ^{85}Kr as diffusible indicator.

The average regional CBF for the whole group was 28.4 ml/100 g/min at an arterial P_{CO_2} of 41.8 mm Hg, compared to 44.7 ml/100 g/min in elderly normals (Fieschi et al., 1966).

The diminution of regional CBF in the acute cerebrovascular group was predominantly due to a decrease of flow rate of the fast component (53.6 vs. 78.2 ml/100

TABLE 4

AVERAGE CBF IN ACUTE CEREBROVASCULAR LESIONS AND IN THE ENTIRE
GROUP OF CEREBROVASCULAR LESION

	Mean flow (ml/100 g/min)	Flow grey (ml/100 g/min)	Flow white (ml/100 g/min)	Weight grey (%)
Acute cerebro-vascular lesion	28.4	53.6	17.1	32.9
Total cerebro-vascular lesion	30.2	51.4	15.8	40.8

g/min) and its relative weight (32.9 *vs.* 43%). The flow rate of the slow component was less markedly reduced (17.1 *vs.* 20.8 ml/100 g/min). With respect to the entire group of cerebrovascular lesions (Table 4) the reduction in the weight of the fast component is the only significant change. When the clearance rate of ^{85}Kr is very slow (with a calculated regional CBF < 20 ml/min) the curve tends to approach a monoexponential decrement and the compartmental analysis becomes problematic; a true "fast" phase has practically disappeared.

The regional findings in "stroke patients", show a marked variability of blood flow

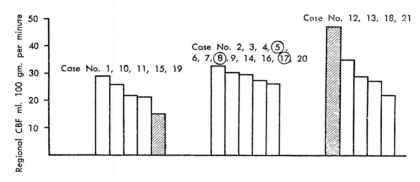

Fig. 2. Distribution of regional CBF in 21 patients with acute stroke: significant regional ischemia (left), uniformly low blood flow (center), reactive hyperemia (right).

between different brain regions. According to the threshold of 35; interregional variations, 9 out of 18 cases with ischemic lesions, and none of the hemorrhages examined within four days of the stroke, had pathological interregional variability of regional CBF.

This nonuniformity of regional CBF may depend on regions with excessively low ("focal ischemia") or excessively high ("reactive hyperemia") blood flow with respect to the adjacent area of the same hemisphere (Fig. 2).

The identification of an area of "reactive hyperemia" or significant "focal ischemia" is based on arbitrary criteria. We have adopted the following: Reactive hyperemia or "luxury perfusion" (Fig. 3): (1) interregional variations of at least 35%; (2) regional CBF > 45 ml/100 g/min, and/or flow of the "fast component" > 100 ml/100 g/min.

Significant focal ischemia (Fig. 4): (1) interregional variations of at least 35%; regional CBF < 20 ml/100 g/min and/or flow of the "fast component" < 35 ml/100 g/min.

Cases with focal ischemia have been observed on each of the four days after the acute episode, while in patients with reactive hyperemia at least forty-eight hours had elapsed since the stroke.

In a patient reexamined fourteen days after the first regional CBF measurement, the reactive hyperemia had disappeared, and it was never observed in cases studied at a later stage than four days (Fieschi *et al.*, 1968).

References pp. 408–410

B.J. No. 154
2 days

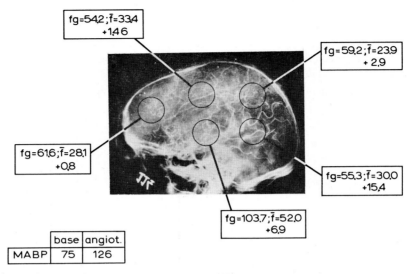

	base	angiot.
MABP	75	126

Fig. 3. Regional CBF two days after a right ischemic softening. fg = flow rate of the fast component, $\bar{f}$ = mean regional flow. Reactive hyperemia ("luxury perfusion") in temporal region. Serioangiography shows early filling of septal, thalamostriate, and internal cerebral veins. During induced hypertension autoregulation is lost in prerolandic and occipital regions. Changes are expressed in ml/100 g/min with respect to mean flow in basal conditions.

D.G.E. No. 152
Same day

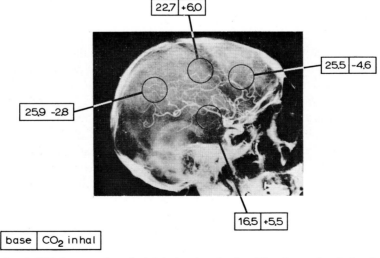

base	CO_2 inhal

Fig. 4. Regional CBF the same day of a left ischemic softening. Flow is very low in basal conditions with a significant focal ischemia in temporal region. During CO_2 inhalation flow slightly increases in temporal and rolandic regions; decreases in parietal and frontal regions (intracerebral steal?). Changes are expressed in ml/100 g/min with respect to basal conditions.

rCBF in other brain disorders

(*a*) *Uniformly low blood flow* This is the most common finding in different types of pathology. In cerebrovascular lesions, we have seen that uniformly low rCBF is observed very frequently in post apoplectic states at a distance from the acute phase, or in chronic ischemic disturbances of cerebral arteriosclerosis (Ingvar 1967) in brain stem lesions and in cases with circumscribed lesions in the contralateral hemisphere (Hoedt-Rasmussen and Skinhoj, 1964, Ingvar *et al.*, 1964). Beside primarily vascular pathology, regional cerebral blood flow is diffusely decreased in organic dementia and in some brain tumor (Cronquist and Agee, 1957) although in most tumors the flow is unevenly distributed.

(*b*) *Uniformly high blood flow* This is a rare condition which may be expected in cases with tissue acidosis and vasomotor paralysis. Thus, a uniformly high blood flow has been hypothesized in some post-concussive syndromes (Lassen, 1966); it has been observed in experimental posthypoxic states (Freeman and Ingvar, 1968, Haggendal *et al.*, 1966), in severe metabolic acidosis of chronic respiratory insufficiency (Fig. 5). In these circumstances the homeostatic mechanisms of tissue and cerebrospinal fluid acid-base equilibrium are disrupted and a diffuse brain syndrome ensues (such as the respiratory encephalopathy), so that the apparent paradox of a disturbance of consciousness combined with an increased blood flow is observed.

(*c*) *Regionally reduced blood flow* We have just seen that cerebral blood flow may be diffusely reduced even with circumscribed cerebral lesions. Yet, differences of perfusion among cerebral regions are often noted, and in some cases they reach a threshold beyond which we may speak of a focal cerebral ischemia, defined as earlier. This has been noted in acute cerebral vascular lesions as well as in cerebral tumors (Cronquist and Agee, 1967) (Fig. 4).

F.C. No. 198/201
Respiratory encephalophaty

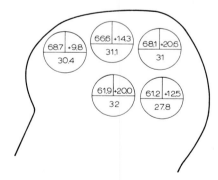

Base I	Hypert.
aP_{CO_2} 73	aP_{CO_2} 79
aP_{CO_2} 65	aP_{CO_2} 68
CSFpH 7.26	MABP 133
MABP 107	
Base II	
aP_{CO_2} 39	
aP_{CO_2} 65	
MABP 100	
CSFpH 7.32	

Fig. 5. In the first determination (Base I), the regional cerebral blood flow is diffusely increased, and its autoregulation is lost. In the second determination (Base II), while aP_{CO_2} and CSF pH have returned to normal limits after prolonged passive hyperventilation and medical treatment, the regional cerebral blood flow is decreased to below normal. Blood flow values and its changes are expressed in ml/100 g/min.

References pp. 408–410

Among tumors, 36 percent of cases have a low flow in the tumor area compared to the surrounding normal tissue, regardless of whether the tumor is avascular or with pathological vessels seen at angiography (Cronquist and Agee, 1967).

(*d*) *Regionally increased blood flow* In the very area, or at the periphery of the area of a focal cerebral lesion (tumor, softening, hemorrhage) the vessels may be dilated and regional cerebral blood flow increased (reactive hyperemia). This abnormality indicates a vasodilatation due to the focal or perifocal tissue acidosis. When the arterial blood is normally oxygenated, the draining veins carry arterialized blood due to increased flow and poor tissue oxygen utilization. Therefore, this condition has been named the red veins syndrome (Feindel and Perot, 1965, Waltz and Sundt, 1967) or the luxury perfusion syndrome (Lassen, 1966).

Thus a regional increase of perfusion rate indicates a functional derangement of vasoregulation and damage to the nervous tissue. In cerebral hemorrhages the paradoxical vasodilatation is "a fortiori" in the tissue surrounding the hemorrhage. It is an infrequent finding, since in most instances the compression of the tissue by the expanding mass increases the vascular resistance and reduces the blood flow. In cerebral softening the reactive hyperemia may be found in the region of ischemia proper, when the circulation is resumed after the acute focal anoxia. Frequently, however, the reactive hyperemia is at the periphery of the softening, where tissue acidosis and vasoparalysis are brought about by diffusion of acid metabolites from the anoxic site, or where an efficient collateral circulation takes place before anoxia has irreversibly damaged the tissue (Fig. 6).

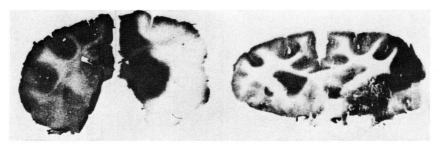

Fig. 6. Autoradiographies in two cats whose middle cerebral artery has been ligated less than 24 h prior to the blood flow measurements. The darkening is proportional to [14C] antipyrine concentration, and its function of the local blood flow. On the left, persistence of a large ischemic focus with perifocal reactive hyperemia. On the right, the circulation has been resumed in the ischemic tissue where, due to postanoxic acidosis and vasoparalysis, the blood flow is paradoxically increased (focal reactive hyperemia or luxury perfusion).

Also in tumor cases a regional increase of blood flow may be observed in the tumor tissue or at its periphery (Fig. 7). (Cronquist and Agee, 1967).

In this last case the situation is similar to that found in brain hemorrhages with perifocal tissue damage and vasoparalysis accompanied by a sufficiently high perfusion pressure. The occurrence of an increased perfusion rate in the tumor vessels is a finding usually coinciding with the angiographic appearance of neoformed vessels (23 out of 28 cases). However, an increased blood flow may be observed over angiographically silent tumors (3 out of 11 cases according to Cronquist and Agee, 1967); the possibility that in these cases the increased blood flow is in the perifocal damaged nervous tissue rather than in the neoplasm is discussed by these authors.

Another instance of regionally increased blood flow with initial "shunt" peak is the vascular malformations with A-V shunts (Cronquist *et al.*, 1966, Haggendal *et al.*, 1965, Oldendorf and Kitano, 1964).

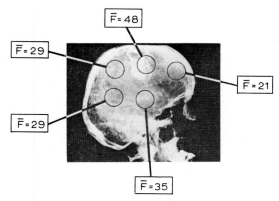

Fig. 7. Hyperemic focus corresponding to the neoformed vessels of a glioblastoma multiformis in rolandic region. Blood flow values are expressed in ml/100 g/min.

Head traumas with contusion of brain tissue may also present a regionally increased blood flow according to the experimental findings of Brock and co-workers (1967), although this has not yet been recorded in man.

Autoregulation of CBF during drug induced hypertension in normal subjects and in patients with cerebrovascular diseases.

The effects of pharmacological or environmental stimuli on cerebral vessels in man have been reexamined on the basis of regional cerebral blood flow methods. Autoregulation, defined as the property of cerebral vessels to respond to changes in perfusion pressure in order to maintain a constant cerebral perfusion rate, has been tested in 15 normotensive healthy subjects and in 24 patients with focal cerebral vascular disease: 21 ischemic infarcts and three T.I.A. (Agnoli *et al.*, 1968).

All patients were normotensive, thirteen patients were studied within the first two days of an ischemic episode, and 11 were studied 15 days to several months after an ischemic episode. Mean arterial blood pressure was raised with intravenous infusion of approximately 40 g/min of angiotensin and was kept at 30 to 40 mm Hg above the resting level.

In the control group the average increase of mean arterial blood pressure produced by angiotensin amide was 34.7 mm Hg. The variations in Pa_{CO_2} were between $\pm$ 1.5 mm Hg. Values for rCBF before and during hypertension were almost identical: mean

References pp. 408–410

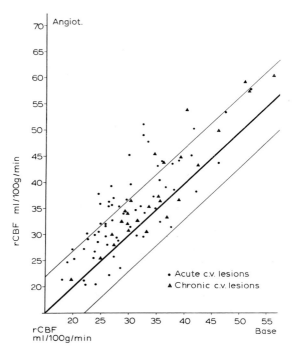

Fig. 8. Changes of regional cerebral blood flow during induced hypertension. On the abscissa are values of rCBF in the resting state and on the ordinate are values of rCBF during a 30 to 40 mm Hg increase of mean arterial blood pressure. The identity line and confidence limits of the normal response to hypertension ($\pm$ 2 S.D.) are drawn. Twenty of 64 regions examined in "acute" cases and four of 26 regions examined in "chronic" cases are above the upper line, indicating loss of auto-regulation.

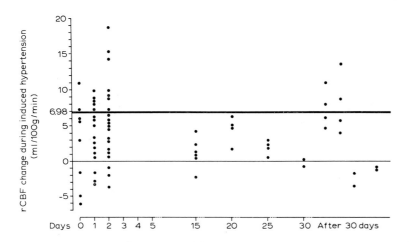

Fig. 9. Response of rCBF to hypertension in patients with cerebral vascular lesions. Points above the upper line indicate regions where autoregulation was lost (increase of rCBF $+$ 7 ml/100 g/min). In the first days after the stroke a greater number of regions had lost autoregulation.

increase during hypertension was 0.26 ml/100 g/min. Also flow rates and relative weight of the fast and slow compartments were practically unchanged.

In patients with cerebral vascular disease we observed slight variations of flow in both the fast and slow compartments with little increase in weight of the fast component. Mean increases in rCBF in patients with cerebral vascular disease were 4.4 ml/100 g/min in the "acute" group and 2.9 ml/100 g/min in the "chronic" group. Analysis with the "t" test for coupled data showed that the difference from the control group was statistically significant in both instances (P < 0.001). In these 24 patients, rCBF was measured in 90 regions; impairment of autoregulation, manifested by an increase in rCBF during hypertension exceeding the 2 S.D. limit of the normal range ($\pm$ 7 ml/100 g/min), was found in 24 regions (26.6%) (Figs. 8 and 9).

It is apparent from figure 9 that autoregulation of rCBF is impaired in a greater number of regions measured in patients with acute cerebral vascular lesions than in "chronic" cases. Ten of 13 patients within 48 hours of a stroke showed a regional loss of autoregulation, but only two of 11 patients studied later, in a nonacute stage, showed an increase of rCBF exceeding 7 ml/100 g/min during hypertension.

Further analysis of the clinical findings in the "acute" group showed that all three patients with preserved autoregulation had transient ischemic attacks. The other 10 patients, who had impairment of autoregulation, had definite brain softenings.

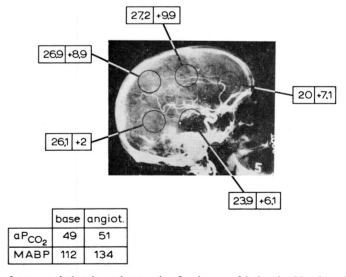

R.R. No. 144
1 day
Right hemiparesis and aphasia

	base	angiot.
aP_{CO_2}	49	51
MABP	112	134

Fig. 10. Loss of autoregulation in and around a focal area of ischemia. Numbers indicate rCBF in the resting state and the change (in ml/100 g/min) during induced hypertension. From the clinical electroencephalographic, and scintigraphic data (Fig. 11), the ischemic focus can be located in the frontal region. Loss of autoregulation was found in the frontal, rolandic, and the parietal regions.

References pp. 408–410

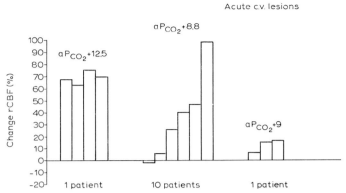

Fig. 13. Frequency of the different types of response of cerebral vessels to hypercarbia in acute cerebral vascular lesions (3 days and later after the stroke). From left to right, homogeneous response, heterogeneous response, lack of vasodilatation. Each column represents one cerebral region.

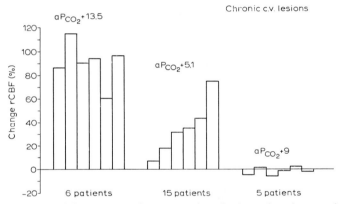

Fig. 14. Frequency of the different types of response of cerebral vessels to hypercarbia in stabilized vascular lesions (15 days and less after the stroke). From left to right, homogeneous response, heterogeneous response, lack of vasodilatation. Each column represents one cerebral region.

Therefore in some chronic as well as in acute cases a dissociation is noted between normal autoregulation and impaired response to CO_2.

A similar dissociation was noted by Fazekas and Alman (1964). These authors reported the occurrence of a normal vasoconstriction during hyperventilation in patients who had lost the vascular reactivity to hypercarbia. One could generalize that in severely atherosclerotic subjects, the cerebral blood flow seems to work at a nearly maximal level so that no further vasodilatation is obtained even with so potent an agent as CO_2.

This form of reduced cerebrovascular reactivity to CO_2 is not attributable to a purely mechanical factor 'such as rigidity of the arteriolar wall') since the vessels are still capable of constricting; rather it is attributable to a reduction or to exhaustion of the available reserve for vasodilatation (maximal vasodilatation).

The major interest of the rCBF studies lies in the groups of Figs. 13 and 14 which include the heterogeneous and the paradoxical responses.

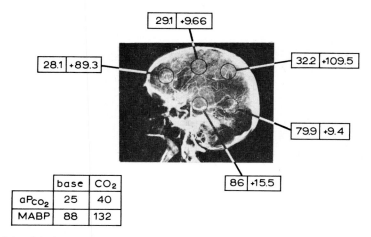

	base	CO₂
aP_CO₂	25	40
MABP	88	132

Fig. 15. Left hemiplegia, studied the day after the stroke (hemorrhage). Luxury perfusion in temporal and occipital regions, where during hypercarbia (aP_{CO_2} 15 mm Hg; MABP + 44 mm Hg) rCBF increased by 15.2 and 9.4%. The reactivity was much higher in the remaining regions (+ 74 to + 110%).

The finding of an uneven vascular reactivity in focal brain disorders is not surprising (Fig. 15) nor is the occurrence of an active redistribution of blood flow, also known as intracerebral steal (Fig. 16).

Fazekas and Alman (1964) had noted already that CO_2 inhalation could lead to a paradoxical decrease of the cerebral blood flow in vascular diseases. About at the same time a phenomenon of intracerebral redistribution of blood flow leading occasionally to regional ischemia was described in special anatomical situations. More recently this "steal" phenomenon was demonstrated quantitatively in cases of

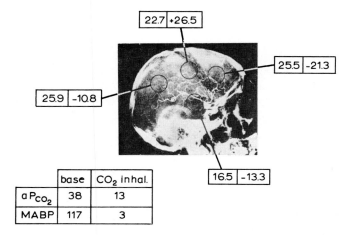

	base	CO₂ inhal.
aP_CO₂	38	13
MABP	117	3

Fig. 16. Right hemiplegia and aphasia, studied the same day of the stroke. During CO₂ inhalation (aP_{CO_2} +13 mm Hg; MABP +3 mm Hg) rCBF increased in rolandic and temporal regions, decreased in frontal (− 21.3%) and parietal (− 10.8%) regions (intracerebral steal).

TABEL 5

CBF REACTIVITY TO HYPERCARBIA IN CVD*

Type of reactivity	No of cases	Middle Cerebral Artery occlusion	Stroke without occlusion	Mild ischemic episodes	TIA
Acute					
Focally reduced	17	5	9	3	0
Paradoxical ("steal")	8	2	5	1	0
Uniform	13	0	5	2	6
After 2 weeks					
Focally reduced	13	3	3	4	3
Paradoxical ("steal")	3	0	3	0	0
Uniform	24	0	4	11	9
Total	78	10	29	21	18

*Combined Copenhagen (40 patients) and Genoa (38 patients) case records.

apoplexy. It was interpreted as the expression of a focal vasoparalysis in a region adjacent to others reacting normally to vasodilating stimuli.

Experimental demonstrations of the same phenomenon in cases of arterial occlusion were subsequently provided.

Table 5 shows the frequency of the steal phenomenon in apoplexy in the combined case records from Genova and from Copenhagen.

In all stroke patients with Middle Cerebral Artery occlusion there are focal impaired reactions to CO_2, two patients of the acute group showing intracerebral steal. In cases of stroke without arterial occlusion at the time of the study, one observes absent or paradoxical regional reactivity to CO_2 inhalation in the majority of acute as well as in stabilized cases.

Steal was never observed in T.I.A. In cases of ischemic episodes with minor residual defects, abnormal focal responses are also rare and decrease in frequency with time; in these cases an intracerebral steal was observed only once, one day after the attack.

In summary, the intracerebral steal produced by CO_2 inhalation is a phenomenon observed in focal brain lesions, and it is especially noted in the acute phase. Since the action of CO_2 on cerebral vessels may be mediated by the extravascular H^+ concentration, the excess of local vasodilator stimuli provided by the post-anoxic metabolic acidosis of the brain explains such an extreme derangement of the regional vasomotor regulation. The vasomotor paralysis of the acute post anoxic brain syndrome may be revealed by a "luxury perfusion", or by paradoxical responses of CBF to changes in MABP or to changes in aP_{CO_2}: all these phenomena are a consequence rather than a cause of the focal ischemia.

Therefore a CO_2 test remains of little value as a screening procedure for hemodynamic disturbance which might lead to ischemic episodes, even now after the introduction of methods for measuring regional CBF. In fact, we never observed an intracerebral steal in T.I.A. and only once in the acute phase of an ischemic episode with minor residual defects. On the other hand CO_2 responses are of major interest from a therapeutic rather than diagnostic viewpoint.

In view of the absent or paradoxical responses of rCBF in many patients with stroke, giving CO_2 as a treatment appears useless or contraindicated. It is probable that areas of impaired CBF regulation are present in the majority of patients with a severe brain damage. Indeed the flow distribution after a vascular occlusion with brain ischemia is quite erratic, much more than the radioactive gas regional clearance technique can show (Fieschi, 1970).

Hyperventilation appears then as a logical procedure in the acute phase of brain ischemia, reversing the potential disadvantages of CO_2 inhalation. However, as already suggested by Meyer *et al.* (1968), in the less severe stroke cases hyperventilation may further impair a situation that is barely compensated and clinical and experimental studies on the effects of hyperventilation in the treatment of acute brain lesions is still controversial.

Discrepancies between autoregulation and CO_2 reactivity of cerebral vessels

While studying rCBF in brain disease, we noted that abnormal reactivities to CO_2 and to changes in blood pressure can be dissociated in the same cerebral region.

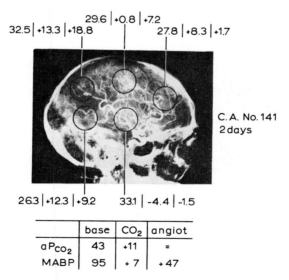

29.6 | +0.8 | +7.2
32.5 | +13.3 | +18.8   27.8 | +8.3 | +1.7

C.A. No. 141
2 days

26.3 | +12.3 | +9.2   33.1 | -4.4 | -1.5

	base	CO_2	angiot
aP_{CO_2}	43	+11	=
MABP	95	+7	+47

Fig. 17. Patient C.A. studied 2 days after onset of a right hemiplegia and aphasia due to hemispheric infarction. The numbers represent the mean regional blood flow (Kr[85] intracarotid injection, compartmental analysis), and its absolute changes during CO_2 inhalation and during angiotensin infusion. Changes in aP_{CO_2} and MABP during tests are indicated at the bottom of the figure. The 5 regions behave unevenly: the parietal and occipital regions react to CO_2 but have lost autoregulation; the temporal region shows preserved autoregulation but reacts to CO_2 in a paradoxical manner; the rolandic region has lost both autoregulation and CO_2 reactivity; finally the frontal region reacts normally.

References pp. 408–410

These discrepancies (Fieschi *et al.*, 1969 a, b) are present in about 40% of the areas of acute focal brain lesions, that show either impaired autoregulation with preserved response to CO_2, or vice-versa (Fig. 17).

Two possible explanations were considered, namely: (1) these discrepancies confute the unitarian theory of the cerebral vasomotor regulation; (2) the "pH" model still holds and these dissociations must be explained as artifacts.

The artifact may depend on the fairly large size of the region explored by our probes (open face $2\frac{1}{2}$ cm), a region that certainly includes vessels in different functional states. For example, the parietal and occipital regions of the patients shown in Fig. 17 may include vessels that are normally regulated, whose response to CO_2 gives a sufficient vasodilatation to simulate a significant increase in the mean flow for the entire region. At the same time, other vessels may be unreacting, thus increasing their "mean" regional flow significantly when the blood pressure is raised.

The opposite type of discrepancy is less frequently observed as shown in the temporal region of Fig. 17 and in the temporal region of Fig. 18, where the response to CO_2 is abolished while autoregulation (by increasing the arterial pressure) is preserved. It is conceivable that autoregulation is only *apparently* preserved: in fact, the increased intracranial pressure due to the vasodilatation in the confining region may increase the extravascular resistance enough to counteract the effect of the increased arterial pressure (Fieschi *et al.*, 1969). In certain extreme cases it is possible to observe in such regions with severe vasoparalysis and brain edema a paradoxical decrease in flow during induced hypertension.

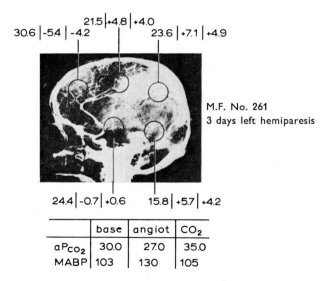

M.F. No. 261
3 days left hemiparesis

	base	angiot	CO_2
aP_{CO_2}	30.0	27.0	35.0
MABP	103	130	105

Fig. 18. Patient M.F. studied 3 days after the onset of a left hemiparesis with occlusion of the right M.C.A. The numbers represent the mean regional blood flow and its absolute changes (in ml/100 g/min) during angiotensin infusion and during CO_2 inhalation. Changes in MABP and aP_{CO_2} during tests are indicated at the bottom of the figure. Dissociated response (preserved autoregulation with lost response to CO_2) in the temporal region.

Nevertheless, our evidence suggests that independent mechanisms may regulate the response of cerebral vessels to CO_2 and to perfusion pressure changes and that these mechanisms may be affected at a different level in disease states.

Cerebral blood flow in metabolic and respiratory coma

The cerebral perfusion rate is classically related to the metabolic and functional activity of the brain. Actually, CBF is reduced in comatose states; this reduction being dependent on the depth of coma rather than on its etiology. On the other hand, to the concentration of H^+ in the ECF of the brain, the role has recently been attributed of the main "signal" or determinant of the tone of the arteriolar smooth muscle of the cerebral vessels: following this hypothesis, a reduction in functional and metabolic activity influences the CBF through a reduction in hydrogen ions in the ECF. This however is a final common pathway, that may be independently effected by several other factors. This is clearly shown among others, by the studies on CBF during adaptation to prolonged hypercarbia (Agnoli *et al.*, 1969). Consequently, any time a disturbing factor of systemic origin affects the acid-base status of the brain monitored, in clinical cases, by the CSF pH, the relationships between flow and state of consciousness, may be lost. The first known example of such uncoupling was reported more than 20 years ago by Kety *et al.* (1948) who in severe acidotic (diabetic) coma (arterial pH 7.00) recorded a CBF 20% higher than normal. This uncoupling was unexplained until the "Severinghaus electrode" theory of CBF control was advanced.

Recently however, a new kind of "uncoupling" has been noted, this time between CBF and CSF pH.

In 20 rCBF determinations in patients with various degrees of coma of metabolic or respiratory origin (Battistini *et al.*, 1969), we have clearly noted both types of uncoupling between depressed consciousness and high CBF and between low CSF pH and low flow in more severe cases. Such a dissociation between low CSF pH and low flow is an indication of brain edema. For practical purposes, any attempt to interpret CBF findings in pathological cases must take into account the fact that an important component of the cerebral vascular resistance in disease may depend on extra vascular factors, such as intracranial pressure and brain edema: the abnormality of vasomotor regulation in such cases, however, is evident from the passive responses to blood pressure changes, and from the lack of response to CO_2.

Relationships between EEG and regional cerebral blood flow

Regional cerebral blood flow measurements in man have allowed a more accurate study of the relationships between tissue perfusion and electrical activity similar to those carried out in animals. The link between these functions is represented by the actual tissue oxygen consumption. It follows that in any instance of decoupling between oxygen consumption and cerebral blood flow (as for instance in severe hypoxemia), the relationship between cerebral flow and EEG is lost.

Also in acute vascular lesions the correlation between regional cerebral blood flow and EEG is poor because there are instances of normal or even increased blood flow with profound EEG slowing and, less frequently, the opposite type of changes (Loeb and Fieschi, 1967). Similar relationships were found by Magnus and coworkers (1967) by the intracarotid injection technique of radioalbumin.

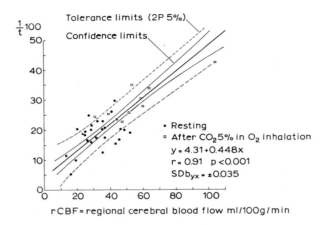

Fig. 19. Inverse of mean transit time of RISA ($1/\bar{t} \cdot 100$) on the ordinate and rCBF calculated from the regional clearance of ^{85}Kr on the abscis. Radioactivity was recorded over the temporo-parietal area, ipsilateral to the injected internal carotid artery. The following values are given in the figure: the equation of the regression line, the standard deviation of the coefficient b(SDb_{yx}), and the coefficient of correlation r. The confidence limits of the regression line of y on x and tolerance limits of y are shown in graphical form.

Relationships between circulation time and regional cerebral blood flow

These have been explored by comparing the transit time (t) of RISA and regional cerebral blood flow in the same region (Fieschi *et al.*, 1966). This study showed a linear regression between RISA transit time and regional cerebral blood flow, although in individual cases a wide range of regional cerebral blood flow can be expected for any observed value of RISA $\bar{t}$ (Fig. 19). For example, a $\bar{t}$ of five seconds tolerates (within 95% of probability) regional cerebral blood flow values ranging from 24–246 ml/100 g/min. As noted by Zingesser and co-workers (1968) circulation time does not yield flow rates unless the volume of vascular bed is known, and its changes are not linear with flow changes unless the cerebral blood volume is constant. The effects of volume variations on RISA transit time have been examined by Fieschi and co-workers (1966) by showing that an increase of flow brought about by hypercarbia is underestimated by changes of RISA $\bar{t}$.

Relationship between rCBF and angiography

In patients with carotid thrombosis the average CBF measured by injecting the ^{85}Kr solution in the contralateral internal carotid artery, was 34 ml/100 g/min; the flow of the fast component was 57 ml/100 g/min and that of the slow component 18.4 ml/100 g/min; these values are reduced with respect to controls, but significantly higher than in the remaining cases with cerebrovascular lesions.

A middle cerebral artery occlusion is associated with a greater reduction of rCBF (20 ml/100 g/min = 36%) in comparison with patients without occlusion that are characterized by a 27% diminution of flow rate of the fast and slow components, and by a 25% diminution of the relative weight of the fast component (Fieschi et al., 1966). In our acute patients (Fieschi et al., 1968) serioangiographic studies performed within twenty-four hours of the regional CBF measurement have also shown in some cases areas of focal ischemia (slow circulation, poor filling of vessels) or hyperemia (capillary blush, early filling veins). When this was observed, there was always a corresponding finding in the regional CBF measurement. However several cases with focal ischemia or hyperemia as revealed by the measurement of regional CBF were not evident at seroangiography. No cases with uniform distribution of regional CBF showed any ischemic or hyperemic area on the seroangiograms.

These data suggest that the radioisotopic measurement of regional blood flow is a more sensitive index of the hemodynamic situation than angiography.

rCBF studies during carotid surgery

Surgical treatment of carotid stenosis requires that the common and internal carotid arteries are temporarily occluded during the endarteriectomy. The clamping may last 12 to 15 minutes, a sufficient length of time to induce a cerebral damage if collateral circulation is not adequate to prevent a severe ischemia in the territory supplied by the stenosed vessel.

Pistolese et al. (1971) and Boysen (1971) studied with CBF measurement how to determine the threshold of regional ischemia that can be safely tolerated for the duration of surgery, and how to prevent such an ischemia by means of a controlled increase in arterial pressure. Patients who showed a decrease in CBF below 30 ml/100 g/min despite induced hypertension where considered too risky to be submitted to endarteriectomy.

We have reexamined this problem by measuring the regional rather than the hemispheric blood flow, and testing its response to CO_2 inhalation and to hyperventilation during a temporary clamping of the artery to be operated upon (Agnoli et al., 1970).

The clamping of the internal carotid artery at normotension and normocapnia reduced rCBF on the average by 42%. This reduction is not uniform in the various regions; consequently the threshold of tolerance by the brain to a 15 minutes clamping is 30 ml/100 g/min when measuring the average CBF, while when measuring the regional CBF a flow as low as 25 ml/100 g/min is well tolerated. Below these limits there are two acceptable choices: either to apply means to increase the rCBF during clamping, or to avoid the operation. Operating despite the recognized risk, is inacceptable in a "prophylactic" type of surgery.

The means are: (a) to give CO_2 or vasodilators; (b) to hyperventilate the patient to a high P_{O_2} and a low P_{CO_2} level; (c) to increase the depth of anesthesia; (d) to increase the arterial pressure; (e) to apply an internal shunt. According to our experience neither of these means has a proven and constant effect of increasing the local CBF. Hypercapnia did not restore the flow that was reduced during clamping in

TABLE 6

rCBF DURING INTRASURGICAL CAROTID CLAMPING, AT VARIOUS LEVELS OF
MABP AND ARTERIAL P_{CO_2}

	Normotensive + normoventilation	Normotensive + hyperventilation	Hypertensive + normoventilation
Base	60.8	33.8	79.7
Clamp.	35.5	21.2	43.2

previous studies of Pistolese *et al.* (1971). These authors found hypertension more helpful under those circumstances, however in our subsequent study (Agnoli *et al.*, 1970) we found little beneficial effect from hypertension. On the other hand rCBF is less reduced by clamping during hyperventilation than in other conditions, except when pre-clamping value is already low. In the last case the final result is often a flow below the threshold value (Table 6). As for the internal shunt, its risks and contra-indications have been pointed out by Pistolese *et al.* Generally speaking, the level of blood pressure is a more relevant factor for preventing an excessive drop of local CBF than the level of Pa_{CO_2}.

REFERENCES

AGNOLI, A., BATTISTINI, N., NARDINI, M., PASSERO, S. AND FIESCHI, C. (1969) Lack of adaption of CBF and CSF pH in hypoxic hypercapnia, in *Cerebral Blood Flow*, Brock *et al.* (Eds.), Springer, New York.

AGNOLI, A., FIESCHI, C., BOZZAO, L., BATTISTINI, N. AND PRENCIPE, M. (1968) Autoregulation of cerebral blood flow. Studies during drug induced hypertension in normal subjects and in patients with cerebral vascular disease. *Circulation*, 38.

AGNOLI, A., FIESCHI, C., PRENCIPE, M., PISTOLESE, G. R., FARAGLIA, V., PASTORE, E., SEMPREBENE, L. AND FIORANI, P. (1970) *Cerebral blood flow studies during carotid surgery*. Reactivity of cerebral circulation to CO2 and hypertension in basal condition and during clamping. International C.B.F. Symposium, London.

AGNOLI, A., PRENCIPE, M., PRIORI, A. M., BOZZAO, L. AND FIESCHI, C. (1969) Measurements of rCBF by intravenous injection of 133 Xe. A comparative study with the intra-arterial injection method. In *Cerebral Blood Flow*, Brock *et al.* (Eds.), Springer, New York.

BATTISTINI, N., CASACCHIA, M., BARTOLINI, A., BAVA, G. AND FIESCHI, C. (1969) Effects of hyper-ventilation on focal brain damage following middle cerebral artery occlusion. In *Cerebral Blood Flow*, Brock *et al.* (Eds.), Springer, New York.

BROCK, M., INGVAR, D. H. AND SEM JACOBSEN, C. W. (1967) Regional blood flow in deep structures of the brain measured in acute cat experiments by means of a new beta-sensitive semiconductor needle detector. *Exp. Brain Res.*, **4**, 126.

CRONQUIST, S. (1967) *La circulation de luxe: données radiologiques et données isotopiques*. VIII Symposium Neuroradiologicum. Paris.

CRONQUIST, S. AND AGEE, F. (1967) *Regional cerebral blood flow in intracranial tumors*. VIII Symposium Neuroradiologicum. Paris.

CRONQUIST, S., INGVAR, D. H. AND LASSEN, N. A. (1966) Quantitative measurements of regional cerebral blood flow related to neuroradiological findings, *Acta Radiol. Diagn.*, **5**, 760.

FAZEKAS, J. E. AND ALMAN, R. W. (1964) Maximal dilatation of cerebral vessels. *Arch. Neurol. (Chic.)*, **11**, 303.

FEINDEL, W. AND PEROT, P. (1965) Red cerebral veins. A report on arteriovenous shunts in tumors and cerebral scars. *J. Neurosurg.*, **22**, 315.

FIESCHI, C. (1970) *Regulation of cerebral blood vessels to CO_2 in acute brain disease and its relevance to therapy.* Conference on cerebrovascular Disease. Princeton.

FIESCHI, C., AGNOLI, A., BATTISTINI, N. AND BOZZAO, L. (1966) Relationships between cerebral transit time of nondiffusible indicators and cerebral blood flow. A comparative study with Krypton 85 and radioalbumin. *Experientia (Basel)*, **22**, 271.

FIESCHI, C., AGNOLI, A., BATTISTINI, N. AND BOZZAO, L. (1966) Mean transit time of a non diffusible indicator as an index of regional cerebral blood flow. An experimental study in man with albumin I 131 and Krypton 85. *Trans. Amer. Neurol. Ass.*, **19**, 224.

FIESCHI, C., AGNOLI, A., BATTISTINI, N. AND BOZZAO, L. (1966) Regional cerebral blood flow in patients with brain infarcts. *Arch. Neurol.*, **15**, 653.

FIESCHI, C., AGNOLI, A., BATTISTINI, N., BOZZAO, L., NARDINI, M. AND PRENCIPE, M. (1969) Vasomotor responses of cerebral vessels in brain disease, in *Pharmakologie der localen Gehirndurchblutung* E. Betz and R. Wullenweber, Verlag Banaschewski, (Munchen) 181.

FIESCHI, C., AGNOLI, A., BATTISTNI, N.. BOZZAO, L. AND PRENCIPE, M. (1968) Derangement of regional cerebral blood flow and of its regulatory mechanisms in acute cerebrovascular lesions. *Neurology*, **18** (12), 1166–1179.

FIESCHI, C., AGNOLI, A., BOZZAO, L., BATTISTINI, N. AND PRENCIPE, M. (1969) Discrepancies between autoregulation and CO_2 reactivity of cerebral vessels. In *Cerebral Blood Flow*. Brock *et al.* (Eds.), Springer Verlag, New York.

FIESCHI, C., AGNOLI, A. AND PRENCIPE, M. (1971) Automatic analysis of cerebral blood flow. *J. Nucl. Biol. Med.*, in press.

FIESCHI, C., AGNOLI, A., PRENCIPE, M., BATTISTINI, N., BOZZAO, L. AND NARDINI, M. (1969) Impairment of the regional vasomotor responses of cerebral vessels to hypercarbia in vascular diseases. *European Neurology*, **2**, 13-30.

FREEMAN, J. AND INGVAR, D. H. (1968) Elimination by hypoxia of cerebral blood flow autoregulation and EEG relationship. *Exp. Brain Res.*. **5**, 61.

HAGGENDAL, E., INGVAR, D. H., LASSEN, N. A., NILSSON, N. I. P., NORLEN, G., WICKBOM, A. AND ZWETNOW, N. (1965) Pre- and postoperative measurements of regional cerebral blood flow in three cases of intracranial arteriovenous aneurysm. *J. Neurosurg.*, **22**, 1.

HAGGENDAL, E., LOFGREN, J., NILSSON, N. J. AND ZWENTOW, N. (1966) *Die Gehirndurchblutung bei experimentellen Likordruckänderungen*. Meeting of Germany Society for Neurosurgeons. Bad Durkheim.

HØEDT RASMUSSEN, K. AND SKINHØY, E. (1964) Transneural depression of the cerebral hemisperic metabolism in man. *Acta Neurol. Scand.*, **40**, 41.

HØEDT RASMUSSEN, K. AND SKINHØY, E. (1966) In vivo measurements of the relative weights of gray and white matter in the human brain. *Neurology*, **16**, 515–520.

HØEDT RASMUSSEN, K., SKINHØY, E., PAULSON, O., EWALD, J., BJERRUM, J. K., FAHRENKRUNG, A. AND LASSEN, N. A. (1967) Regional cerebral blood flow in acute apoplexy. The luxury perfusion syndrome of brain tissue. *Arch. Neurol.*, **17**, 271.

KETY, S. S., POLIS, L. D., NADLER, C. S. AND SCHILIDT, C. F. (1948) The blood flow and oxygen consumption of the human brain in diabetic acidosis and coma, *J. Clin. Lab. Invest.*, **27**, 500.

INGVAR, D. H. (1967) *The pathophysiology of the stroke related to findings in EEG and to measurements of regional cerebral blood flow in stroke.* Thule International Symposia. Nordiska Bokhaundelns Ferlag, p. 105.

INGVAR, D. H., CRONQUIST, S., EKBERG, R., RISBERG, J. AND HØEDT RASMUSSEN, K. (1965) Normal values of regional cerebral blood flow in man, including flow and weight estimates in gray and white matter. *Acta Neurol. Scand., Suppl.*, **14**, p. 72.

INGVAR, D. H., HAGGENDAHL, E., NILSSON, N. J., SOURAUDER, P., WUCKBONNE, J. AND LASSEN, N. A. (1964) Cerebral circulation and metabolism in a comatose patient. *Arch. Neurol.*, **11**, 13.

LASSEN, N. A. (1966) The luxury perfusion syndrome and its possible relation to acute metabolic acidosis localized within the brain. *Lancet*, ii, 1113.

LASSEN, N. A., HØEDT RASMUSSEN, K., SORENSEN, S. C., SKINHØY, E., CRONQUIST, S., BODFORSS, B. AND INGVAR, D. H. (1963) Regional cerebral blood flow in man determined by Krypton. *Neurology*, **16**, 719.

LOEB, C. AND FIESCHI, C. (1967) Electroencephalograms and regional cerebral blood flow in cases of brain infarction. In: WIDEN, L. (Ed.), Recent advances in clinical neurophysiology, *Electroencephalogr. Clin. Neurophysiol., Suppl.*, **25**, 111. Elsevier Amsterdam.

MAGNUS, O., VAN DEN VERG, B. AND VANDEN DRIFT, A. (1967) EEG and cerebral circulation. Isotope technique in recent advances in clinical neurophysiology. WIDEN, L. (Ed.), *Electroencephalogr. Clin. Neurophysiol., Suppl.*, **25**, 107. Amsterdam.

OBRIST, W. D., THOMSON, H. K., KING, C. H. AND WANG, H. S. (1967) Determination of regional cerebral blood flow by inhalation of 133 Xenon. *Circulat. Res.*. **20**, 124.

OLDENDORF, W. H. AND KITANO, M. (1964) The free passage of 131 I antipyrine through brain as an indication of AV shunting. *Neurology*, **14**, 1078.

PAULSON, O. B. (1969) Regional cerebral blood flow at rest and during functional tests in occlusive and non-occlusive cerebrovascular disease. In: *Cerebral Blood Flow*, BROCK, M., FIESCHI, C. *et al.* (Eds.), Springer-New York, 111.

PISTOLESE, G. R., CITONE, G., FARAGLIA, V., BENEDETTI-VALENTINI, F. JR., PASTORE, E., SEMPREBENE, L., DE LEO, G., SPERANZA, V. AND FIORANI, P. (1971) Effects of hypercapnia on cerebral blood flow during the clamping of the carotid arteries in surgical management of cerebrovascular insufficiency. *Neurology*, in press.

VEAL, N. AND MALLET, B. L. (1966) Regional CBF determination by ^{133}Xe inhalation and external recording the effect of arterial recirculation. *Clin. Sci.*, **30**, 352.

WALTZ, A. G. AND SUNDT, T. M. (1967) The microvasculature and microcirculation of the cerebral cortex after arterial occlusion. *Brain*, **90**, 681.

WILKINSON, I. M. S., BULL, J. W. D., DU BOULAY, G. H., MARSHALL, J., ROSS, R. W. AND RUSSEL, L. (1969) The heterogeneity of blood flow through the normal cerebral hemisphere. In: *Cerebral Blood Flow*, BROCK *et al.* (Ed.), Springer, New York.

Concepts of Cerebral Perfusion Pressure and Vascular Compression During Intracranial Hypertension*

J. DOUGLAS MILLER, ALBERT STANEK AND THOMAS W. LANGFITT

Division of Neurosurgery University of Pennsylvania

INTRODUCTION

Continuous monitoring of intracranial pressure (ICP) has become an increasingly common practice in neurosurgical units. Intracranial hypertension is produced by a variety of pathological states, and the increased pressure rather than the underlying disorder may be primarily responsible for death in these patients. There is general agreement that the intracranial hypertension disturbs brain function by reducing cerebral blood flow (CBF) and causing brain herniation with brainstem compression or displacement.

We have measured ICP continuously in patients with severe head injury, brain tumor, subarachnoid hemorrhage, hydrocephalus, cerebral hypoxia, pseudotumor cerebri, or encephalitis, and regional CBF has been measured in some of these patients using the ^{133}Xe clearance technique (unpublished observations). In addition, several models have been developed in an attempt to simulate clinical conditions in the laboratory animal (Langfitt *et al.*, 1965; Marshall *et al.*, 1969; Miller and Ledingham, 1971). This report describes observations in one of these animal models.

In recent reports on the effects of increased ICP on CBF (Zwetnow, 1970; Jennett *et al.*, 1970) increasing emphasis has been placed on the concept that changes in ICP affect CBF through alterations in cerebral perfusion pressure (CPP), and that in this respect they may be compared with changes in systemic arterial pressure (SAP) by considering CPP to be the difference between SAP and ICP. The purposes of this study were to test: (1) the effects of changes in ICP and SAP on CBF in the same animal, with intact and defective autoregulation, as a means of further evaluating several proposed mechanisms of autoregulation; (2) the sensitivity of autoregulation to raised ICP; (3) the response of CBF to a concomitant increase in SAP and ICP at a constant CPP, with intact and defective autoregulation.

MATERIALS AND METHODS

Small unselected mongrel dogs were used for the experiments. Anesthesia was induced

* Supported by the John A. Hartford Foundation, Incorporated.

References pp. 431–432

and maintained with pentobarbital sodium or chloralose. The animals were paralyzed with gallamine triethoxide and artificially ventilated. CBF was measured from the cerebral venous outflow using a modification of preparations described by Rapela and Green (1964) and D'Alecy (1971). The cerebral venous drainage in the dog leaves the skull by paired retroglenoid veins, extensions of the lateral and temporal sinuses, which exit from the skull base in front of the auditory meatus to join the maxillary vein, and by paired sigmoid sinuses which traverse the occipital bone to empty into the vertebral venous plexus. In this preparation blood was shunted from the torcular Herophili, using a cannulating screw, to the external jugular vein after ligating the retroglenoid veins flush with the base of the skull. The sigmoid sinuses were then unroofed using a dental drill, entered and packed with heparinized cotton wool. The flow of blood along the torculo-jugular shunt was measured by electromagnetic flowmeter and by injecting small air bubbles into the shunt distal to the flow probe and measuring the transit time along tubing of known volume.

SAP was measured from a catheter in the brachial artery and ICP from a needle in the cisterna magna. Cerebral venous outflow pressure was measured at the proximal end of the shunt. Arterial blood gases and pH were measured intermittently using direct reading electrodes, and end-tidal CO_2 was monitored continuously using an infra-red CO_2 analyzer. Blood gases were maintained within normal limits by altering the rate and stroke volume of the respirator. Body temperature was kept constant by a heating lamp connected by a feedback circuit to a thermistor probe in the rectum. ICP, SAP, CBF (flowmeter), and end tidal CO_2 were recorded continuously on an 8-channel polygraph. Heparin and intravenous bicarbonate and 5% glucose were administered during the experiment.

EXPERIMENTAL PROTOCOL

After control measurements of CBF, SAP was either elevated by intra-arterial infusion of norepinephrine or reduced by withdrawal of blood. After SAP had returned to control values, ICP was increased by infusion of Ringer's solution or mock CSF into the lumbar subarachnoid space. The effect of increased SAP on CBF during elevated ICP was studied in some preparations by injection of norepinephrine. In other animals a marked increase in ICP induced an arterial pressure response.

CPP is defined in this study as the difference between mean SAP and mean ICP (the diastolic pressure plus one third the difference between the diastolic and systolic pressures). CBF is expressed in ml/min. Brain weights were measured, but expression of CBF as ml/100 g/min was thought not to be justified because of uncertainty about the proportion of total cerebral blood flow measured with this technique. Intact autoregulation, determined by the response of CBF to a change in SAP of more than 15 mm Hg, was arbitrarily defined as a change in CBF of less than 1 ml/min at 3 min after the onset of the pressure change. Any change in CBF due to a change in SAP which exceeded these criteria was defined as defective autoregulation.

RESULTS

The mean CBF value for this preparation in 14 dogs at arterial P_{CO_2} levels between 36 and 40 mm Hg was 21.9 ml/min; when corrected for total brain weight, CBF was 29.5 ml/100 g/min.

The goal of each experiment was to compare the response of CBF to changes in CPP produced first by a decrease in SAP and second by an increase in ICP. The data presented was obtained from 27 runs in 16 animals in which the two types of pressure changes were performed in succession.

Based on the definition of autoregulation used in these studies, the 27 runs were divided into 11 where autoregulation was intact and 16 where autoregulation was defective. In those 11 runs where a change in SAP within the autoregulatory range produced no change in CBF, there was no change in CBF when ICP was increased within the autoregulatory range. In the 16 runs where autoregulation was found to be defective to a change in SAP, elevation of ICP caused an immediate fall in CBF. Fig. 1 illustrates two runs in the same animal in which CPP was reduced, first by

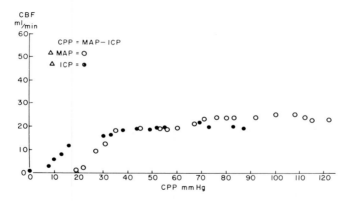

Fig. 1. Effect of altering cerebral perfusion pressure in a dog with intact autoregulation to changing arterial pressure (open circles). Increasing intracranial pressure (closed circles) causes no change in cerebral blood flow until CPP falls below 40 mm Hg in these circumstances.

lowering SAP, then by elevating ICP. Autoregulation is intact in both instances, demonstrated by normal CBF values until CPP falls to 40 mm Hg. Following return of ICP to normal, SAP was reduced, and autoregulation was now defective; CBF follows CPP passively (Fig. 2). When SAP was returned to normal and ICP was increased, autoregulation was again defective to the change in CPP produced by this method.

Changes in CBF produced by the two methods of altering CPP were then compared in order to determine if there was any difference in the efficiency of autoregulation according to whether CPP was reduced by lowering SAP or raising ICP. Mean values were obtained for CBF at fixed levels of CPP determined by visual inspection of those pressure/flow graphs for which adequate data was available over the range of CPP from 0 to 100 mm Hg. When autoregulation was intact (Fig. 3), CBF remained

References pp. 431–432

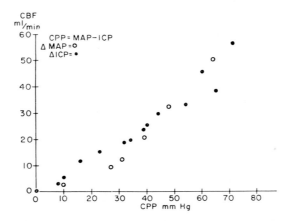

Fig. 2. Effect of altering cerebral perfusion pressure in the same dog after autoregulation to changing arterial pressure (open circles) has been lost due to a preceding period of severe intracranial hypertension with cessation of CBF. At this stage increasing ICP (closed circles) caused marked changes in CBF.

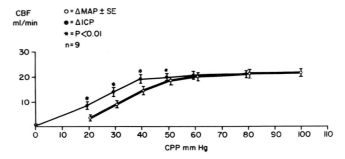

Fig. 3. Effect of altering cerebral perfusion pressure by decreasing arterial pressure (open circles) and by increasing intracranial pressure (closed circles) in dogs with intact autoregulation. Significance between changes assessed by paired *t*-test.

constant with both methods to a CPP of 50 mm Hg. CBF then fell when CPP was reduced below 50 mm Hg by lowering SAP; but increasing ICP did not cause CBF to decline until the CPP fell below 40 mm Hg. CBF was significantly higher at CPP levels of 40, 30, and 20 mm Hg ($p < 0.01$) when CPP was reduced by increasing ICP compared to decreasing SAP. This same relationship at low levels of CPP was observed in the non-autoregulating runs (Fig. 4), although to a lesser extent.

In several dogs data was available to study the effect on CBF of increasing SAP when ICP increased in parallel, so that CPP remained constant. When autoregulation was intact or only mildly impaired CBF remained constant at 20 ml/min at a CPP of 60 mm Hg whether SAP was 65 (and ICP 5) mm Hg or SAP was 120 (and ICP 60) mm Hg (Fig. 5). When autoregulation was markedly defective, however, there was a definite increase in CBF as SAP rose (Fig. 6). Since CPP was unchanged this might imply that vascular distention was taking place, to explain the increase in CBF. The problems raised by this observation will be discussed.

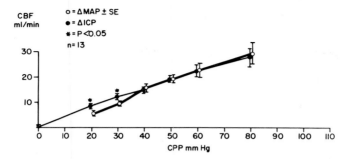

Fig. 4. Effect of altering cerebral perfusion pressure by decreasing arterial pressure (open circles) and increasing intracranial pressure (closed circles) in dogs with defective autoregulation. Significance between changes assessed by paired *t*-test. Note that scatter of flow values above CPP of 50 mm Hg is increased, indicated by increasing value for standard error of the mean.

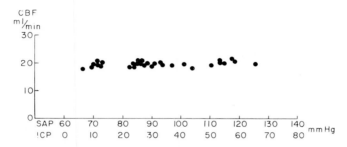

Fig. 5. Effect of increasing arterial pressure but constant cerebral perfusion pressure of 60 mm Hg (*i.e.* concomitant increase of intracranial pressure) in a dog with intact autoregulation.

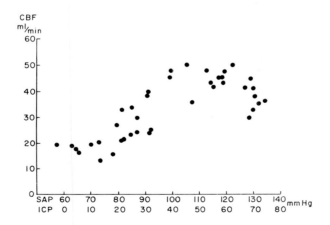

Fig. 6. Effect of increasing arterial pressure but constant cerebral perfusion pressure of 60 mm Hg (*i.e.* concomitant increase of intracranial pressure) in 4 dogs with markedly impaired autoregulation.

References pp. 431–432

TABLE 1

Stimulus	Response	Autoregulation	
		Intact	*Defective*
(a)	CBF decreased	12	22
MAP decrease	CBF unchanged	0	0
	CBF increased	0	0
(b)	CBF decreased	0	20
ICP increase	CBF unchanged	1	2
	CBF increased	9	7

Transient responses of cerebral blood flow (first 20 seconds) to (a) decreasing arterial pressure and (b) increasing intracranial pressure. Numbers refer to observations made when autoregulation was known to be intact (22) and defective (51). Significance of difference in responses assessed by χ^2 test (see text).

The transient response of CBF, the change that occurred during the initial 20 seconds following the change in CPP, was noted during each run (Table 1). A reduction of SAP invariably caused a transient reduction of CBF no matter whether autoregulation was intact (12 instances) or defective (22 instances) (Fig. 7). The response to increases of ICP was quite different. When autoregulation was intact, an increase in ICP caused a transient increase in CBF in 9 instances and no change in

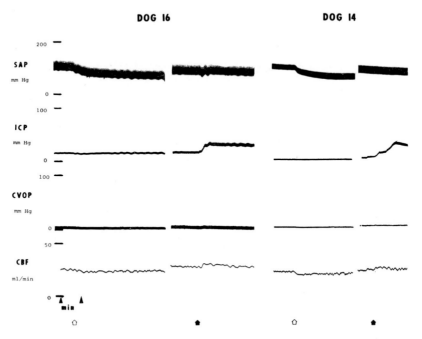

Fig. 7. Chart recordings from 2 dogs to demonstrate differing transient CBF responses to decreasing arterial pressure (open arrows) and increasing intracranial pressure (closed arrows).

one; CBF never decreased (Fig. 7). When autoregulation was defective, an increase in ICP caused an immediate reduction of CBF in 20 instances, no change in 2, and a transient increase in CBF followed by a later decrease in 7. These differences in CBF response with changes in SAP and ICP were highly significant (for all runs χ^2 22.38, $P < 0.001$; autoregulation intact χ^2 22.10, $P < 0.001$; autoregulation defective χ^2 7.64, $P < 0.02$), and the difference in response to ICP change in autoregulating and non-autoregulating runs was also highly significant (χ^2 14.87, $P < 0.001$).

There was a marked difference in CBF values at the same CPP when autoregulation was defective. This difference existed among animals and among runs within the same animal at a constant arterial P_{CO_2}. In Fig. 8 the data from 13 runs is expressed as

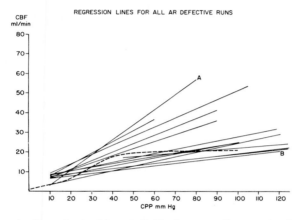

Fig. 8. Plot of regression lines obtained from individual pressure/flow graphs obtained from animals with defective autoregulation to show wide variation in CBF values with increased CPP. The dashed line indicates the mean flow for dogs with intact autoregulation.

regression lines derived from the pressure/flow graph for each run and the variation in CBF can be expressed as the range of gradients, which was from 0.092 to 0.771. Autoregulation was defective in all instances. A and B are different dogs. Comparing the animal with the steepest slope (A) with the animal with the flattest slope (B) it is seen that at a CPP of 70 mm Hg dog A has a CBF of 50.0 ml/min while dog B has a CBF of 14.0 ml/min. At a CPP of 30 mm Hg the CBF in dog A is 18.5 ml/min and in dog B 9.0 ml/min. CBF in dog A is therefore hyperemic at a normal perfusion pressure.

To this point autoregulation has been considered to be either present or absent. The present data suggests, however, that autoregulation is a quantitative phenomenon that becomes more defective with increasing insult to the brain. If one defines the degree of defective autoregulation as a change in CBF per unit change in CPP, it is clear that autoregulation is more defective in dog A than in dog B. The dashed line in Fig. 8 is the pressure/flow graph in normal autoregulation. At a CPP of 30 mm Hg, dog B with defective autoregulation has a CBF of 9.0 ml/min compared to 12.0 ml/min in an animal with normal autoregulation. But dog A that began at hyperemic levels has a CBF of 18.5 ml/min at 30 mm Hg, higher than the normal animal, even though

References pp. 431–432

autoregulation is more defective in this preparation. Whenever hyperemia was present, autoregulation was defective, but contrariwise, 7 animals had defective autoregulation without hyperemia. The data suggests that in this preparation hyperemia is a stage of damage to vasomotor reactivity beyond defective autoregulation.

An explanation for defective autoregulation was sought in each preparation. Of the 16 runs in which autoregulation was defective, 7 were first runs (change in SAP); ICP had not been deliberately increased beforehand. Defective autoregulation was thought to be due to periods of arterial hypotension during the surgical preparation (2 dogs) or subdural hematomas with elevated ICP (2 dogs). None of these animals regained autoregulation during the remainder of the experiment (up to 4 hours). No explanation for defective autoregulation was found in the remaining 3 animals. Among 9 runs in which autoregulation was defective and ICP had been intentionally increased beforehand, the increase in ICP had reduced CBF by more than 50% in 3 runs and by 25–50% in 2 runs. Most importantly, an increase in ICP that was insufficient to reduce CBF nevertheless damaged autoregulation on 4 occasions. Thus, no satisfactory explanation for defective autoregulation was found in 7 of the 16 runs.

CLINICAL OBSERVATIONS

In analyzing data from continuous measurements of ICP from a ventricular cannula, we have been impressed by the occasional observation of patients in whom ICP increases to levels close to SAP, yet no signs of gross neurological dysfunction appear. Two such patients are described in whom ICP approached the SAP on one or more occasions. Despite a CPP that was virtually nil, the patients were alert and well oriented indicating adequate CBF.

V.M. was a 24-year-old woman who presented with a 2-month history of headache and a 1-week history of neck pain, diplopia, and paresthesias in both hands. She was alert and well oriented. Fundoscopy showed severe bilateral papilledema with hemorrhages. The remainder of the neurological examination was normal except for intermittent horizontal nystagmus. Roentgenograms of the skull, brain scan, cerebrospinal fluid examination, bilateral carotid angiograms, vertebral angiogram, and complete myelogram were normal. EEG showed moderate generalized slowing. A pneumo-encephalogram revealed small lateral ventricles with no other abnormalities. An extensive search for evidence of infection, infestation, or a toxic etiologic agent was unproductive. The diagnosis was pseudotumor cerebri.

ICP was recorded continuously from a cannula in the right lateral ventricle for 3 days. Mean ICP ranged from 55 to 90 mm Hg. She remained alert, and there was no change in her neurological status except occasional severe headache at the pressure peaks. At a time when mean ICP was 90 mm Hg (115/78), mean arterial pressure recorded from a brachial cuff was 89 mm Hg (124/72). Although true arterial pressure was undoubtedly higher than the cuff pressure, CPP in this patient must have been very low.

E.L. was a 27-year-old woman with a 6-month history of diffuse frontal-occipital headaches and increasing cerebellar ataxia for several weeks. The neurological

examination was normal except for ataxia. Vertebral angiography revealed a hem-
angioblastoma of the left cerebellar hemisphere with obstructive hydrocephalus.
ICP was recorded from a cannula in the right lateral ventricle for 3 days, and CSF
was drained periodically in preparation for surgery. SAP was recorded continuously
from a catheter in the radial artery. Initial ICP was elevated and was punctuated by
large pressure waves. On one occasion she developed a transient reduction in vision
at the peak of a pressure wave. Otherwise, she was alert and well oriented throughout
the recording period. Fig. 9 illustrates the relationship of ICP to SAP. At 3 pressure
peaks CPP was 10, 6, and 16 mm Hg respectively. There was no change in her neurological status throughout this period.

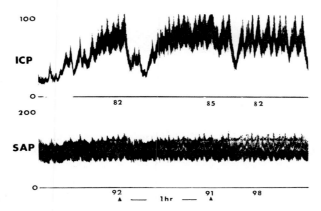

Fig. 9. ICP recorded from a lateral ventricle and SAP from the radial artery in patient E.L. during
spontaneous pressure waves. ICP and corresponding SAP are indicated at peaks of pressure waves.

Regional CBF studies were not performed in these two patients because another
puncture of the carotid artery for the sole purpose of injecting Xenon was considered
to be unjustified.

DISCUSSION

In studies of the effects of increased ICP on CBF the main difference in the results
has been the response of CBF to the initial increase in ICP. In some studies a decrease
of CBF occurred as soon as ICP was raised (Langfitt *et al.*, 1965; Bloor, personal
communication; Lewis, personal communication), and in other studies a moderate
increase of ICP, up to 30 mm Hg, was tolerated with no reduction in CBF (Kety
et al., 1948; Greenfield and Tindall, 1965; Rapela and Green, 1964; Shulman and
Verdier, 1967; Kogure and Scheinberg, 1970). These differences may be explained
by the method used to increase ICP, the rate of increase of ICP, and as suggested by
the results of the present study, by the autoregulatory status of the subject determined
by changes of SAP.

In considering the possible mechanisms responsible for the effect of an increase
in ICP on CBF, two viewpoints may be taken which depend on the definition of CPP.

References pp. 431–432

Theory of constant cerebral perfusion pressure. Organ perfusion pressure is ordinarily defined as inflow pressure minus outflow pressure; in the case of the brain CPP is the carotid/vertebral artery pressure (at the point of penetration of the dura) minus jugular bulb pressure. During an increase in ICP of extravascular origin there is no change in jugular venous pressure, hence no change in CPP if SAP remains constant. According to Ohm's law, applied to the circulation

$$CBF = \frac{CPP}{CVR} \qquad (1)$$

where CVR = total cerebrovascular resistance. Thus, if CBF and CPP remain constant during increasing ICP, total CVR must remain the same. In cranial window studies, however, pial arterial dilatation has been observed during increasing ICP (Wolff and Forbes, 1928; Fog, 1933). If total CVR can be regarded as a series of resistances along the cerebral vascular bed,

$$CVR = R \text{ arteries} + R \text{ arterioles} + R \text{ capillaries} + R \text{ veins} + R \text{ dural sinuses} \qquad (2)$$

then it follows that a drop in arterial resistance must be balanced by an increase in resistance downstream if CVR is to remain constant. According to this view, then, constant CBF during increasing ICP may be explained by a progressive increase in venous resistance as cerebral veins are compressed by rising ICP, balanced by a corresponding reduction in arterial resistance. Resistance in vascular beds, as in rigid tubes, is primarily a function of vascular radius (Peterson, 1966). From Poiseuille's equation governing the laminar flow of Newtonian fluids through small caliber rigid tubes, flow (Q) is yielded by:

$$Q = \frac{\pi R^4 (P_1 - P_2)}{8 \, \eta \, l} \qquad (3)$$

where
R $\qquad$ = tube radius
$P_1 - P_2$ = perfusion pressure
η $\qquad$ = viscosity of fluid
l $\qquad$ = length of tube

Since flow is a function of the 4th power of the radius, the change in radius due to compression or dilatation need not be great to exert a marked effect on flow. Caution has to be exercised, however, in extrapolating Poiseuille's equation to explain the hemodynamics of the cerebrovascular bed. Since the vessels are distensible, radius is a function of the distending or transmural pressure and the thickness and the stiffness of the vascular wall which determine how the radius varies with the distending pressure. If, in addition, an increase in vascular distension produces an active response in the form of decreasing radius, this further complicates the relationship between pressure and radius.

Much of this hypothesis hinges on evidence for venous compression during increasing ICP. Wright (1938) noted that bridging cerebral veins observed through a cranial window collapsed only when ICP exceeded SAP, at which point blood was forced proximally, indicating that outflow resistance now exceeded resistance in the proximal vascular bed. Wright postulated that increased ICP caused constriction of veins at their junction with the sagittal sinus; this has been supported by the work of Hedges *et al.* (1964) and Greenfield and Tindall (1965). We studied the problem in Rhesus monkeys by measuring ICP and dural sinus pressures during expansion of an extracerebral balloon and during the development of experimental brain swelling (Langfitt *et al.*, 1966; Shapiro *et al.*, 1966). The relationship of sagittal sinus pressure to ICP seemed to be best explained by a combination of compression of cerebral veins proximal to the sinus and compression of the sinus itself distal to the recording catheter. In the animals with severe brain swelling coronal sections of heads frozen at the time of sacrifice showed collapse of cortical veins and near collapse of the sagittal and straight sinuses (Shapiro *et al.*, 1966). A recent study by Osterholm (1970) demonstrated constriction of the sagittal sinus with increased ICP. Shulman and Verdier (1967) measured CBF and sagittal sinus wedge pressure, which approximates cerebral venous pressure (Shulman, 1965), maintaining sagittal sinus outflow pressure at zero during increasing ICP. They observed that wedge pressure increased with rising ICP and CBF remained the same, leading to the conclusion that autoregulation maintaining constant CBF despite rising ICP was accompanied by a decrease in prevenous resistance and concomitant increase in venous resistance.

If the definition of CPP as SAP minus jugular venous pressure is used, it is necessary to explain maintenance of CBF during rising ICP by a finely adjusted compensatory link between venous compression and arterial dilatation. There are two main problems with such a hypothesis. First, evidence for progressive venous compression at lower levels of increased ICP is scanty. In nearly all studies venous compression has been observed when ICP is at levels close to SAP; *e.g.* Wolff and Forbes' (1928) data shows venous compression occurring at a mean pressure difference of 23 mm Hg (Table 2); in such cases apparent venous compression may really be venous collapse due to diminishing cerebral blood volume from decreased CBF. Fog (1933) stated

TABLE 2

SAP	ICP		CPP
mm Hg	mm H$_2$O	mm Hg	mm Hg
88	1000	74	14
72	1600	118	−46 (0)
140	1800	132	8
96	700	51	45
142	1400	103	39
105	1050	77	28
185	2200	162	23
130	1400	103	27
200	2400	177	23

Arterial, intracranial and cerebral perfusion pressure levels at which persistent cerebral venous compression was observed. Data taken from Wolff and Forbes (1928).

References pp. 431–432

"increase in the intracranial pressure produces first a compression of the vein, and then the vein dilates again to its normal size or a little more . . . and it appears to keep this size throughout the rest of the experiment". Wolff and Forbes (1928) commented also on the temporary venous compression immediately upon rapidly increasing ICP and distinguish this from the more protracted venous collapse observed at high levels of ICP. In other studies in which venous compression has been demonstrated, brain swelling and distortion have been present, in which situation local factors, independent of ICP, may be responsible for venous compression.

The second difficulty with the venous compression hypothesis is that it implies some type of feedback from the compressed veins to the arterial resistance vessels; if increasing intravascular pressure proximal to the site of venous constriction is transmitted back across the capillary bed, the increased pressure is more likely to cause reflex arterial constriction rather than dilatation. If it is the increased extravascular pressure (ICP) at the arterial end of the bed which causes the compensatory increase in arterial radius, observed through the cranial window, it is difficult to postulate a mechanism responsible for a decrease in arterial resistance equal to the increase in venous resistance produced by the compression so that CBF remains constant.

Theory of diminishing cerebral perfusion pressure.   One of the most important features of the cerebral circulation, emphasized since the writings of Alexander Monro (1783), is that it is confined within a rigid space. If compressible vessels in such a space are submitted to an increasing extravascular pressure, according to Permutt and Riley (1963) the hydrodynamics of the system become analogous to those of a sluice or waterfall. According to their hypothesis, as long as intravascular pressure remains above extravascular pressure, perfusion pressure is accurately defined as the arterial minus the venous outflow pressure; as soon as extravascular pressure increases above intravascular pressure constriction develops just proximal to the outflow orifice, the point of lowest pressure in the tube. Fluid entering the tube now tends to back up behind the region of constriction, and the resultant increase in pressure dilates the constricted portion of the tube to its previous diameter. Flow increases, but at the same time pressure in the tube falls below the external pressure, and the distal end of the tube is again constricted. The hydrodynamic situation at the outflow orifice shows some analogy with Torricelli's principle for fluid leaving a container with a hole in its side, where flow (Q) is given by

$$Q = A \sqrt{\frac{2(Pc - Po)}{\rho}} \tag{4}$$

where
A = area of orifice
Pc = pressure in container
Po = outside pressure
ρ = density of fluid
It can be seen from this equation that if the area of the orifice can vary, a change in flow need not imply a change in pressure, and pressure drop can be independent of flow.

The model may be applicable to the cerebral circulation when ICP is increased. Normally cerebral venous pressure is higher than ICP. As ICP rises above venous pressure, constriction occurs near the junction of a cerebral vein with the dural sinus. Blood then continues to enter the vein proximally, increases venous pressure that rises transiently above ICP, and the vein opens. Thus, the diameter of the vein at the site of constriction flutters as ICP continues to rise. Since the difference between venous pressure and ICP must at all times be minimal

$$CPP = SAP - ICP \qquad (5)$$

Another important feature of the vascular waterfall hypothesis is that the total resistance to flow is only the sum of vascular resistances proximal to the point where external and internal pressures are equal. Thus, as ICP rises to equal the pressure in veins, then capillaries, then arterioles, the vessels distal to the region of equal pressures no longer contribute to the total resistance. Total resistance decreases, and according to equations (1) and (2) normal CBF with rising ICP is explained by a decrease in resistance that matches the fall in CPP. If the vascular waterfall hypothesis can be applied to the cerebral circulation, compression of the cerebrovascular bed need not be invoked to explain the effects of increased ICP on CBF. But it is difficult to visualize no flow when, for example, carotid artery pressure and ICP are 100 mm Hg, jugular venous pressure is 5 mm Hg, and the cerebral vascular bed from the carotid artery to the jugular vein is patent. A pressure head of 95 mm Hg exists across an open system of tubes. Furthermore, one of the criticisms of the venous compression hypothesis may be applied here. By what precise mechanism is the distal to proximal loss of resistance, that occurs with increasing ICP, adjusted to the fall in CPP so that CBF remains constant?

Using the definition of CPP as SAP minus ICP, Zwetnow (1970) and Häggendal *et al.* (1970) have shown that CBF in the dog remains constant over a wide range of levels of increased ICP (0–100 mm Hg) until CPP falls below 40 mm Hg. This has been confirmed in the baboon by Jennett *et al.* (1970) and in the present studies. Thus, in empirical terms, the validity of the concept of decreasing CPP with increasing ICP is supported, since in these three studies the effect of increasing ICP on CBF was related to the level of arterial pressure, which may vary greatly during increasing ICP. Vascular compression, if it exists, must be demonstrated by observations through a transparent water-tight calvarium and measurements of small artery and vein pressures so that the appearance of the vessels can be correlated with changes in resistance measured by pressure drops across segments of the cerebrovascular bed.

Definitions of intracranial pressures. Because of the special hemodynamic situation created by increased ICP, it is necessary to define several intracranial pressures before discussing possible regulatory mechanisms for the cerebral circulation. Transmural pressure at the arterial end of the system (P_{TMA}) is defined as:

$$P_{TMA} = SAP - ICP \qquad (6)$$

This is identical with CPP as defined in equation (5). Mean intravascular pressure

References pp. 431–432

$(P_{\overline{IV}})$ has been defined by Burton and Stinson (1960) as the average of inflow and outflow pressure:

$$P_{\overline{IV}} = \frac{SAP + JVP}{2} \tag{7}$$

but according to the vascular waterfall concept this should be amended to:

$$P_{\overline{IV}} = \frac{SAP + ICP}{2} \tag{8}$$

Mean transmural pressure $(P_{\overline{TM}})$ is the difference between $P_{\overline{IV}}$ and extravascular pressure (ICP) and this becomes:

$$\begin{aligned} P_{\overline{TM}} &= \left(\frac{SAP + ICP}{2} \right) - ICP \\ &= \frac{SAP - ICP}{2} \end{aligned} \tag{9}$$

Two points are pertinent at this stage; the relevant SAP in all of these definitions is the arterial pressure in the subarachnoid space; in most studies aortic or large artery pressure is used for this measurement. Although this may be a reasonable approximation at normal levels of SAP the error of this assumption may increase as SAP falls. The second point concerns the significance of measurements of mean intravascular and transmural pressures. These are mathematical abstractions, and the anatomical locus of the mean pressures is unknown. In other words, the information required for a full explanation of the pressure/flow relationship in the cerebral circulation is the profile of pressure distributions along the length of the vascular bed and how it is altered by increased ICP.

Autoregulation of cerebral blood flow. The term autoregulation is applied to the mechanism by which CBF maintains constancy despite changes of perfusion pressure. This term involves an assumption which has yet to be proven, namely, that CBF adapts to changing CPP by mechanisms which are entirely independent of systemic influences. Several mechanisms have been proposed to explain this type of flow regulation, and although a detailed description of the arguments for and against each theory is beyond the scope of this discussion they will be briefly described with emphasis on how the present data on the effect of increased ICP on CBF relates to each hypothesis.

A neurogenic mechanism has been proposed. Although there is evidence that neurogenic factors (sympathectomy and sympathetic stimulation) may influence the CBF level at which autoregulation occurs (James *et al.*, 1969) there is no firm evidence as yet that the mechanism itself is neurogenic in origin.

The metabolic theory of autoregulation to CPP changes proposes that alterations in CPP cause temporary passive changes in CBF which then alter the concentration of extracellular vasoactive substances so as to return CBF to control levels by an appropriate resetting of vascular radius. Recently Ekstrom-Jodal (1970) has presented evidence that neither oxygen nor carbon dioxide tension changes in the extracellular space can account for cerebral autoregulation to SAP changes. Zwetnow (1970) concluded that changes in cerebral extracellular pH cannot be responsible for the autoregulation which occurs to rising ICP. One essential feature of the metabolic hypothesis is that a stimulus in the form of a passive change of CBF has to be present in order to excite the appropriate regulatory response. In the present experiments there was no reduction in CBF when CPP was reduced by increasing ICP when auto-regulation was intact; thus, no stimulus was present for the production of a vasodilator metabolite or inhibition of a vasoconstrictor metabolite. Similar observations have been made by Kogure et al. (1970). If the mechanisms for autoregulation to changes of both SAP and ICP are the same, then it is hard to envisage the metabolic theory as being responsible, unless a selective regional reduction of CBF in some vital area is postulated, too small to be manifest in a total CBF measurement but causing autoregulation in the whole brain.

According to the tissue pressure theory, proposed by Rodbard (1971) the changes in resistance which constitute autoregulation take place in the capillary bed, not the arterioles. An increase in arterial pressure is communicated to the capillaries causing a net exchange of fluid towards the tissues. The increase in extravascular fluid volume is limited by the distension of the organ, causing an increase in tissue pressure, capillary compression and increased resistance, thus restoring flow to control levels. A decrease in arterial pressure results in decreased capillary pressure, enlargement of the capillary bed by inflow of fluid from the tissues and decreased resistance. This mechanism, however, fails to account for maintenance of normal CBF when there is a primary increase in ICP and presumably also in cerebral pericapillary tissue pressure.

The fourth mechanism advanced to explain autoregulation is the myogenic theory, originally proposed by Bayliss (1902) and extensively studied in hindlimb preparations by Folkow (1948, 1956). According to this hypothesis, resistance vessels have a high degree of resting vasoconstrictor tone due mainly to smooth muscle contraction in the walls. An increase in intraluminal pressure stimulates a further increase in tone by first stretching the muscle causing a reactive shortening of radial fibers and reduction of vascular radius. A decrease in intraluminal pressure has the opposite effect, passive constriction results followed by an increase in vascular radius. The effective pressure is not intraluminal pressure per se but the difference between intravascular and extra-vascular pressure, transmural pressure. Since transmural pressure at the arterial end of the bed is the same as CPP (equations 5 and 6) the myogenic mechanism is consistent with the existence of autoregulation to increasing ICP as demonstrated by Zwetnow (1970) and Jennett et al. (1970), and also with the co-existence of auto-regulation, both intact and impaired, to changes of both SAP and ICP, as seen in the present study.

Some further light on the relationship between CPP and P_{TMA} has been shed by the experiments of Ekstrom-Jodal (1970) who has shown that increasing cerebral venous pressure in the absence of increasing ICP caused a reduction in CBF in dogs in which autoregulation to changing SAP was present; CBF then remained constant as SAP was elevated. These findings have been confirmed in our laboratory (un-published observations) and may be interpreted in two ways. First, if the vascular segment responsible for autoregulation is entirely precapillary, mild elevation of cerebral venous pressure with no rise in ICP results in a fall of CPP but no change in P_{TMA} assuming that the rise in venous pressure is not transmitted as far upstream as the arterioles. CBF is therefore reduced due to the reduction of CPP in the absence of any stimulus to autoregulation. The second possibility is that the increased venous pressure is transmitted back to the vasoactive portion of the cerebrovascular bed increasing $P_{\overline{TM}}$ (or P_{TMA}). If autoregulation is intact this increase in $P_{\overline{TM}}$ will cause vasoconstriction so that CBF is reduced even more than it would be due to a decrease in CPP alone. The flow reductions observed by both Ekstrom-Jodal and ourselves appear to be greater than could be accounted for by a reduction in CPP alone. This point could be clarified by elevating cerebral venous pressure when autoregulation is intact and when it is markedly impaired. If the second explanation is correct, the fall in CBF should be greater when autoregulation is intact because of active vaso-constriction to the increase in P_{TMA}.

A rather philosophic objection to the transmural pressure-myogenic theory of autoregulation is that it seems unlikely that such a vital homeostatic function should be in the form of an intrinsic vascular reflex and if it is, that such a mechanism should be so vulnerable to ischemia (Lassen and Paulson, 1969), hypoxia (Häggendal, 1968), and brain trauma (Reivich *et al.*, 1969). In the present study there were several instances where autoregulation was found to be impaired following periods of in-creased ICP during which there had been no reduction of CBF.

Cerebral blood flow at low perfusion pressures   One of the observations from the present study which requires further explanation, particularly as it has important implications for the clinical situation, is the finding that at low levels of CPP, CBF appears to be significantly greater when ICP has been elevated than when SAP has been decreased at the same level of CPP. Several factors have to be taken into con-sideration. The most important is the validity of the blood pressure recording. In calculating CPP, SAP was measured from the aorta at the origin of the carotid artery, assuming that the pressure drop along the artery to the point where it enters the skull is insignificant. Although this may be acceptable when aortic pressure is normal, during arterial hypotension the pressure drop along the carotid artery may increase due to hydrodynamic factors and possibly also to an increase in sympathetic tone elicited by the hypotension. Thus, the values of CPP obtained during arterial hypo-tension may be overestimated. This possibility is indirectly supported by comparing data from Harper (1966) who showed CBF to fall when SAP, measured from the aorta, fell below 60 mm Hg, and from Machowicz *et al.* (1961) showing that CBF was constant down to an SAP of 30 mm Hg when this was measured from the vertebral artery at the base of the skull. Furthermore, even under normotensive conditions, Kanzow and Dieckhoff (1969) found that 20% of cerebrovascular resistance is located between the aorta and the major branches of the middle cerebral artery. A second factor to be considered is the contribution of increases in kinetic energy to CBF, when the energy of pressure is constant, and the contribution of pulsatile flow. When

ICP is increased and SAP is normal, cardiac output and pulse pressure are greater than when SAP is reduced; both of these factors could theoretically increase CBF even when CPP is constant.

Variations in cerebral blood flow at constant perfusion pressure. In dogs with markedly impaired autoregulation, CBF was found to increase with rising SAP but constant CPP (*i.e.* when ICP was increasing in parallel with SAP). In this situation P_{TMA} and $P_{\overline{TM}}$ also remain constant during the rise of SAP but intravascular pressure increases. On theoretical grounds increasing pulsatility and kinetic energy might account for the increased CBF, but the fact that this was not observed when auto-regulation was intact suggests that at constant CPP non-autoregulating vessels distend with increasing intravascular pressure. This raises considerable hemodynamic problems because it suggests that although intravascular pressure and extravascular pressure are rising in concert, the force tending to distend the vessel is greater than that tending to compress the vessel. Clearly this area merits further study.

Transient responses of cerebral blood flow to changes of arterial and intracranial pressure. The differing responses of CBF immediately following changes of SAP and ICP are of interest in that they may shed further light on the mechanisms involved in autoregulation. The immediate reduction of CBF following a decrease in SAP may be explained by the following sequence of events: SAP is reduced while ICP and cerebral venous pressures are essentially unchanged; CPP, P_{TMA}, $P_{\overline{TM}}$, and $P_{\overline{IV}}$ are simultaneously reduced. The immediate reduction in CBF is due to the fall in CPP perhaps augmented by a passive reduction in calibre of the arterial end of the vascular bed and/or by an increase in sympathetic tone elicited by the fall in SAP. CBF begins to return to normal as the radius of the resistance vessels increases, possibly due to a Bayliss effect triggered by the fall in P_{TMA}. Thus, we postulate that during a fall in SAP, the rate of change of CPP at first exceeds the rate of increase in arteriole radius, and CBF falls; when flow begins to return toward control (auto-regulation) this dynamic relationship has been reversed. Thus,

$$\frac{dCPP}{dt} > \frac{dr}{dt} \rightarrow \frac{dr}{dt} > \frac{dCPP}{dt}$$

The sequence of events following an increase in ICP is more difficult to interpret. When ICP is increased and SAP is unchanged, P_{TMA} is reduced immediately and CPP is reduced, though not immediately, because some finite time must be required for intracranial venous pressure to equilibrate with ICP. Landis (1930) demonstrated that when venous pressure in the forearm was abruptly increased by inflation of an upper arm cuff, it took 15–45 seconds for capillary pressure to rise beyond cuff pressure. $P_{\overline{TM}}$ is reduced and $P_{\overline{IV}}$ increases, again with the same time requirement as for CPP. The immediate effect of increasing ICP might be a small reduction in CBF due to compression of capacitance vessels before compensatory dilatation of resistance vessels takes place. This statement assumes that venous compression occurs with rising ICP. A reduction in CBF was never seen in autoregulating animals, but since venous outflow was being measured, a transient decrease in CBF could have been obscured due to squeezing blood from the veins into the recording system. Even if

References pp. 431–432

cerebral blood volume in the dog is as much as 10% of brain volume, and if it is postulated that as much as one half could be expelled, this would amount to 3–4 ml of blood in the dogs using the present study; at a CBF rate of 20 ml/min, this factor could account for an increase in CBF lasting at most 12 seconds. Thus, the increases of CBF lasting up to 1 minute seen in autoregulating dogs when ICP was increased cannot be explained entirely on this basis. The fact that such transient increases were less frequent when autoregulation was defective suggests that the increase in flow is due to active vascular dilatation (Bayliss effect) which initially is in excess of that required for maintenance of CBF at the reduced CPP. This interpretation is supported by Fog's (1933) observations of pial artery diameter during increasing ICP. An immediate well-marked dilatation was seen lasting 2 minutes; the vessel then constricted but to a diameter still above control levels. In the situation of increasing ICP with intact autoregulation the relationship between CPP and vascular radius may be expressed by:

$$\frac{dr}{dt} > \frac{dCPP}{dt} \rightarrow \frac{dCPP}{dt} > \frac{dr}{dt}$$

These rate changes may then be considered as resultants of several different directional changes of CBF.

Similar responses of blood flow to changes of arterial and extravascular pressures have been demonstrated in the renal circulation by Nash and Selkurt (1964) who showed that when extravascular (ureteral) pressure was increased, renal blood flow increased when autoregulation to arterial pressure was intact but decreased when autoregulation was absent.

Analysis of changes in rate and direction of CBF during changes in SAP and ICP in situations where autoregulation is intact and defective should yield further information on the latency of autoregulation and perhaps its mechanisms.

Cerebral blood flow with impaired autoregulation. The marked differences in slope of the pressure/flow graphs in non-autoregulating animals bears comment, particularly as it might relate to the interaction of CBF and CPP in patients with disorders of cerebral autoregulation. With CPP levels in the autoregulatory range CBF was more often above normal levels than below in non-autoregulating animals, suggesting a decrease in resting vasoconstrictor tone of the resistance vessels. This condition has been variously entitled (reactive) hyperemia, luxury perfusion (Lassen, 1966), and vasomotor paralysis (Langfitt *et al.*, 1965). In the absence of reactive changes in vascular radius, flow increases linearly with perfusion pressure, the gradient depending on the vascular caliber. If, in addition, passive distension of vessels occurs, the curve becomes convex to the pressure axis; isolated examples of this were seen in the present study, particularly during sudden sharp increases in arterial pressure. This may represent the same phenomenon as increasing CBF with rising SAP when CPP is constant and again raises questions about the relative effects of intra- and extravascular pressures in determining flow.

It can be stated that when autoregulation is impaired, it is the response to changes of CPP which is abnormal; no particular level of CBF at any level of CPP is implied.

In the study of Reivich *et al.* (1969) in which CBF autoregulation was impaired by mechanical trauma to the brain, CBF remained normal at normal levels of SAP; it was only by altering SAP that the flow disorder became apparent. Vasomotor paralysis (or paresis) represents a stage beyond defective autoregulation wherein CBF is increased at normal SAP. In the present experiments autoregulation was more impaired in the presence of vasomotor paresis because there was a greater change of CBF for each change in CPP; yet the brain was better "protected" from ischemia due to decreasing SAP or increasing ICP, since even at low levels of CPP, CBF was higher in the animals with vasomotor paresis than in those with normal autoregulation.

Applications to clinical studies. The experiments described have utilized a simple model of increased ICP, and obviously caution has to be exercised in interpreting the results in terms of clinical abnormalities of ICP. In particular, the model does not take into account local CBF changes such as might be produced by expanding intracranial masses. The latter type of lesion introduces another factor into pressure/flow relationships, one which is highly relevant to the clinical situation, namely local distortion of cerebral vessels which may act on local CBF independent of ICP. In the two patients presented, however, the causes of the intracranial hypertension were diffuse cerebral edema and obstructive hydrocephalus. Thus, it appears justified to seek an explanation from the animal experiments for the observation that these patients were alert and well oriented with a CPP of 10 mm Hg or less. The following mechanisms bear discussion:

(1) In dog A in Fig. 8, CBF is 11 ml/min at a CPP of 20 mm Hg. This is approximately 50% of the normal mean CBF (21.9 ml/min) in this series. If the patients had defective autoregulation and vasomotor paresis, comparable to dog A, CBF even though reduced could have been adequate to maintain consciousness and intellectual function.

(2) SAP and CPP may have been higher than they appear to be. This explanation is supported by the fact that cuff pressures are lower than intra-arterial pressure measurements (patient V.M.). In patient E.L., however, SAP was recorded from the radial artery which is equivalent in diameter to the internal carotid artery as it enters the skull.

(3) Additional factors may have increased resting CBF or decreased the vulnerability of the brain to low CPP. Hypothermia protects the brain from ischemia by a reduction in cerebral metabolism, even though CBF declines passively with $CMRO_2$ (Meyer and Hunter, 1957). Body temperature was normal in both of our patients. Hypercapnia and hypoxia increase CBF and impair autoregulation (Harper, 1965; Häggendal, 1968) perhaps creating a situation that again is analogous to dog A in Fig. 8. Blood gases were normal in both patients except for hypocapnia in patient E.L. The findings in these patients must be contrasted with the observations that in other patients CBF ceases when mean ICP equals mean SAP. We described previously three such patients (two with postoperative brain swelling, one with a spontaneous intraventricular hemorrhage) who were comatose and being ventilated following spontaneous respiratory arrest (Langfitt and Kassell, 1966). At the time when ICP equalled SAP, opaque injected into the carotid-vertebral system failed to enter the

References pp. 431–432

intracranial space. Perhaps CBF is adequate to maintain function until CPP falls from 5–10 mm Hg to zero. Alternatively the cause of the intracranial hypertension may be as important as the height of ICP in determining CBF; for example, edema might create an increase in local tissue tension that is sufficient to collapse the micro-circulation without a comparable increase in ICP. Finally, brainstem displacement and compression, a difficult diagnosis to make clinically, may be independent of the level of ICP (Weinstein *et al.*, 1968).

Answers to these questions await serial measurements of regional CBF in patients with a variety of intracranial lesions at different levels of ICP and correlation of the results with neurological status. This will not be feasible until an isotope inhalation technique, or another method that is comparably inocuous, is developed for measuring regional CBF in man.

CONCLUSION

CBF was measured from the cerebral venous outflow in dogs with intact and defective autoregulation during alterations in CPP produced by lowering SAP or increasing ICP. When autoregulation was intact, CBF did not fall until CPP was reduced to 40–50 mm Hg by either method. Autoregulation was significantly more effective when CPP was reduced by raising ICP compared to lowering SAP. When auto-regulation was defective, CBF followed CPP passively with both methods of changing CPP.

When autoregulation was intact, raising SAP and ICP together, so that CPP remained constant, had no effect on CBF. But when autoregulation was defective, CBF increased steadily even though CPP was constant. These observations suggest that increasing intravascular pressure dilates cerebral vessels even though transmural pressure remains constant.

CBF always decreased transiently when SAP was lowered but nearly always increased transiently when ICP was increased. This is most likely due to a difference in the relationship between CPP and vascular radius with the two methods of lowering CPP.

Some animals demonstrated vasomotor paresis, an increase in the resting vaso-constrictor tone of the resistance vessels, in addition to defective autoregulation. In these dogs, CBF was in the normal range at very low CPP's because the initial CBF was so high, even though autoregulation was quantitatively more defective.

In some animals autoregulation was very sensitive to elevated ICP. Even though CBF was not decreased below normal with an initial increase in ICP, autoregulation was demonstrated to be defective when ICP was increased a second time.

Patients may be neurologically normal at a time when mean intraventricular pressure is within 10 mm Hg or less of mean SAP. Since CBF must be adequate in these patients, the observations suggest that in some clinical situations CBF can autoregulate to increased ICP even better than in the animal preparations.

REFERENCES

BAYLISS, W. M. (1902) On the local reactions of the arterial wall to changes of internal pressure. *J. Physiol. (London)*, **28**, 220–231.

BLOOR, B. M. (personal communication).

BURTON, A. C. AND STINSON, R. H. (1960) The measurement of tension in vascular smooth muscle. *J. Physiol. (London)*, **153**, 290–305.

D'ALECY, L. G. (1971) *Sympathetic control of the cerebral circulation.* Ph. D. Thesis, University of Pennsylvania.

EKSTROM-JODAL, B. (1970) On the relation between blood pressure and blood flow in the canine brain with particular regard to the mechanism responsible for cerebral blood flow autoregulation. *Acta Physiol. Scand., Suppl.* **350**, 1–61.

FOG, M. (1933) Influence of intracranial hypertension upon the cerebral circulation. *Acta Psychiat. Neurol. Scand.*, **8**, 191–198.

FOLKOW, B. (1948) Intravascular pressure as a factor regulating the tone of small vessels. *Acta Physiol. Scand.*, **17**, 289–310.

FOLKOW, B. AND LÖFVING, B. (1956) The distensibility of the systemic resistance vessels. *Acta Physiol. Scand.*, **38**, 37–52.

GREENFIELD, J. D. AND TINDALL, G. T. (1965) Effect of acute increase in intracranial pressure on blood flow in the internal carotid artery of man. *J. Clin. Invest.*, **44**, 1343–1351.

HÄGGENDAL, E. (1968) Elimination of autoregulation during arterial and cerebral hypoxia. *Scand. J. Lab. Clin. Invest., Suppl.* **102**, VD.

HÄGGENDAL, E., LÖFGREN, J., NILSSON, N. J. AND ZWETNOW, N. N. (1970) Effects of varied cerebrospinal fluid pressure on cerebral blood flow in dogs. *Acta Physiol Scand.*, **79**, 262–271.

HARPER, A. M. (1965) The inter-relationships between aP_{CO_2} and blood pressure in the regulation of blood flow through the cerebral cortex. *Acta Neurol. Scand., Suppl.* **14**, 94–103.

HARPER, A. M. (1966) Autoregulation of cerebral blood flow, influence of the arterial blood pressure on the blood flow through the cerebral cortex. *J. Neurol. Neurosurg. Psychiat.*, **29**, 398–403.

HEDGES, T. R., WEINSTEIN, J. D., KASSELL, N. F. AND STEIN, S. (1964) Cerebrovascular responses to increased intracranial pressure. *J. Neurosurg.*, **21**, 292–297.

JAMES, I. M., MILLAR, R. A. AND PURVES, M. J. (1969) Observations on the extrinsic neural control of cerebral blood flow in the baboon. *Circ. Res.*, **25**, 77–93.

JENNETT, W. B., HARPER, A. M., MILLER, J. D. AND ROWAN, J. O. (1970) Relation between cerebral blood flow and cerebral perfusion pressure. *Brit. J. Surg.*, **57**, 390.

KANZOW, E. AND DIECKHOFF, D. (1969) On the location of vascular resistance in the cerebral circulation. *Cerebral Blood Flow*, M. BROCK, C. FIESCHI, D. H. INGVAR, N. A. LASSEN AND K. SCHÜRMANN (Eds.), Springer-Verlag, Berlin and New York, pp. 96–97.

KETY, S. S., SHENKIN, H. A. AND SCHMIDT, C. F. (1948) The effects of increased intracranial pressure on cerebral circulatory functions in man. *J. Clin. Invest.*, **27**, 493–499.

KOGURE, K., SCHEINBERG, P., FUJISHIMA, M., BUSTO, R. AND REINMUTH, O. M. (1970) Effects of hypoxia on cerebral autoregulation. *Amer. J. Physiol.*, **219**, 1393–1396.

LANDIS, E. M. (1930) Micro-injection studies of capillary blood pressure in human skin. *Heart*, **15**, 209–228.

LANGFITT, T. W. AND KASSELL, N. (1966) Non-filling of cerebral vessels during angiography: Correlation with intracranial pressure. *Acta Neurochir.*, **14**, 96–104.

LANGFITT, T. W., KASSELL, N. F. AND WEINSTEIN, J. D. (1965) Cerebral blood flow with intracranial hypertension. *Neurology*, **15**, 761–773.

LANGFITT, T. W., WEINSTEIN, J. D. AND KASSELL, N. F. (1965) Cerebral vasomotor paralysis produced by intracranial hypertension. *Neurology*, **15**, 622–641.

LANGFITT, T. W., WEINSTEIN, J. D., KASSELL, N. F., GAGLIARDI, L. J. AND SHAPIRO, H. M. (1966) Compression of cerebral vessels by intracranial hypertension. I. Dural sinus pressures. *Acta Neurochir.*, **15**, 212–222.

LASSEN, N. A. (1966) The luxury-perfusion syndrome and its possible relation to acute metabolic acidosis localized within the brain. *Lancet*, **ii**, 1113–1115.

LASSEN, N. A. AND PAULSON, O. B. (1969) Partial cerebral vasoparalysis in patients with apoplexy. In: *Cerebral Blood Flow*, M. BROCK, C. FIESCHI, D. H. INGVAR, N. A. LASSEN AND K. SCHÜRMANN (Eds.), Springer-Verlag, Berlin and New York, pp. 117–119.

LEWIS, H. P. (personal communication).

MACHOWICZ, P. P., SABO, G., LIN, G., RAPELA, C. E. AND GREEN, H. D. (1961) Effect of varying cerebral arterial pressure on cerebral venous flow. *Physiologist*, **4**, 68.

MARSHALL, W. J. S., JACKSON, J. L. F. AND LANGFITT, T. W. (1969) Brain swelling caused by trauma and arterial hypertension. *Arch. Neurol.*, **21**, 545–553.

MEYER, J. S. AND HUNTER, J. (1957) Effects of hypothermia on local blood flow and metabolism during cerebral ischemia and hypoxia. *J. Neurosurg.*, **14**, 210–227.

MILLER, J. D. AND LEDINGHAM, I. McA. (1971) Reduction of increased intracranial pressure: Comparison between hyperbaric oxygen and hyperventilation. *Arch. Neurol.*, **24**, 210–216.

MONRO, A. (1783) *Observations on the Structure and Function of the Nervous System*. Creech and Johnson, Edinburgh.

NASH, F. D. AND SELKURT, E. E. (1964) Effects of elevated ureteral pressure on renal blood flow. *Circ. Res.*, **14/15**, Suppl. 1, 142–146.

OSTERHOLM, J. L. (1970) Reaction of the cerebral venous sinus system to acute intracranial hypertension. *J. Neurosurg.*, **32**, 654–659.

PERMUTT, S. AND RILEY, R. L. (1963) Hemodynamics of collapsible vessels with tone: The vascular waterfall. *J. Appl. Physiol.*, **18**, 924–932.

PETERSON, L. H. (1966) Physical factors which influence vascular caliber and blood flow. *Circ. Res.*, **18/19**, Suppl. 1, 3–13.

RAPELA, C. E. AND GREEN, H. D. (1964) Autoregulation of cerebral blood flow. *Circ. Res.*, **15**, 205–211.

REIVICH, M., MARSHALL, W. J. S. AND KASSELL, N. (1969) Loss of autoregulation produced by cerebral trauma. *Cerebral Blood Flow*, M. BROCK, C. FIESCHI, D. H. INGVAR, N. A. LASSEN AND K. SCHÜRMANN (Eds.), Springer-Verlag, Berlin and New York, pp. (05–208.

RODBARD, S. (1971) Capillary control of blood flow and fluid exchange. *Circ. Res.*, **28**, Suppl. **1**, 51–58.

SHAPIRO, H. M., LANGFITT, T. W. AND WEINSTEIN, J. D. (1966) Compression of cerebral vessels by intracranial hypertension. II. Morphological evidence for collapse of vessels. *Acta Neurochir.*, **15**, 223–233.

SHULMAN, K. (1965) Small artery and vein pressures in the subarachnoid space of the dog. *J. Surg. Res.*, **5**, 56–61.

SHULMAN, K. AND VERDIER, G. R. (1967) Cerebral vascular resistance changes in response to cerebrospinal fluid pressure. *Amer. J. Physiol.*, **213**, 1084–1088.

WEINSTEIN, J. D., LANGFITT, T. W., BRUNO, L., ZAREN, H. A. AND JACKSON, J. L. F. (1968) Experimental studies of patterns of brain distortion and ischemia produced by an intracranial mass. *J. Neurosurg.*, **28**, 513–521.

WOLFF, H. G. AND FORBES, H. S. (1928) The cerebral circulation. V. Observations of the pial arteries during changes in intracranial pressure. *Arch. Neurol. Psychiat.*, **20**, 1035–1047.

WRIGHT, R. D. (1938) Experimental observations on increased intracranial pressure. *Aust. N.Z.J. Surg.*, **7**, 215–235.

ZWETNOW, N. N. (1970) Effects of increased cerebrospinal fluid pressure on the blood flow and on the energy metabolism of the brain. *Acta Physiol. Scand.*, *Suppl.* **339**, 1–31.

Author Index

Subject Index